Foreword

Sir Eric Stroud
Hon. Medical Director, Children Nationwide Medical Research Fund.
Emeritus Professor of Child Health, King's College Hospital, University of London.

There is probably no subject in which major advances in scientific medicine of the last few years have had such an impact as in the practice of paediatrics.

The annual scientific conference which is the basis of this publication is of great importance, bringing together the knowledge of these advances and discussing the ways in which they can be used to improve our care of children and their families. Children are very different from the adults which they will become. The whole field of growth and development is one which is unique to them and also one which affects nearly every special interest in research and clinical practice. During this period of childhood the effect of social environment is of immense importance as is the quality of the family into which the child is born.

The work reported is not restricted to laboratory and clinical advances but also deals with the delivery of health care and the epidemiology of childhood disease and its prevention. As should be expected, new advances in genetics, immunology and oncology are also highlights because it is these subjects as much as any which have reduced the isolation and esoteric nature of organ specialisation in paediatrics.

All of this is of course incomplete unless a lead is offered in pointing the way to proper care of children in their communities and at the same time bringing us up to date on serious social illnesses such as child abuse. The practice of paediatrics attempts to help all children to achieve the advantageous genetic potential with which they were endowed at conception. This principle is well illustrated in each of the various chapters.

Acknowledgement

The Royal College of Physicians is grateful to the Children Nationwide Medical Research Fund for contributing so willingly and substantially towards the cost of this publication.

Paediatric specialty practice for the 1990s

Papers based on a conference held at the Royal College of Physicians

Edited by
Janet Eyre DPhil MRCP
Department of Child Health, The Medical School, University of Newcastle-upon-Tyne
and
Robert Boyd FRCP
Department of Child Health, University of Manchester

1991

ROYAL COLLEGE OF PHYSICIANS OF LONDON

Royal College of Physicians
11 St Andrews Place, London NW1 4LE

ISBN 1 873240 19 8

Typeset by Oxprint Ltd, Aristotle Lane, Oxford OX2 6TR
Printed by Cathedral Press Ltd, Salisbury, Wilts.

Editors' Preface

An important feature of paediatric practice over the last decade has been the increasing specialisation of paediatrics into sub-specialty areas mainly in referral centres. Within specialty practice it is sometimes difficult to distinguish which changes in clinical habits are based on good data and which on fashion. It is also sometimes difficult for those referring to such services to decide when the disadvantages of referral: distance, potential loss of continuity, lack of familiarity with local support and, on occasion, fragmentation in the care of the whole child, are outweighed by genuine clinical need and advantage.

The present volume, based on papers initially delivered at the 1990 Annual Paediatric Conference at the Royal College of Physicians, attempts to address some of these problems. Individuals from a wide range of paediatric sub-specialties, many chosen with the help and advice of the specialty groups and societies affiliated to the British Paediatric Association, were asked to address two questions. First, what was the evidence justifying changes in the specialty's practice over the last five years. Second, which of the changes are likely to be of most importance for the next decade. The results of our contributors addressing this difficult brief are in the chapters which follow. Almost all commented on the difficulty of covering their development in the space available but most have done so with skill. We are most grateful, for without their efforts there would be no volume. Neonatology was not addressed specifically; it would have expanded the volume beyond reasonable limits. Nevertheless, neonatal aspects of individual sub-specialties are an important element of many of the chapters. The non-tertiary specialty of community paediatrics is however considered in depth.

The overall picture is one of consolidation, elaboration, sometimes simplification, and evolution. The revolution of the new biology has not yet impinged heavily on clinical paediatric practice. As it does so, it will be of great importance that paediatrics continues its tradition of providing good quality child and family centred applications of the scientific advances across the broad range of clinical practice. We must also recruit and train enough able young clinical scientists to allow paediatrics to contribute its share of fresh ideas to the dramatic applications of bioscience to medicine that, together with social factors, appears likely to dominate paediatric practice in the remaining years of the century and beyond.

JANET EYRE and ROBERT BOYD
Editors

Contributors

Barbara Ansell CBE MD FRCS FRCP *Consultant Rheumatologist, previously Head of Division of Rheumatology, Northwick Park Hospital, Harrow, Middlesex HA1 1UJ.*

J. David Baum MSc MD FRCP *Professor of Child Health, Royal Hospital for Sick Children, St Michael's Hill, Bristol BS2 8BJ.*

Alan Craft MD FRCP *Director of Paediatric Oncology, Department of Child Health, The Medical School, University of Newcastle-upon-Tyne, Framlington Place, Newcastle-upon-Tyne NE2 4HH.*

Dian Donnai MB BS FRCP DCH *Consultant Clinical Geneticist, Department of Medical Genetics, St Mary's Hospital, Manchester M13 0JH.*

Ian Hann MD MRC(Path) FRCP *Consultant Haematologist, Department of Haematology and Oncology, Hospital for Sick Children, Great Ormond Street, London WC1N 3JR.*

Alan Jackson MD FRCP *Professor of Human Nutrition, Department of Human Nutrition, University of Southampton, Bassett Crescent East, Southampton SO9 3TU.*

David Jones MB ChB MRCPsych DCH *Clinical Lecturer, Consultant Child Psychiatrist, Park Hospital for Children, Old Road, Headington, Oxford OX3 7LQ.*

Fotini-Heleni Karachaliou MB BS *Research Fellow, Royal Hospital for Sick Children, St Michael's Hill, Bristol BS2 8BJ.*

Michael Levin FRCP *Professor of Paediatrics, Department of Paediatrics, St Mary's Hospital Medical School, South Wharf Road, London W2 1NY.*

Roland Levinsky BSc MD FRCP *Professor of Immunology, Hugh Greenwood Department of Immunology, Institute of Child Health, 30 Guilford Street, London WC1N 1EH.*

Aidan Macfarlane MB BChir FRCP *Consultant Paediatrician with special interests in Child Health, Consultant in Public Health Medicine, Department of Public Health Medicine, Radcliffe Infirmary, Woodstock Road, Oxford OX2 6AG.*

Peter Milla MSc FRCP *Senior Lecturer in Child Health, Institute of Child Health, 30 Guilford Street, London WC1N 1EH.*

Niall O'Donohoe MD FRCPI *Professor of Paediatrics, Department of Paediatrics, National Children's Hospital, Harcourt Street, Dublin 2, Republic of Ireland.*

Richard Olver BSc MBBS FRCP(Lon) FRCP(Ed) *James MacKenzie Professor of Child Health, Department of Child Health, Ninewells Hospital and Medical School, University of Dundee, Dundee DD1 9SY.*

Denis Pereira Gray OBE FRCGP FRSA *General Practitioner, Professor of General Practice, Director Postgraduate Medical School, Royal Devon and Exeter Hospital, Gladstone Road, Exeter EX1 2ED.*

Richard Robinson FRCP *Consultant Paediatric Neurologist, Department of Paediatrics, Guy's Hospital, St Thomas' Street, London SE1 9RT.*

Michael Silverman MD FRCP *Reader in Paediatric Respiratory Medicine, Department of Paediatrics, Royal Postgraduate Medical School, Hammersmith Hospital, Du Cane Road, London W12.*

Penelope Thompson MB MRCPsych DCH *Senior Registrar in Child and Adolescent Psychiatry, Park Hospital for Children, Old Road, Headington, Oxford OX3 7LQ.*

John Wagget MBBS FRCS *Consultant Paediatric Surgeon, Department of Paediatric Surgery, Royal Victoria Infirmary, Queen Victoria Road, Newcastle-upon-Tyne.*

Richard White MD FRCP DCH *Professor of Paediatric Nephrology, Consultant Paediatrician, Renal Department, The Children's Hospital, Ladywood Middleway, Birmingham B16 8ET.*

Christopher Wren MB ChB MRCP *Senior Lecturer in Paediatric Cardiology, Department of Paediatric Cardiology, Freeman Hospital, Freeman Road, High Heaton, Newcastle-upon-Tyne NE7 7DN.*

Contents

1 | Community paediatrics

Aidan Macfarlane
Oxfordshire District Health Auhtority

Introduction

This chapter will examine the major changes in community paediatrics that have occurred over the past five years, and predict what major changes will occur over the next five years. The concept of giving some kind of priority to the importance of these changes is incorporated, as giving priorities assumes increasing importance as resources are continually limited. All the developments outlined are interlinked, and are only artificially separated here for the sake of clarity.

The most significant developments of the past five years

1. Establishment of the post of Consultant Community Paediatrician

The innovation of the post of consultant community paediatrician, frequently with overall responsibility for the organisation of child health services within a district, has instigated certain processes, such as:

(a) the definition of the health needs of the whole population of children and of subpopulations of children, within the community;
(b) the development of information systems for recording these needs;
(c) planning effective interventions to meet these needs;
(d) measuring the outcomes of these interventions.

Also crucial is having a person in each district with an interest in *prevention* of illness and *promotion* of health, rather than crisis intervention when illness has occurred. Exemplary of this approach has been the work of Dr Alan Colver[1] in Northumberland, who began working there in 1983. Two examples of developing information systems, planning effective interventions, and being able to show improved outcomes, using his own information, are: (i) improvements in immunisation uptake in his district compared with other districts in the Region (Fig. 1); (ii) improvements in the age at which children in the district were diagnosed as having sensori-neural hearing loss and were fitted with hearing aids (Fig. 2). To produce these figures Alan Colver has not only developed the appropriate computer software system for data collection but also suggested a minimal data set that could be used to evaluate the child health surveillance programme. The data set is too extensive to go into in detail but a few examples are demonstrated in Table 1. Other examples of similar developments around the country could also be given.

2. Definition of the services covered by the child health services

One of the benefits of having community paediatricians responsible for the child health services for a district is that they can define exactly what these services are. The community child health services are a complex, interlinked series of district health authority (DHA) provisions for children in the community. They are provided for all children in co-operation with the family practitioner services, the hospital services, social services, and the local education authority. Careful planning of co-ordinated services has enabled us to use to maximum effect the minimal resources provided.

This planning has to take account of the fact that 80% of all

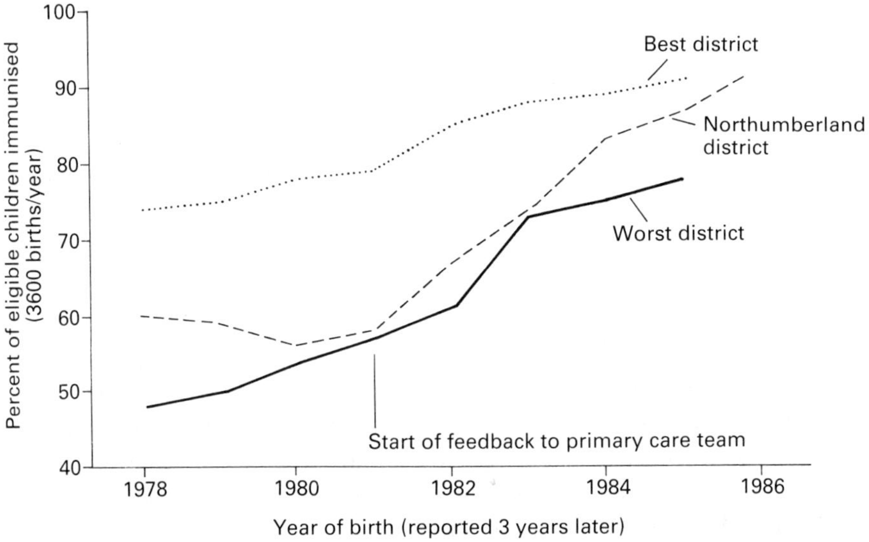

Fig. 1. *Comparison of uptake of immunisation against measles in Northumberland district and other districts in the northern region. From 1978–1986.*

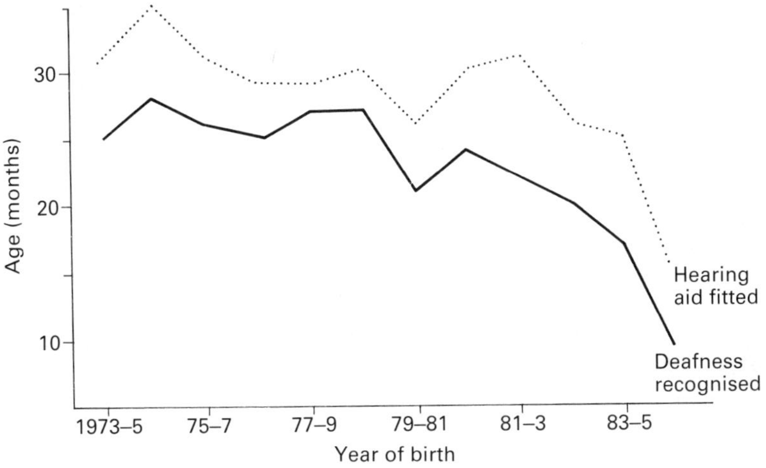

Fig. 2. *Age of children in Northumberland district at detection of congenital deafness and when hearing aids were fitted. Figures are three-year rolling averages. Deafness > 60 dB in better ear.*

Table 1. Data set that could be used to evaluate health surveillance schemes.

Developmental guidance and health education
Immunisation uptake
Accident and emergency department attendance for injuries
Hospital admissions for injuries
Screening and assessment
Uptake of screening test
Average age at diagnosis of congenital deafness
Average age at which children with cerebral palsy start therapy
Average age at which children with congenital dislocation of the hip are diagnosed
Proportion of boys undergoing orchidopexy before the age of 6 years
Number of children starting school with unidentified squint
Average age at which children are referred for severe growth hormone deficiency

illnesses in children are treated and managed by the parents without referral to the primary health care team. Of the 20% of children who are taken to see a member of the primary health care team,[2] only 3% are referred to the hospital.[3] The community child health services are therefore concerned with the 99%-plus of all childhood health problems that never go near a hospital.

All the services provided by community child health services are carried out in conjunction with the primary health care teams, including general practitioners, community nurses, health visitors, district nurses, community paediatric nurses, and practice nurses. The services comprise:

(a) provision of parental support, clinical cover, health promotion, immunisations, surveillance, and management and treatment of health problems to all preschool and school-children;
(b) responsibility for the early identification, assessment, management, and treatment of all children with impairments, disabilities, and handicaps;
(c) provision of clinical care in the community for children with acute and chronic illnesses;
(d) provision of specialised health services to all families who may have difficulties gaining access to medical services (eg children from homeless families, travellers' families, ethnic minority families);
(e) provision of diagnostic, assessment, support, and management services to all children who have been subjected to physical and sexual abuse;
(f) provision of initial medical assessment and continuing medical supervision to all children who are adopted, fostered, or taken into care;
(g) liaison with all the acute hospital services concerned with the care of children, with the primary health care teams, with the Family Health Service Authority and Local Medical Committee, with the local education authorities, with the local county council, and with social services;
(h) planning, monitoring, managing, administering, and auditing all these services;
(i) provision of training for staff working in all the above services.

The services having been defined, many districts have been able to set their 'Aims and Objectives and Standards'.

3. The development of information systems

Crucial to the developing concept of child health services in the community has been taking on responsibility for the health of every child within a population—a concept of 'whole-population paediatrics' —with concern for every child, whether that child is at home, in care, in hospital, or at school. The Fifth Report to the Secretary of State by the Steering Group on Health Services Information, the so-called 'Korner Report',[4] has certainly not found favour with everyone. However, it did highlight the need for Child Health Information Systems:

> Screening and surveillance of children, as well as immunisation, require a level of administration and co-ordination which cannot be undertaken effectively without a computer-based system. As most programmes directed towards children are intended for every child, there is agreement on the need to develop a single integrated administrative system in each district designed to schedule appointments and ensure an accurate record of immunisation, surveillance, screening tests, and action in relation to special educational needs. (Paragraph 8.12)

The result has been a proliferation of child health computer systems run on anything from personal computers (PCs) used by individual consultants to main-frame computers running the National Child Health Computer System at regional level. In most districts, some health information is being collected on computer on every child. In most cases this concept of having epidemiological information on every child is only just beginning. One-hundred-and-thirty-seven of the 192 health districts are now using the national system for their Imm and Vac data, 63 are using it for preschool information data, and 27 are using it for school health information. The developments of the system have gone to real-time interactive systems with access to information on visual display units out in the community in health centres and in hospitals. Other invaluable information for the community child health services has been provided by epidemiologists: for example, the information on the 13,135 children born in 1970 and followed up in the Child Health and Education Study—reported in the book *From Birth To Five*[5]—and yet more information will come from the new 'Children of the 90s' study based in Avon but involving 32,000 children in five countries.

4. Immunisations

The recent increase in immunisation rates has been one of the most significant developments in community paediatrics (Fig. 3), and we are well on our way to reaching the 90% target for the uptake of all immunisations. How far this can be attributed to developments in community paediatrics is arguable, but it has emphasised the importance and the benefits of central organisation. Dr David Salisbury at the Department of Health manages the service nationally via designated immunisation officers with overall responsibility for the immunisation

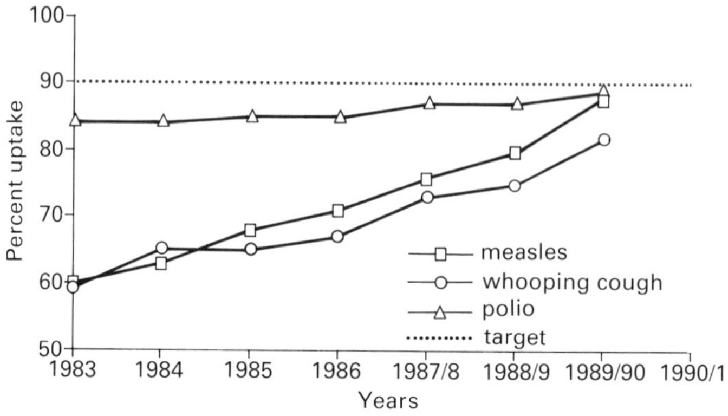

Fig. 3. *Yearly immunisation uptake in England from 1983–1989/90.*

rates in each district. These immunisation officers meet regularly to discuss, among other things, methods of increasing immunisation rates, new immunisations, new schedules, etc. With the present emphasis on resource management, it must also be acknowledged that the two triple vaccines—diphtheria, tetanus, and pertussis (DPT) and measles, mumps, and rubella (MMR)—have both been found to show very considerable cost-benefit ratios.

However, although immunisation rates show great improvements, we also have information showing that 'outcomes' have also changed dramatically in the reported cases of measles (Fig. 4), and in the reported cases of mumps (Fig. 5). The latter is of particular interest as the mumps vaccine was only introduced in the form of the triple measles-mumps-rubella vaccine in the autumn of 1988. Projected into 1991, it leads to the exciting prospect of 30,000 to 40,000 fewer cases of mumps resulting in 100 fewer cases of meningo-encephalitis, five fewer cases of sensori-neural deafness, and two fewer deaths, quite apart from the other burdens of misery the disease brings.

5. A comprehensive review of child health surveillance

In 1983 a review of who did what, and how much, in the preschool health services in England[6] revealed that each district seemed to have a different health surveillance programme based more on the historical factors and the whim of the person running the services rather than on any research evidence of effectiveness. In 1986 a joint working party between the Health Visitors Association, the Royal College of General Practitioners, the British Medical Association, and the British Paediatric Association was set up to review the field. Its report *Health For All Children: A Programme for Child Health*

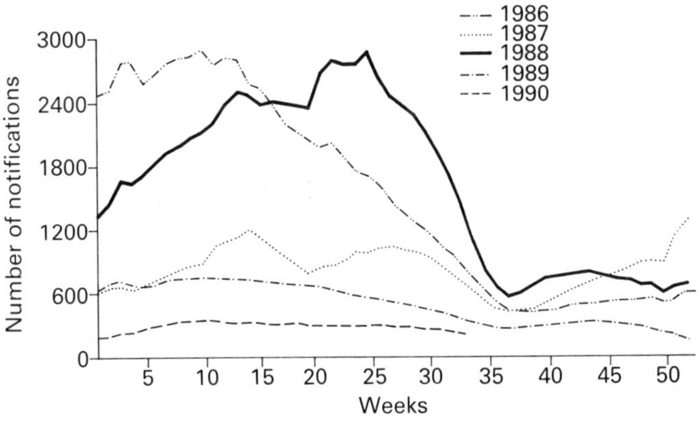

Fig. 4. *Measles notifications to Department of Health (England and Wales) from 1986 to August 1990. (Five week moving average).*

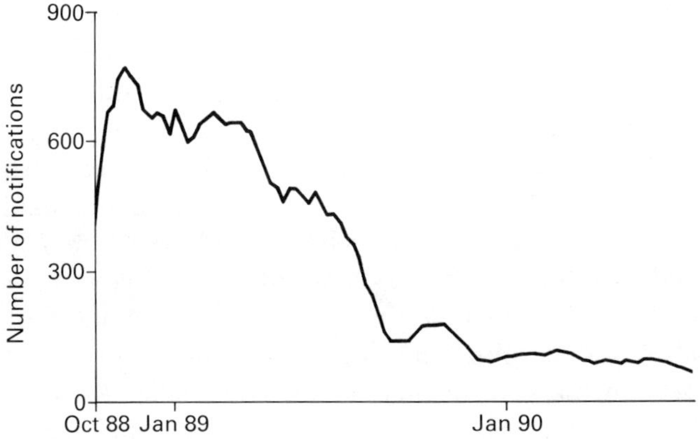

Fig. 5. *Mumps notifications to Department of Health in England and Wales from October 1988 to August 1990. (Five week moving average). NMR vaccine was introduced in October 1988.*

Surveillance, was published in 1989,[7] reviewed over 300 papers on various child health surveillance programmes and suggested a basic national standard. Since that time a 'circus' of speakers has toured the country lecturing on the programme to GPs, health visitors, and clinical medical officers. In September and October 1990, a brief audit as to how far the new child health surveillance programme was actually being used around the country was carried out by two Dutch doctors; and seemed to indicate that implementation was far from complete.[8] The study was carried out because the Dutch wish to perform a similar exercise, and rather than re-invent the wheel they would like to learn from our experience. Such international co-operation must be one way of increasing our efficiency in the future.

Such international co-operation must be one way of increasing our efficiency in the future.

6. Acknowledgement of the essential role played by parents in child care

As already mentioned, there is research showing that parents deal with 80% of illness in their children without referring to a medical professional. Before consulting a medical professional the average parent consults at least three other non-medical people,[3] usually a relative, friend, or neighbour. It is therefore essential that parents are provided, via the media and published material of all kinds, with information which helps them make informed decisions over what action they should take when their child does become ill.

One major move towards this objective in the UK has been the development of a national parent-held 'Personal Child Health Record'.[9] This record will be given to every mother having a baby. It is in loose-leaf form, so that it can start with information about antenatal care, and sections can be added to follow the child through the preschool and school years into adulthood. It is designed to be used not only by health professionals but also by all those concerned with the care of the child. Thus it contains extensive sections for the parents' observations of their child's health and development, sections for the child's preschool teachers, and additional sections for therapists and others involved in the child's care. Giving the parents responsibility for keeping the record acknowledges the parents' essential role in the care of their child, and makes the appropriate information available at whatever point the parents seek help for their child, whether at home, at an accident-and-emergency department, at an outpatient department, or at a GP's surgery; and to whomever is providing the care for the child, whether this be the parent, a relative, a childminder, a nurse, or a doctor. The 'Personal Child Health Record' is also used to provide health education messages particularly concerned with accident prevention.

Parents of 'special needs' children can also gain access to further information about their children through assessment centres, many of which now ensure that a copy of their final report goes to the parents. Part of the philosophy of the Education Act 1981 is also to encourage more involvement with, and information for the parents.

Health education and preventive medicine are not simple. We do not simply decide on a method of preventing a health problem one day and expect it to work the next. People's behaviour is changed by a highly complex mix of influences, perhaps the most effective being legislation. However, there frequently remains a gap between knowledge of a health hazard and changing behaviour to avoid it. A recent survey of schoolchildren[10] showed that 98% knew that smoking was harmful to their health, and 21% smoked. We are however, beginning to learn just how complex are the issues that guide people's decision-making when behaving in certain ways, and how dangerous it may be to interfere with their informed decisions. Certain general principles based on careful research have evolved. One is that feeding back specific information about a person's health, such as the serum cholesterol level, is more likely to be effective in changing behaviour than is providing general information. Another is that where information is provided on the media, such as a television programme about preventing injury to children, follow-up with direct professional input—for example, a visit from a health visitor to discuss the programme—is much more likely to have an effect.

7. Integration of community paediatrics, hospital paediatrics and public health medicine

Integration has been slow in coming, and the emphasis will be more on what should happen in the future than on what has happened in the past. However, one area of significant development has been the employment of clinical community paediatric nurses. An example of the workload of one such nurse, as assessed in Oxford, is given in Table 2.

Table 2. Workload of one community paediatric nurse in Oxford for one year.

Colostomy care and anal dilations	56 visits
Suprapubic catheter care	34 visits
Tracheo-oesophageal fistula care	40 visits
Intermittent catheterisations	60 visits
Changing burns dressings	36 visits
Care of cardiac problems	56 visits
Asthma care	40 visits
Care of epilepsy medications	40 visits
Home oxygen dependency	60 visits
Bowel care	70 visits
Care of handicapping conditions	50 visits
New diabetics	420 visits
Established diabetics	480 visits

The following facts demonstrate the effect on hospital admissions of this particular nurse in the district where she works. In 1983, 46 children were admitted with a diagnosis of diabetes or a complication of diabetes. In 1985 the community paediatric nurse was employed to work with diabetic children, and by 1988 the number of admissions of children with diabetes or complications of diabetes had dropped to 14. This represents a saving of £25,000 pa on the hospital budget, which makes the community paediatric nurse extremely cost-effective.

Other examples of integration could be given by highlighting the number of community paediatricians who are also working in hospital paediatric departments. Integration is, however, a two-way process and there are still too few hospital paediatricians who are willing to come and work part-time in the community.

8. Child development teams and comprehensive care of children with impairments, disabilities, and handicaps

Developments in the care of children with special needs have not been extensive over the past few years. A number of studies have continued to indicate how poor is provision for most of these children —especially young adults—and their families.[11] However, the overall situation has been helped by associated developments, including the total population computer systems which allow for the services provided for these children to be monitored, and the formation of local child development teams and district handicapped teams. The fact that these are multidisciplinary has allowed for better use of integrated resources between the various services contributing to the care of children. With the implementation of the Education Act 1981, there has been increased emphasis on the educational needs of handicapped children and less on their medical needs. Further future developments may take place in providing for the needs of these children and their families with the implementation in 1991 of the Children's Act 1989.

9. Identification and management of children suspected of being sexually abused

Although this subject is dealt with in a later chapter, it is also an area of much concern to community paediatricians. Of particular interest are: (a) what is the normal development pattern of sexuality in children; (b) what can be done about prevention of child sexual abuse; (c) which, if any, interventions have been shown to improve long-term outcome; and (d) could legislation not be enacted by which the suspected perpetrator be denied access to the child for a limited period of time, rather than the child being denied access to its family?

Where community paediatrics is going over the next five years

First, there is a dichotomy: community paediatrics appears to be going in two directions. One direction is towards what can be termed 'total population paediatrics'—that is, concerned with maintaining the optimal health and wellbeing of every child within a population using an integrated approach combining hospital paediatrics, community/social paediatrics, and public health medicine. This perspective views and uses hospital paediatrics as just one of many facilities in helping to maintain the health of a whole population of children in the optimal state available, in the light of current knowledge. It is also a concept that puts increasing emphasis on: (a) recognising the parents as the primary health care-givers to their children; (b) the tools of health promotion and prevention of illness, rather than crisis intervention in disease processes that have already occurred; (c) an advocacy role for children and their families both in the media and politically.

The second direction in which community paediatrics is going is towards a greater role for the 'developmental' paediatrician, with greater integration with educational and social services, in carrying out statutory obligation work concerned with the Education Act 1981 and the Children's Act 1989. In the future they may head up a 'local' child development team, covering a population of between 50,000 and 100,000. Other members of the team would include psychologists/psychiatrists, therapists, community nurses, and professionals from education and social services. The team could be responsible for all children of whatever age in the patch who had physical or mental impairments/disabilities/handicaps, and take over part of the role of the school health services. The team would have the responsibility for ensuring that local services for children with special needs and their families were clearly identified and met, and could also have local involvement with children suspected of being abused. Such local teams should lead to the more efficient use of integrated resources and cut down on inappropriate hospital outpatient referrals.

Other areas of future development

1. Research

The quality and quantity of research carried out in the community has greatly improved over the past few years, but much more needs to be done. The first essential step is to get agreement on a number of valid basic outcome measures by which we can judge the health of a population of children. We have the beginnings in mortality data, and data concerning notifiable diseases. These need to be added to by further research involving case/control studies to look at the effectiveness of different interventions, including different methods of service provision. We have made some progress, with the recent document published by the British Paediatric Association,[12] but more discussion needs to take place at national and international level. Much valid research concerning child health is also available from other countries, and rather than taking an isolationist view and trying to 're-invent the wheel', if the research is well carried out and appears applicable then it should be used.

2. Further integration between community paediatrics, hospital paediatrics, primary health care, and public health medicine

Some community paediatricians already also hold the title of consultants in public health medicine. Public health has much to teach us, and the areas in which we might co-operate[13] are shown in Table 3.

Table 3. Public health medicine/community paediatric interface.

Monitoring screening programmes
Organisation of immunisation programmes
Liaison with social services and education services
Organisation of health promotion programmes
Health advocacy (especially political)
Community approaches to prevention
Training other health professionals
Planning and developing children's services
Developing outcome measures for child health

Integration between hospital paediatrics and community paediatrics is also vital. A study from Nottingham[14] showed that, on average, a first-born child had 26.7 contacts with health professionals during its first year of life. These included an average of 12.9 visits to the child health clinic, 6.5 visits to the GP's surgery, 0.8 visits to the hospital inpatient and outpatient services, and 0.5 home visits by the GP. The balance is made up of visits by the health visitor and midwife to the child's home.

Integration could be developed so that both nurses and doctors are trained to feel comfortable working in either setting, and also actually work in both settings. The possible areas of integrated work are shown in Table 4.

Table 4. Hospital paediatric/community paediatric interface.

Developing day care for a wide variety of surgical and medical paediatric problems with the resulting cost benefits for the services and emotional benefits for parents and child
Working to achieve the aim that no child should be admitted to hospital unnecessarily
Developing joint protocols for the care of specific conditions in the community and in the accident and emergency departments
Monitoring of accident and emergency department attendances
Monitoring hospital admissions
Monitoring referrals from primary health care teams
Developing a clinical paediatric community nursing service for children with chronic clinical problems, specifically in the fields of oncology, neonatology, and respiratory diseases
Developing an integrated service for the care of handicapped children

Integration between community paediatrics and primary health care operates on many different fronts, as follows.

(a) With Family Health Services Authorities
Setting standards: both the standards of training and clinical practice that the GP should have before being admitted to the child health surveillance list, and the professional standards as to what should be included in a child health surveillance programme. This should be done in conjunction with others involved in child health surveillance, ie health visitors.

(b) Over quality assurance
We are entering a new age of professional accountability, where clinical freedom for individual doctors will have to be integrated with certain accepted professional standards. As an example, a recent study of hysterectomies carried out in women in the USA found that 81% of the hysterectomies were carried out on grounds that did not meet the most up-to-date professionally accepted standards.

We have been fortunate in England to have available a set of standards both for immunisations[15] and for child health surveillance.[7] The question now remains how best to audit the services provided both by the district health authority and the primary health care doctors in order to meet these standards. Some suggestions that are being explored are:

(i) visiting clinics using a group of professionals including GP, health visitor, and community paediatrician, to observe not only individual practice but also working relationships. Should a parent also be included?

(ii) using the 'non-carbonated' copies from the parent-held Personal Child Health Record.

(c) With the Local Medical Committee and postgraduate general practice training

Training comprises: (a) initial training in child health for GPs (in Oxford, there are now two Senior House Officers in community paediatrics, both as part of the local GP training scheme); (b) update courses for GPs as part of their postgraduate medical training in child health; (c) courses for practice nurses concerning primary prevention, including immunisation and child health surveillance; (d) combined update courses for all those involved in child health, including health visitors.

(d) Directly with individual practices

The district health authority is obligated to provide child health surveillance for children where GPs do not wish to carry out this procedure or are not suitably qualified to do so. In the 130 practices in Oxfordshire, only one is not at present undertaking child health surveillance for the children in their own practice.

3. Immunisations

There are two advances that are possible in the future. First, the introduction (hopefully within the next two or three years) of the vaccine against *Haemophilus influenzae*. It is estimated that there is a cumulative incidence of one systemic infection with Hib for every 600 children before their fifth birthday, with a 5% mortality rate. Extrapolating from these results, there are 1300 systemic cases nationally with 65 deaths.[16] The introduction of this vaccine is a good example of co-operation between specialists in the field of community paediatrics and infectious diseases.

Secondly, as already suggested, enormous strides have been made in achieving high immunisation uptake rates, with very significant reductions in the incidence of the relative infectious diseases. The aim of the 'Health for All 2000' programme to manage over 90% uptake rates looks achievable. Already organisations are working to persuade manufacturers towards the next goal of developing vaccines that are even more polyvalent, so that a single injection might protect a child against, say, six or seven infectious diseases. The second advance is that such vaccines should be made thermostable, so that the cold chain will no longer be the vital and vulnerable link that it is at present.

4. Increasing the role of the parent

The move to make information more accessible to the parent by providing every parent with a Personal Child Health Record now needs to be extended to all new births in the country, and should be followed by allowing parents full access to all other medical records kept on their children.

5. Prevention of injury

Injuries remain the single commonest cause of death in children aged from one to nineteen years. In 1989 there were 1,020 deaths due to injuries in children and young adults (from the age of nought to twenty-four), and an estimated 3,000 were left permanently disabled. American research suggests that for each death there are 45 children who need admission to hospital, and 1,300 who require medical treatment.[17] It has also been estimated that 29% of deaths in children could be prevented by instituting 12 preventive measure at present available.[18] The major causes of severe injuries and death are motor vehicle accidents involving both car occupants and pedestrians, drowning and near drowning, and burns.

Injuries to children require special consideration because children depend on society to protect them from harm and to minimise their vulnerability from both unintentional and intentional injury. Most injuries result from complex interactions of the environment, the

Occupants of motor vehicles

- better in car restraints with legislation on usage
- vehicle design improvements
- alcohol abuse prevention programmes

Pedestrian and cycle injuries

- control of toddlers using restraints
- parental knowledge of children's abilities on the road both on foot and on bicycle
- use of cycle helmets
- alcohol abuse prevention programmes
- better traffic control systems

Fire and burns

- smoke detectors
- controlling temperature of tap water
- fire guards

Drowning and near drowning

- regulations concerning surroundings of pools

Fig. 6. *Interventions for injury prevention and control.*

host, and the energy source. No single intervention will normally be wholly effective but many opportunities for accident prevention exist, some of which are shown in Fig. 6.

The role of community paediatrics in preventing injury is a varied one, but the priority is to obtain information concerning injuries in children in the local district, from local accident and emergency departments, the police, and the road safety officer of the local county council. Many districts are now setting up joint planning committees on injury prevention between health services, local county council, education authority, and police.

Conclusions

Community paediatrics is the most rapidly expanding branch of paediatrics as a whole. With the new provider/purchaser arrangements, increasing flexibility and co-operation is needed between community paediatrics, other paediatric specialities, and the education and social services. Community paediatricians should be involved in defining the 'health' and 'illness' services required for all children within a district. In order to do this the most important 'future needs' to be considered are, the development of valid outcome measures by which the effectiveness of interventions can be judged, the increasing involvement of parents, the better use of resources for the care of 'special needs' children and their families, and the development of better methodologies for preventing illness and injury in children.

References

1. Colver, A. (1990) Health surveillance of preschool children: four years' experience. *British Medical Journal*, **300**, 1246–1248.
2. Spencer, N.J. (1984) Parent's recognition of the ill child. In *Progress in child health* (vol 1) Macfarlane, J.A. (ed.). Edinburgh and London: Churchill Livingstone, pp. 100–112.
3. Cartright, A., Anderson, R. (1981) *General practice revisited.* London: Tavistock Publications.
4. Steering Group on Health Services Information (1984) Fifth Report to the Secretary of State. London: HMSO.
5. Butler, N., Golding, G. (1986) *From birth to five.* Oxford: Pergamon Press.
6. Macfarlane, J.A., Pillay, U. (1984) Who does what, and how much, in the preschool health services in England. *British Medical Journal*, **289**, 851–852.
7. Hall, D. (ed.) (1989) *Health for all children; a programme for child health surveillance.* Oxford: Oxford Medical Publications.
8. Donkers, L., Merkx, J. (1990) *How to arrange less.* Report for Dutch Committee on Child Health Surveillance.
9. BPA, HVA, RCGP, BMA (1989) *Parent and professional held records used in child health surveillance. Report of a joint working party.* London: British Paediatric Association.

10. Macfarlane, A., McPherson, A., McPherson, K., Ahmed, L. (1987) Teenagers and their health. *British Medical Journal*, **62**, 1125–1129.
11. Thomas, A., Bax, M., Smyth, D. (1989) *The health and social needs of physically handicapped young adults*. Oxford: Blackwell Scientific Publications.
12. BPA (1989) *Measurement of child health: Report of a working party of the Executive Committee of the Community Paediatric Group*. London: British Paediatric Association.
13. BPA (1990) *Together for Tomorrow's Children: Report of joint working party from the Faculty of Public Health Medicine and the British Paediatric Association*. London, British Paediatric Association.
14. Polnay, L. (1990) Personal communication.
15. DoH (1990) *Immunisation against infectious disease*. London: HMSO.
16. Tudor-Williams, G., Frankland, J., Isaacs, D. (1989) Haemophilus influenzae type b disease in the Oxford Region. *Archives of Diseases in Childhood*, **64**, 517–519.
17. Guyer, B., Ellers, B. (1990) Childhood injuries in the United States. *American Journal of Diseases in Children*, **144**, 649–652.
18. Gallagher, S.S., Messenger, K.P., Guyer, B. (1987) State and local responses to children's injuries: The Massachusetts statewide childhood injury prevention programme. *Journal of Social Issues*, **43**, 149–162.

2 | Children's sexual experience – normal and abnormal

David P. H. Jones and Penelope J. Thompson
Park Hospital for Children, Oxford

Children's sexual knowledge and behaviour ranges from normal to abnormal. Paediatricians and others involved in the health and social services frequently have to decide whether a particular child may have been abused or not. It is clear from the wide variety of definitions used in various epidemiological studies[1] that there is lack of agreement as to what constitutes abuse or exploitation in childhood. We do know, however, that abusive and exploitative experiences are relatively common during childhood. Some cases involve exposure of the genitals or single touching experiences, and others, extensive penetrative sexual acts over an extended period. The term 'normal' may describe what happens to the majority of children, but it is already clear that within a single society the range of normality is wide. It is within this context of inadequate information that practitioners have to work with potentially abused children. An aim of this chapter is to describe the range of normal sexuality in relation to childhood, particularly its place in the assessment and management of abuse. It is apparent that the crisis in Cleveland[2] had many different aspects, but a notable one was the variability between different professionals' preparedness to recognise and respond to child sexual abuse. Recent issues in the assessment and treatment of child sexual abuse will then be considered.

Psycho-sexual development and the recognition of abuse

Despite the enormous interest in child sexual abuse shown in recent years there has been little corresponding concern with 'normal' psycho-sexual development in children. This deficiency is especially important for those who have to decide if a child's sexual understanding, knowledge, or experiences are normal or not. There is in any case great controversy over the use of the term 'normal'. Should 'normal' be considered in the sense of customary or usual practices, or in the sense of what is morally acceptable? Any view of what is normal (in the sense of customary or usual) has to take into account children of different genders at different developmental stages and ages. There is great difficulty in developing this information due to the continuing taboos about sexuality in general.

The Kinsey Report[3] is still one of the best sources of information about the range of common activities, thoughts, and feelings in relation to sex among adult men and women. There is no equivalent report relating to childhood sexuality. Goldman and Goldman[4] have gone some way towards remedying this. Their research included a wide range of questions about sexuality. It involved 838 children and looked at boys and girls from four different countries and five different age-bands. Thus, in each cell there were only approximately 40 boys and girls from each country in the age-band in question. Furthermore, the range of topics considered was very broad, being concerned with sex role, sexual identity, and knowledge about birth control, marriage, childbirth etc., with less accent upon the children's own sexual feelings and experiences. However, it is an important study which helps to emphasise the range of considerations necessary for the practitioner when considering psycho-sexual development in children. As with adults,[3] studies of childhood sexuality have to deal with the differences between what is said publicly and what actually happens behind the closed doors of the family. The Kinsey Report was extremely helpful in emphasising the great variability of sexual knowledge and experience in the community, yet currently there is no similar bank of knowledge relating to childhood sexuality.

Components of childhood sexuality

By considering psycho-sexual development in children we are concerning ourselves with the knowledge which children have at different ages, their experience of sex, including their sexual behaviour, and what parents know about their children in relation to these three areas. Considering children's knowledge of sexuality first, we need to distinguish between their self-knowledge, their knowledge about other children of both genders, and their knowledge about adults of both genders. We must also be concerned with considerations about sex role, identification, and aspects of procreation. Furthermore, we are interested in children's knowledge about abuse and inappropriate sexual activities at different ages. Recent work has examined the sexual knowledge of non-abused children aged from two to seven years, and demonstrated significant age and social class differences in sexual knowledge.[5] Younger children know significantly less than older ones about sexual body parts and their function, sexual behaviour, pregnancy, birth, and the prevention of sexual abuse. Children from higher socio-economic backgrounds have more knowledge than those from lower backgrounds. Most seven-year-olds only had a limited understanding of adult sexual behaviour such as intercourse.

Goldman and Goldman[4] found that children aged five and seven years were very unrealistic about sex differences, but by nine years of age a realistic view of sexual differences between children and prepubertal changes had emerged. Swedish children were approximately two years ahead of those from Australia, England, or the USA, possibly reflecting the impact of different cultural attitudes within the family and education towards discussion of sexual matters with children. While most children did not know the origin of babies until about eleven years of age, Swedish children showed this ability at around the age of nine. Additionally, about one-quarter of Swedish children at the age of five had some idea of the physical basis of procreation. As for gestation and birth, most children had a realistic response by the age of eleven, whereas the vast majority of children at the ages of five and seven thought that babies emerged from the anus. Nevertheless, one-fifth of eleven-year-olds thought that babies came from the anus. With regard to sexual intercourse, children aged nine and ten years were already beginning to relate the production of babies to intercourse, while those aged five and seven had no apparent knowledge of this. After the age of nine, children began to say that intercourse had other functions beside procreation, such as enjoyment or the expression of love; boys indicating pleasure responses, and girls tending towards notions of romantic love. Contraception was rarely known about until the age of thirteen, though at an earlier age in Sweden. Children from higher socio-economic groups demonstrated better knowledge of contraception, though class effects were rarely demonstrated with regard to other aspects of children's knowledge. Most children knew what was meant by the word 'rape' by the age of eleven, with fully appropriate responses given by most children at the age of thirteen. These data provide a broad perspective, but 'cell' size and methodological problems do limit the applicability and clinical usefulness of the findings.

When children are deliberately taught about the possibility of sexual assault, most successfully learn the prevention content.[6,7] In the short term there is some evidence that their skill in preventing abuse is also increased.[8] However, qualitative work with offenders indicates that there are many gaps, especially with regard to identifying vulnerable children, and preventing the abuse through coercion and the desensitisation of children.[9] Even if these latter problems could be overcome by prevention programmes, the concern remains that children will learn the content and presume that it applies to other children rather than to themselves. A similar process has been noted in relation to AIDS knowledge in nine-year-old children,[10] where children felt the knowledge acquired was not relevant to them.

By contrast, we have very little information about children's experience of sex, and there are few large, epidemiologically sound samples which enable us to draw conclusions about what may be described as 'normal'. Very little information is available about experimentation between children. To what degree and extent are showing, touching, and variations on the game of 'doctors and nurses', the norm for children in our society? Does such activity vary with age, gender, social class, etc? What is the normal degree and extent of sexual experimentation between children within families or in residential settings?

It has been generally assumed that there is little touching activity in sexual areas between children and their parents. However, a study by Rosenfeld *et al.*[11] showed that in the majority of families studied there was looking at and touching of genitals between the adults and children, usually of an accidental nature or in the context of bathing, dressing, and normal family intimacy.

Turning to the play and the drawings which non-abused children produce, we have even less information. The lack of normative data for the free play of children exposed to anatomically correct dolls has been put forward as a reason for caution in their use.[12] Nevertheless, professionals tend to deduce a great deal from the free play of children with such dolls. There is, however, considerable individual and between-group variation in professionals' interpretation of the meaning of children's play with anatomical dolls.[13]

Children's modesty at different ages has received little attention. The Goldmans[4] reported their findings on children's thoughts about nakedness. Rosenfeld *et al.*[14] examined parental perceptions of their children's modesty, and found that a gradual increase in modesty feelings about being seen without clothes, or on the toilet, occurred between the ages of two and ten years, with few sex differences. First-born children showed markedly less modesty than those born later. Unfortunately, the variability (see below) in these findings was not highlighted in the results, despite being referred to in the discussion.

An English study by Smith and Groche, from the Institute of Child Health, London, has remedied many of the shortcomings of previous work.[15] They studied 148 children aged from four to sixteen years, and their mothers, comparing them with an abused group of children. A small but significant number of the non-abused children were relatively frequently exposed to pornographic materials and sexually explicit videos. They also discovered that behaviours considered by some authorities to be indicative of abuse, such as drawing of genitalia and masturbation, occurred relatively commonly in the non-abused. Age and class differences did exist. These important findings will enable British clinicians to develop guidelines which neither over- nor under-estimate the range of normal in children of different ages.

Variability in psycho-sexual development

Many of the results reported above have indicated the variability in both knowledge and experience that is dependent upon social class, gender, or the attitudes and approach to education as in the Swedish children in the Goldmans' study. However, there are other factors which can have an effect on both knowledge and experience. For example, having a sibling of the opposite sex resulted in an increased knowledge about sex differences when compared with children with siblings of the same sex only.[4] The effect of large families, overcrowding, and sharing bedrooms has not been examined to date. Recent reports from the family therapy literature reveal that in newly reconstituted families there may be more evidence of an expression of sexual feeling between adults, and it could be that this too would influence children's understanding and knowledge of sex. The family's viewpoint and attitude towards personal nudity, as well as exposure to sexually explicit material such as video tapes and its influence on children's knowledge and experience, have received very little attention until recent work by Smith and Groche[15] and Friedrich.[16] Friedrich[16] examined the responses of three groups of children to anatomically correct dolls, and their free drawings of human figures. The three groups were a sexually abused group, a non-abused group, and a group who, although non-abused, had been exposed to excessive personal nudity in the home or had watched explicit videos. The abused group more frequently drew genitalia and played in a sexual manner with anatomically correct dolls than the non-abused. However, the third group had responses more in keeping with the abused than with the non-abused children.

There have been several studies of the play of young, non-abused children with anatomical dolls.[17,18,19] These large-scale studies have indicated how few children exhibit explicit sexual play. However, Everson and Boat[19] illustrate that within a sub-group of their sample, who were poor, black, male, and aged five years or more, rates of sexually explicit play with anatomically correct dolls was in excess of 20%. Such variabilities are crucial for practitioners to keep in mind when they are interpreting play. In one small-scale study,[20] a group of abused and non-abused children were re-interviewed with a standard protocol utilising anatomically correct dolls, where the interviewer was blind to the subject condition. Interviewers achieved a barely greater than chance correct categorisation on assessment of the children's spontaneous remarks and behaviour, with both false positives and negative diagnoses. However in this study, for ethical reasons, specific inquiry about sexual abuse was not undertaken, which limits the applicability of the study to general clinical situations.

Leventhal *et al.*[21] in a retrospective survey of 83 children under seven years old, found that when anatomically correct dolls were used the children were able to convey significantly more information. However, the sub-group of children who did not use dolls contained eleven children who were considered too young to use them. This figure probably affected the results obtained. Nevertheless, the study is one of the first to explore the potential *benefit* of anatomically correct dolls as opposed to concern with their misuse.[22]

Comparison of abused and non-abused children

Turning to the development of children who have been sexually abused compared with those who have not, several studies have shown an increased rate of sexualised behaviour following abuse.[23,24] Few studies have examined abused children's sexual knowledge and understanding in comparison to that of non-abused children. Einbender and Friedrich[25] are an exception, and demonstrated in their study higher rates of sexual preoccupation in the abused compared with the non-abused. By contrast, Gordon *et al.*,[26] in a matched comparison sample, showed no difference between abused and non-abused children regarding knowledge of sexuality. Interestingly, many of the abused children gave unusual emotional responses or made spontaneous utterances suggestive of abuse in response to the questions asked. This finding confirms the impression of other researchers[19] and clinicians[27] that the type of response as well as the accompanying verbal utterances may be more significant than the simple nature of play or response to questions.

In summary, then, we can say that there is a wide range of 'normal' psycho-sexual understanding and experience among children. Additionally, it appears that children are 'sexual' throughout their childhood and do not seem to demonstrate a latency period. The conclusion that one type of understanding or behaviour is normal and another abnormal must, therefore, be made with great care by professionals, who must themselves bring into the equation their own experience, knowledge, and attitudes to sexuality. Perhaps one of the best ways of understanding whether a particular behaviour represents abuse or not is to consider if it is exploitative when first initiated.[27] For example, was the activity unwanted when it first started, and/or involved a misuse of conventional age, authority, or gender differentials to obtain the co-operation of the child. Further, when determining whether 'normal' family intimacy is exploitative or abusive, one should consider the extent to which the child's own feelings and sensitivities were respected or not.

Child sexual abuse is defined[27] as the occurrence of a sexual act(s), involving a child, which is committed by a person who is five or more years older or who, in initiating the sexual act, exploits the child in question.

The term 'sexual acts' includes the following:

acts of genital exposure;

genital or anal sexual contact (child's or adult's);

penetration (oral, vaginal, or anal);

other acts which involve the child as the object of sexual gratification.

The term 'exploitation' refers to the balance of power between the child and the other person at the time the sexual activity first occurred.[28] Thus exploitation is considered to have occurred if the activity was unwanted when first started, and if it involved a misuse of conventional age, authority, or gender differentials.

In general, the 'five or more years' age-gap is part of this definition. However, in children less than five years old, all activities falling into the above categories constitute child sexual abuse. Also, in cases where a possible victim and abuser are less than five years apart in age, the situation is examined for signs of exploitation (cases of brother–sister incest are thus often included despite an age-gap of less than five years if exploitation was present at the initiation of activities).

Recognition of child sexual abuse

The importance of clear and agreed working arrangements between professionals has been stressed by many recent documents.[2,29] However, trust cannot be prescribed. Nevertheless a feasible context can be organised to enable trust between professionals to develop. While the national guidelines are helpful, they are worthless without local interpretation, and area child protection committees (ACPCs) need to take the lead by establishing realistic practical procedures. Nevertheless, creating arrangements for joint working between paediatricians and police surgeons may be difficult. Sometimes there is a similar difficulty in the working relationship between community and hospital-based paediatricians. The relationship of medical services to social services and police departments needs to be clearly worked out. Controversy exists as to what is the appropriate training for a doctor intending to examine potential victims of child sexual abuse, and although a joint statement has been produced, police surgeons tend to emphasise the importance of the forensic base to their work with children, whereas paediatricians emphasise the need for a 'whole child' approach. At this stage there seems no substitute for effecting local agreements about the requisite training and continuing-education requirements, as well as direct working arrangements.

Locally in Oxfordshire, occasional meetings of front-line practitioners—social services, police, and medical practitioners—have been helpful to enable practical policies to be agreed by managers. It is useful for doctors to remember that whereas senior medical practitioners are also managers of the service they provide, in the police and social services this is not the case. In these latter two services there is a significant divide between practitioners and managers of services. This has major implications for the working of area child protection committees, to ensure that the experience of direct practitioners is brought into the forum where procedures are agreed.

Presentation

Jones and McQuiston[27] have reviewed how sexually abused children present to professional attention. There appear to be five main routes:

1. through an account by the child;
2. through disturbed behaviour exhibited by the child;
3. through physical signs and symptoms;
4. through an association with another form of maltreatment;
5. by allegations arising from parents, relatives, or other adults.

The most common route is through the direct statement of the child.[30] The child usually tells another child of the same age, who subsequently raises the alarm by telling his or her parent. The second commonest route is for the child to tell a parent or trusted adult. A presentation through physical signs or symptoms is relatively unusual (less than 10%).

Medical issues of recognition and diagnosis

Much controversy has arisen in recent years over the importance attached to physical findings in the diagnosis of child sexual abuse. Although there is a general consensus that physical examination is usually only an adjunct to the child's account, much research has centred on trying to find definitive measurements and pathognomonic signs. Unfortunately, this has been compounded by pressures from the legal system to provide 'concrete' evidence for the courts.

Some of the controversy has arisen because of the diversity of examination techniques employed and in the interpretation of the findings. White and Ingram[31] have concluded from their study of 242 girls that measurements of vaginal introital diameter can be highly diagnostic of child sexual abuse. However, these findings have been criticised by other workers.[32] Some workers have recommended the use of the paediatric otoscope and the colposcope.[33] In their prospective study of genital findings in sexually abused girls, these workers found the otoscope and colposcope useful in detecting findings in one-third of these girls. In contrast, Muram[34] studied 205 prepubertal female victims of child sexual abuse. He found that in the vast majority (96%) of these girls the abnormalities were observed with unaided examination, ie without colposcopic examination. Of the remaining 4% examined by colposcopy the abnormal findings were detected on repeated unaided examination.

In both these studies the genitalia of the majority of the sexually abused girls were normal. Another interesting study by Muram[35] compared the findings observed in victims of sexual abuse with the sexual acts to which the perpetrator subsequently admitted. Although specific findings were more commonly observed when the perpetrator admitted to vaginal penetration, 39% of the 'penetrated' girls showed either normal genitalia or only non-specific abnormalities.

Anal examination and the importance and specificity of anal dilation has also been the subject of much discussion, especially since the Cleveland Inquiry. The Inquiry concluded that 'the sign of anal dilation is abnormal and suspicious and requires further investigation. It is not in itself evidence of anal abuse'.[2] The importance of assessing the child and family as a whole was stressed; the evidence from a physical examination should also be assessed within this context.

Recent studies of anal examination in non-abused children have produced interesting results. McCann and colleagues in the USA[36] selected 267 non-abused children by questionnaire and found a large range of physical findings on anal examination. These were erythema, pigmentation, anal dilation, venous congestion, and tags. Interestingly, none had fissures or tears, haematomas, abrasions, or haemorrhoids. Forty-nine percent had some degree of anal dilation; however, only 1.2% had anal dilation greater than 2cm. Muram[34] has looked prospectively at peri-anal findings of 310 victims of child sexual abuse and found that 66% had normal perinea on examination. Stanton and Sutherland,[37] in a study of 200 children from outpatient clinic populations, found a degree of anal dilation in 6% to 43% of children attending clinic. The reason for this large difference in frequency is unclear.

In contrast, Hobbs and Wynne[38] have described their findings on anal examination of 337 children likely to have been sexually abused. Between 42% and 60% of these children had one or more anal finding, and 86% of those with multiple anal findings showed anal dilation. The implication of the diversity of findings underlines the importance of full assessment of the child and family in suspected cases of child sexual abuse, and lays particular emphasis on what the child says.[39] Undue reliance on physical findings alone can be misleading. Many studies have looked for the presence of sexually transmitted disease in sexually abused children. By far the most common of these is gonorrhoea, although syphilis, trichomoniasis, chlamydia, genital herpes and genital mycoplasma may also be found. A high incidence of mixed infections has also been reported.[40] There is no agreement on the question of screening victims of child sexual abuse for HIV, even where they are clearly at raised risk.[41] In recent years studies have examined the relationship between anogenital warts and sexual abuse in young children.[42] It has been shown that anogenital warts often co-exist with other infective agents or with other anogenital abnormalities. These studies leave little doubt that in many cases the children are victims of sexual abuse. Transmission from an infected mother during birth is a possible exception, but even young children with infected mothers should be thoroughly assessed. The oncogenic nature of some of the Human papillovirus types means that treatment and long-term follow-up are needed with these children. Most authors advocate that the presence of warts is sufficient grounds to pursue an assessment for child sexual abuse.[42]

It is also important to remember that other conditions can very occasionally present as child sexual abuse. Jenny *et al.*[43] described two cases of genital lichen sclerosis in girls which were mistaken for child sexual abuse. Hay *et al.*[44] described Crohn's disease, with perianal and vulval involvement, presenting with physical signs which could easily have been misdiagnosed as child sexual abuse. In cases such as these, mistaken diagnoses could have a devastating impact on the family, and once again the importance of the child's word and psychological assessment must be stressed, with the emphasis on a more holistic approach to diagnosis.

The psychological process of abuse

It is important to understand the context in which child sexual abuse takes place, not only to give a clearer picture of both victims' and abusers' perspectives, but also to be able to increase the efficacy of prevention programmes. Until recently little was known about the abuser's perspective of abuse; however recent studies have shown how subtle and infiltrative the victimisation process of abuse can be.

Berliner and Conte[45] interviewed 23 victims of child sexual abuse aged under 18 years, and identified three stages of this process: the gradual sexualisation of the relationship; justification of the sexual contact using cognitive distortions; and maintenance of the child's co-operation, often by coercion and exploitation of vulnerability. In a complementary study Conte, Wolfe, and Smith[9] interviewed 20 sexual offenders about the methods used to select and groom their victims. The offenders were able to identify vulnerable children and then manipulate their weaknesses to gain sexual access. Again, they illustrated the sophisticated way in which the offenders gradually desensitised their victims to touch, while increasing the sexualisation of the touching as the relationship developed. Abel *et al.*[46] have shown that the beliefs and cognitions of child abusers about their behaviour differ from those of non-abusers. They are able, therefore, repeatedly to justify their actions through their distorted cognitions.

Less common aspects of child sexual abuse

Although the majority of child sexual abuse takes place between a male abuser and a female victim, more research is becoming available on female abusers, male victims, and children who abuse.

Relatively little is known about females who abuse. However, it has been suggested that the incidence is under-estimated. This may be partially due to unwillingness to accept that females can commit such acts. Such prejudices can lead to difficulty in decision-making about the management of such cases.[47] Krug[48] gives an interesting description of eight male children sexually abused by their mothers. All of the mothers were experiencing marital difficulties, and half were still married at the time of the abuse. None of the mothers were psychotic, although 25% were abusing drugs. In a long-term follow-up of the abused sons, all had problems with long-term relationships, 88% became depressed as adults, 75% were promiscuous, 63% were abusing drugs, and 38% had sexual identity problems. Although the sample is small, the wide range of psychopathology in these males is striking.

The accepted view has been that female abusers perpetrate less serious acts and that they do so as a result of coercion by male partners. It has also been thought that the effects on the victim are less severe than when the abuser is male. The above findings, taken in combination with the evidence emerging from the field of multiple abuse, emphasise the range of severity of acts perpetrated by women, together with the serious long-term effects on victims.

The available research on male victims has been reviewed by Vander-May.[49] Male children seem more likely to be abused by non-family members than by family members. The risk of non-familial abuse appears to be increased if the family is neglectful or if a mother heads the household. The risk of familial sexual abuse is increased if the father has been previously sexually abused, if other siblings are being abused, or if the parents have personality and/or social adjustment problems. An important effect of abuse on boys seems to be a sexualisation of their behaviour, including in some cases abuse of other children.[50] Both male and female children who abuse are becoming increasingly recognised. Cavannagh-Johnson[51] described thirteen female child abusers between four and thirteen years of age, all of whom had been sexually abused. Of these, 85% were abused by a family member, and 37% had been physically abused. Seventy-seven percent of the children who abused chose a victim within their family, the remainder having no family members available. The mean age at the first perpetration was six years nine months; the average number of victims was 3.5, with a range of 1–15. The girls victimised twice as many boys as girls. This and other studies illustrate the need for children's sexualised play to be carefully assessed for evidence of exploitation.

The abuse of groups of children has received much media attention. Jones[52] has made interim proposals for policy, practice, and research of this problem, while noting the absence of adequate data and police corroboration. Meanwhile, cases do present to clinicians in which the abuse of children seems to involve a total immersion in a deviant value and belief system. In these cases sexual abuse is but one aspect of a child's experience. Clinically such cases pose enormous problems in terms of therapy time and skill as well as the personal resources of the staff involved.

Psychological effects of child sexual abuse

The major effects on children who have experienced sexual or physical violence have been collectively described as 'post-traumatic stress disorder'.[53,54] This disorder has also been found in those who have witnessed sexual violence.[55] The characteristics of post-traumatic stress disorder include flashbacks of the traumatic experience. These may occur spontaneously or as a result of non-sexual touching or affection, and may give the victim the sense of re-experiencing the abuse. Other characteristics include withdrawal, detachment, and a sense of heightened anxiety and alertness which may result in insomnia and nightmares. Other indicators may be memory impairment, blankness, irritability, or depression.

Psychosomatic responses may occur in children who have been sexually abused. These include abdominal pain, headache, weakness, and hysterical seizures.[56,57] Other psychological effects of sexual abuse in children include a pervasive loss of self-esteem which may result in a failure of self-care, and in self-neglect.[58] This poor esteem in older children may result in severe depressive feelings, self-mutilation, suicidal attempts, and absconding from home.

The long-term effects into adulthood of child sexual abuse are becoming increasingly recognised. Adult female victims have been shown to have many more psychological symptoms than non-abused females including, in particular, substance addiction, self-destructive behaviour, and re-victimisation experiences.[59] It is becoming increasingly recognised that women with anorexia nervosa and bulimia have a high incidence of previous sexual abuse. One study has shown that half of the sample of 72 women presenting with anorexia nervosa or bulimia had been sexually abused.[60]

There also seems to be a 'dose dependent' effect of the abuse in producing psychological symptoms. For example, if the abuse involves multiple perpetrators, long-term sexual abuse, bizarre acts, and concomitant physical abuse, more psychological symptoms are produced.[59] It has also been shown that psychological symptoms following sexual abuse evolve and change over time.[61]

Treatment issues

Treatment of both victims and abusers is important, not least in order to prevent further abuse. Although the majority of children abused do not become abusers themselves, it is recognised that this can happen and can be prevented if timely and appropriate treatment takes place.[62] It is very important to direct treatment not only at victim and abuser but also at other members of the family, if necessary. Contrary to previous belief, it is not true that most women with abusing partners collude with the abuse, and mothers often need a great deal of support and help after abuse has been disclosed.[63] There is no single successful way of treating abused children, and most authors believe that an eclectic approach should be used. The range of treatments available includes individual psychotherapy, play therapy, group treatment, family work, and behaviour management.

Group work has become popular in recent years because it is economical, provides peer support for the children, and makes the children feel less isolated. Many descriptive accounts of group work have appeared in the literature.[64,65] However, evaluation of the outcome has been anecdotal. Kitchur and Bell[66] have written a comprehensive review of the various types of approaches to group treatment. They have also measured outcome in their group of pre-adolescent girls who did favourably as a result of group treatment. Studies of group treatment of adult women sexually abused as children have also shown favourable results.[67] More long-term studies of the outcome of treatment are needed.

In a carefully designed yet small-scale study, Deblinger *et al.*[68] demonstrated a significant improvement, using standardised measures, in a group of children who underwent a cognitive behavioural treatment programme specifically designed for sexually abused children. Their intervention was aimed at both the child and the non-offending parent, based on other research that has demonstrated that child behavioural treatments are more effective when child and parent components are combined. This research approach is particularly welcome and, as the authors note, further work with larger samples and longer follow-up periods, and, we would add, different treatment approaches, are now particularly needed.

It is important to remember that not only should the index child and family be treated, but help and advice should be also available to substitute carers of these children, who can be extremely difficult to manage. Timely support may help to prevent placement breakdown.

Conclusion

In this chapter we have highlighted the complexity and scope of the term 'normal' sexuality in childhood. Based upon this background the paediatrician faces specific diagnostic issues, but few findings are pathognomic of child sexual abuse and each case has to be seen in context. The assessment of the child and family is all-important. Sexually abused children are subjected to subtle coercive pressures which have substantial implications for prevention and treatment. So far, recognition concerns tend to have overshadowed those of treatment. Now treatment and management issues are being considered, and studies of specific treatment approaches are starting to emerge.

The Children Act 1989, when introduced in October 1991, will require a thorough appraisal of cases to examine the degree and extent of harm posed to the child. In addition the likely benefit of different remedies will be examined. A child protection plan involving the simple removal of the child into care will no longer be sufficient. Practitioners will be required to present arguments to support proposed courses of action. It is to be hoped that the process of treatment planning will now be accorded the importance it deserves. The necessary research findings to educate such decision-making will be crucial.

References

1. Markowe, H.L.J. (1988) The frequency of childhood sexual abuse in the U.K. *Health Trends*, **20**, 2–6.
2. Butler-Sloss, Lord Justice (1988) *Report of the inquiry into child abuse in Cleveland in 1987*. London: HMSO.
3. Kinsey, A.C., Pomeroy, W.B., Martin, C.E., Gebhard, P.H. (1948) *Sexual behaviour in the human female*. Philadelphia: Saunders.
4. Goldman, R., Goldman, J. (1982) *Children's sexual thinking; a comparative study of children aged 5–15 in Australia, North America, Britain, and Sweden*. London: Routledge & Kegan Paul.
5. Gordon, B.N., Schroeder, C.S., Abrams, J.M. (1990) Age and social-class differences in children's knowledge of sexuality. *Journal of Clinical Child Psychology*, **19**, 33–43.
6. Conte, J. (1988) Research on prevention. In *Coping with family violence*. (Ed, G. Hotaling) Newbury Park: Sage.
7. Wurtelle, S. (1987) School-based sexual abuse prevention programs. A review. *Child Abuse and Neglect*, **11** (4), 483–495.
8. Fryer, G.E., Kraizer, S.K., Miyoshi, T. (1988) Measuring actual reduction of risk to child abuse: A new approach. *Child Abuse and Neglect*, **11** (2), 173–179.
9. Conte, J., Wolfe, S., Smith, T. (1989) What sexual offenders tell us about prevention strategies. *Child Abuse and Neglect*, **13**, 293–301.
10. Fassler, D., McQueen, K., Duncan, P., Copeland, L. (1990) Children's perception of AIDS. *Journal of the American Academy of Child and Adolescent Psychiatry*, **29**, 459–602.
11. Rosenfeld, A., Bailey, R., Siegel, B., Bailey, G. (1986) Determining incestuous contact between parent and child: frequency of children touching parents genitals in a non-clinical population. *Journal of the American Academy of Child Psychiatry*, **25**, 481–484.
12. Wescott, H., Davies, G., Clifford, B. (1989) The use of anatomical dolls in child witness interviews. *Adoption and Fostering*, **13**, 6–14.
13. Boat, B.W., Everson, M.D. (1988) The use of anatomical dolls among professionals in sexual abuse evaluations. *Child Abuse and Neglect*, **12**, 171–179.
14. Rosenfeld, A., Siegel-Gorelick, B., Haavik, D., *et al.* (1984) Parental perceptions of children's modesty: A cross-sectional survey of ages 2–10 years. *Psychiatry*, **47**, 351–365.
15. Smith, M., Groche, M. Normal family sexuality and sexual knowledge in children (in press).
16. Friedrich, W.N., Bielke, R.L., Purcell, J. (1988) Child sexual behaviour inventory; preliminary normative data. *The Advisor*, 9–11.
17. Glaser, D., Collins, C. (1989) The response of young, non-sexually abused children to anatomically correct dolls. *Journal of Child Psychology and Psychiatry*, **30**, 547–560.
18. Sivan, A.B., Shore, D.P., Coeppl, G.K., Noble, L.D. (1988) Interaction of normal children with anatomical dolls. *Child Abuse and Neglect*, **12**, 295–304.
19. Everson, M.E., Boat, D.W. (1990) Sexualised doll play among young children: Implications for the use of anatomical dolls in sexual abuse evaluations. *Journal of the American Academy of Child and Adolescent Psychiatry*, **29**, 736–742.
20. Realmuto, G.M., Jensen, J.B., Wescoe, S. (1990) Specificity and sensitivity of sexually anatomically correct dolls in substantiating abuse: a pilot study. *Journal of the American Academy of Child and Adolescent Psychiatry*, **29**, 743–746.
21. Leventhal, J.M., Hamilton, J., Rekedal, S., Tebano-Micci, A., Eyster, C. (1989) Anatomically correct dolls used in interviews of young children suspected of having been sexually abused. *Pediatrics*, **84**, 900–906.
22. Jones, D.P.H. (1989) Some reflections on the Cleveland Affair. *Association of Child Psychology and Psychiatry Newsletter*, **11**, 13–18.
23. Browne, A., Finkelhor, D. (1986) Initial and long-term effects: A review of the

research. In *A Sourcebook on Child Sexual Abuse* (Ed, D. Finkelhor). Beverley Hills: Sage.
24. Friedrich, W.N., Urquiza, A.J., Beilke, R.L. (1986) Behaviour problems in sexually abused young children. *Journal of Pediatric Psychology*, **11**, 47–57.
25. Einbender, A.J., Friedrich, W.N. (1989) Psychological functioning and behaviour of sexually abused girls. *Journal of Consulting and Clinical Psychology*, **57**, 155–157.
26. Gordon, B.N., Schroeder, C.S., Abrams, J.M. (1990) Children's knowledge of sexuality: A comparison of sexually abused and non-abused children. *American Journal of Ortho-Psychiatry*, **60**, 250–257.
27. Jones, D.P.H., McQuiston, M.G. (1989) *Interviewing the sexually abused child*. London: Gaskell, 2–4.
28. Russell, D.E.H. (1986) *The secret trauma: Incest in the lives of girls and women*. New York: Basic Books.
29. DHSS (1988) *Working together; A guide to arrangements for inter-agency cooperation for the protection of children from abuse*. London: HMSO.
30. Conte, J.R., Berliner, L., Schurmann, J.R. (1987) *The impact of sexual abuse on children: Final technical report*. Bethesda, Maryland: National Institute for Mental Health.
31. White, S.T., Ingram, D.L., Lyna, P.R. (1989) Vaginal introital diameter in the evaluation of sexual abuse. *Child Abuse and Neglect*, **13**, 217–224.
32. Paradise, J.E. (1989) Predictive accuracy and the diagnosis of sexual abuse – a big issue about a little tissue. *Child Abuse and Neglect*, **13**, 169–176.
33. Emans, S.J., Woods, E., Flagg, N., Freeman, A. (1987) Genital findings in sexually abused symptomatic and asymptomatic girls. *Paediatrics*, **79**, 778–785.
34. Muram, D. (1989) Child sexual abuse – genital direct findings in prepubescent girls. *American Journal of Obstetrics and Gynaecology*, **160**, 328–335.
35. Muram, D. (1989) Child sexual abuse relationship between sexual acts and genital findings. *Child Abuse and Neglect*, **13**, 211–216.
36. McCann, J., Voris, J., Simon, M., Wells, R. (1989) Perianal findings in prepubertal children selected for non-abuse: A descriptive study. *Child Abuse and Neglect*, **13**, 179–193.
37. Stanton, A., Sunderland, R. (1989) Prevalence of reflex anal dilatation in 300 children. *British Medical Journal*, **298**, 802–803.
38. Hobbs, C.J., Wynne, J.M. (1989) Sexual abuse of English boys and girls: The importance of anal examination. *Child Abuse and Neglect*, **13**, 195–210.
39. Jones, D.P.H. (1990) Talking with children. In *Understanding and managing child sexual abuse* (Ed, R. K. Oates). London: Balliere Tindall.
40. White, S.T., Loda, F.A., Ingram, D.L., Pearson, A. (1983) Sexually transmitted diseases in sexually abused children. *Paediatrics*, **72**, 16–21.
41. Gellert, G.A., Durfee, M.J., Berkowitz, C.D. (1990) Developing guidelines for HIV antibody testing victims of paediatric sexual abuse. *Child Abuse and Neglect*, **14**, 9–17.
42. Hanson, R.M., Grasson, M., McCrossin, I. *et al.* (1989) Anogenital warts in childhood. *Child Abuse and Neglect*, **13**, 225–233.
43. Jenny, C., Kirby, P., Fuquay, D. (1989) Genital lichen sclerosis mistaken for child sexual abuse. *Paediatrics*, **83**, 597–598.
44. Hay, F., Buchan, P.C., Littlewood, J.M., Hall, R.I. (1987) Differential diagnosis in child sexual abuse, *Lancet*, **1**, 283.
45. Berliner, L., Conte, J. (1990) The process of victimisation: The victim's perspective. *Child Abuse and Neglect*, **14**, 29–40.
46. Abel, G.G., Hall, D.K., Holland, C.L., Camp, W. (1989) The measurement of the cognitive distortions of child molesters. *Annals of Sex Research*, **2**, 135–153.
47. Banning, A. (1989) Mother son incest confronting a prejudice. *Child Abuse and Neglect*, **13**, 563–570.
48. Krug, R. (1989) Adult male report of childhood sexual abuse by mothers: Case descriptions, motivations and long-term consequences. *Child Abuse and Neglect*, **13**, 111–119.

49. Vander-May, B.J. (1988) The sexual victimisation of male children – a review of previous research. *Child Abuse and Neglect*, **12**, 61–72.
50. Friedrich, W.N., Beilke, R.L., Urquiza, A.J. (1988) Behaviour problems in young sexually abused boys, a comparison study. *Journal of Inter-personal Violence*, **3**, 21–28.
51. Cavannagh-Johnson, T. (1989) Female child perpetrators. Children who molest other children. *Child Abuse and Neglect*, **13**, 571–585.
52. Jones, D.P.H. (In press). Ritualism and child sexual abuse. *Child Abuse and Neglect.*
53. Kiser, L.J., Ackerman, B.J., Brown, E. *et al.* (1988) Post-traumatic stress disorder in children – a reaction to purported sexual abuse. *Journal of the American Academy of Child and Adolescent Psychiatry*, **27**, 645–649.
54. McClear, S.V., Deblinger, E., Atkins, M.S., *et al.* (1988) Post-traumatic stress disorder in sexually abused children. *Journal of the American Academy of Child and Adolescent Psychiatry*, **27**, 650–654.
55. Pynoos, R.S., Nader, K. (1988) Children who witness the sexual assault of their mothers. *Journal of the American Academy of Child and Adolescent Psychiatry*, **27**, 567–572.
56. Gross, M. (1979) Incestuous rape: A cause of hysterical seizures in 4 adolescent girls. *American Journal of Ortho-Psychiatry*, **49**, 704–708.
57. Goodwin, J., Simms, M., Bergman, R. (1979) Hysterical seizures: A sequal to incest. *American Journal of Ortho-Psychiatry*, **49**, 697–703.
58. Goodwin, J. (1982) *Sexual abuse, incest victims and their families.* Bristol: John Wright.
59. Briere, J. (1988) The long-term clinical correlates of childhood sexual victimisation. *Annals of New York Academic Science*, **528**, 327–334.
60. Hall, R.C.W., Tice, L., Beresford, T.P. *et al.* (1989) Sexual abuse in patients with anorexia nervosa and bulimia. *Psychosomatics*, **30**, 1.
61. Friedrich, W.N., Reams, R.A. (1987) Course of psychological symptoms in sexually abused young children. *Psychotherapy*, **24**, 160–170.
62. Ryan, G. (1989) Victim to victimiser: Rethinking victim treatment. *Journal of Inter-personal Violence*, **4**, 325–341.
63. Hilderbrand, J., Forbes, C. (1987) Group work with mothers whose children have been sexually abused. *British Journal of Social Work*, **17**, 285.
64. Furniss, T., Bingley-Miller, L., Van Elburg, A. (1988) Goal-orientated group treatment for the sexually abused adolescent girl. *British Journal of Psychiatry*, **152**, 97–106.
65. Friedrich, W.N., Berliner, L., Urquiza, A.J., Beikle, R.L. (1988) Brief diagnostic group treatment of sexually abused boys. *Journal of Inter-personal Violence*, **3**, 331–343.
66. Kitchur, M., Bell, R. (1989) Group psychotherapy with pre-adolescent sex abuse victims, literature review and description of an inner-city group. *International Journal of Group Psychotherapy*, **39**, 285–310.
67. Alexander, P.C., Neimeyer, R.A., Follette, V.M. *et al.* (1989) A comparison of group treatments of women sexually abused as children. *Journal Consulting and Clinical Psychology*, **37**, 479–483.
68. Deblinger, E., McVeer, S.V., Henry, D. (1990) Cognitive behavioural treatment for sexually abused children suffering post-traumatic stress; preliminary findings. *Journal of the American Academy of Child and Adolescent Psychiatry*, **29**, 747–752.

3 | Nutrition in childhood

Alan A. Jackson
School of Biological Sciences, University of Southampton

Introduction

Normal growth and development

During childhood, growth is the normal state which allows for physical and intellectual maturation and development. Growth, as a regular if not continuous process, requires the input of nutrients, substrate and cofactors, in the form of food, and is fuelled by the energy derived from food. For any individual, growth is canalised with the particular growth channel being determined by a combination of genetic and environmental factors. By failing to grow or develop a child falls progressively further behind its peers and recovery requires accelerated or catch-up growth, which involves an additional input of energy and nutrients.[1,2]

Nutritional considerations impact across the entire breadth of paediatric practice. Characteristically, both growth and development represent modulated genetic expression, a process which is driven and finely co-ordinated by the substrate and cofactors available from the diet. Any combination of specific nutrient deficiencies, unbalanced losses, unusual demands, or an inadequate or excessive intake must invariably influence the overall processes associated with growth in the short term. One question of overriding importance is the extent to which a limitation in the short term is necessarily associated with a definable and identifiable impairment of function in the long term. On a global scale the ravages of childhood malnutrition still feature as the single most important direct or indirect cause of death. Vitamin A deficiency is still the most common cause for the loss of sight. The mental impairment associated with a dietary deficiency of iodine only serves to emphasise that underdevelopment at the national level must be a natural consequence of significant underdevelopment at the personal level. The general principles which are demonstrated so starkly in a consideration of nutritional problems in the developing world are no different, fundamentally, from the problems faced by paediatricians in the developed world. Once time is taken to ask the question: 'Does the food intake of an infant or child exert any influence upon its behaviour, growth, development, or function?', the answer is invariably: 'Yes, it does'. The only outstanding question is how gross or how subtle the manifestation of impairment might be.

Nutrition and inflammation

The body seeks to maintain its integrity by the deployment of a range of sophisticated processes of which the specific immune response and the non-specific inflammatory response are the most extensively investigated and most clearly understood. The specific immune response, both humoral and cell mediated, is characterised by cellular multiplication, cellular differentiation, and increased levels of protein synthesis. As the substrate demands for the process are, in general, the same as those for normal growth, an immune response is competitive for the supply of nutrients. The limitations imposed upon immune responsiveness by nutrient deficiencies have been well characterised over the years.[3,4]

The nutritional impact upon the local or generalised inflammatory response has been less extensively studied. It is now apparent that the general inflammatory response, the acute phase response, is complex, being co-ordinated at the level of the whole body by chemical mediators, cytokines, released from macrophage populations around the body. The full-blown response induces a major shift in the distribution of nutrients and cofactors available to the different tissues of the body. The inflammatory response not only functions competitively with the demands for growth of the body, but also creates unbalanced nutrient demands and losses from the body. It is becoming increasingly apparent that nutritional considerations interact fundamentally with cytokine responses at all levels, influencing the sensitivity of macrophages to a range of stimuli, the ability of macrophages to release cytokines, the sensitivity of end organs to the effects of cytokines, and the ability of the body to co-ordinate a generalised response to either individual or combinations of cytokines.[5] The potential implications of different diets for the ability of children of different ages to mount an effective inflammatory response is only now becoming appreciated.

There are many issues related to nutrition in childhood and inevitably one has to be selective. Examples of problems have been chosen, either because they illustrate important general principles, or because they represent problems of major public health significance. In order to be able to handle the topic I have divided the problems rather arbitrarily into:

(i) acute effects;

(ii) short-term effects;

(iii) long-term effects;
(iv) therapeutic options.

The grouping is far from perfect, but it serves a purpose.

Acute effects of feeding patterns in infancy

Human milk

For many years paediatricians have acknowledged the particular and peculiar advantage of ensuring that newborn infants are fed naturally on the milk provided by their own mothers. The World Health Organisation insists that the single most important approach to preventive health care in childhood should be the promotion of breast feeding. It is sad, therefore, to note that in the UK, following a bout of enthusiasm for breast feeding in the early 1980s, there has been slippage so that now fewer than 50% of mothers are likely to establish effective breast feeding at this time. It is against this background that the study of Howie *et al.*[6] from Dundee takes on great importance. These investigators have shown that for mothers who breast feed their children for at least 13 weeks there is a substantial health benefit in terms of a decreased risk of gastrointestinal (2% to 6% versus 17% to 20%) and respiratory tract infections (23% to 25% versus 32% to 40%). Even partial breast feeding conferred an advantage relative to the infants who were fed with a formula from a bottle. There were a number of surface infections, of the mouth, eyes, and skin, for which breast feeding did not seem to confer any advantage. Similarly there was no benefit in terms of colic, eczema, or nappy rash.

It has always been considered that the advantage conferred by breast feeding is primarily related to the complex series of factors which it contains that inhibit bacterial growth. Therefore, the demonstration by Pabst and Spady[7] that breast-fed infants are able to mount a more intense antibody response to immunisation with *Haemophilus influenzae b* is of considerable interest. In 57 breast-fed infants the antibody response at 7 and 12 months (29.8 μg/ml and 4.8 μg/ml) was significantly higher than in 24 formula-fed infants (17.5 μg/ml and 3.0 μg/ml), suggesting that the benefits conferred by breast milk are more subtle, and may be more extensive than previously recognised. The important role of breast feeding for the welfare of infants has been taken very seriously by the Department of Health,[7A] which at the present time is mounting a National Breastfeeding Initiative to encourage mothers to breast feed.

Diarrhoea: oral rehydration fluid: supplementation

Around the time of weaning the single biggest risk to health is acute diarrhoeal disease. It is more than a decade since the World Health Organisation adopted the use of oral rehydration fluids as the cornerstone of the approach to management of this potentially lethal condition. During the early years of its promotion this simple but effective approach was slow to catch on. Even at this time it is estimated that less than 25% of those who could benefit from the therapy are treated with appropriate oral rehydration.[8] Diarrhoea has been associated with later stunting,[9] and stunting has been associated with impaired mental development.[10] Recent studies have suggested that dietary supplementation might completely offset the deleterious effects of diarrhoea on linear growth.[11,12]

Vitamin A

Publications from field studies, clinical trials, and laboratory investigations provide an accumulating body of evidence which emphasises the important role played by vitamin A in resistance to intercurrent infection. This is particularly true for infections which directly affect the mucosal surfaces. In addition to the studies in which vitamin A therapy has been used prophylactically to reduce the incidence of gastrointestinal and respiratory infections, there have been others in which the efficacy of therapeutic doses of vitamin A at the time of infection has been assessed. One of the more recent of these studies has demonstrated yet again that vitamin A may have a particularly important role to play in the management of severe measles.[13] In this study 200 children under 13 years of age with measles severe enough to justify admission to hospital were randomly assigned to either treatment or placebo. The treatment group received retinyl palmitate, 120mg, in divided doses over the first two days of admission. In the treated group there was a significant reduction in the severity of diarrhoea and respiratory infections and significantly fewer children died or required intensive care. One important feature of the study is that it was carried out in an area where florid vitamin-A deficiency is not generally recognised to be a problem, so raises the question whether all children with severe measles would benefit from therapeutic doses of vitamin A.

Vitamin K

There has been a series of cases of haemorrhagic disease of the newborn over the recent past. Virtually all the affected infants had received inadequate therapeutic doses of vitamin K during the neonatal period.

This has prompted the British Paediatric Association to provide policy guidelines on vitamin-K prophylaxis for haemorrhagic disease of the newborn.

1. All newborn infants should be given vitamin K.
2. Intramuscular vitamin K, 1mg, ensures adequate prophylaxis in normal-term infants.
3. One dose of 1mg vitamin K orally is adequate prophylaxis for the majority of normal-term infants. Further doses should be considered for breast-fed infants.
4. Infants with jaundice suggestive of cholestasis, and infants with unexplained bleeding, should receive further vitamin K, preferably parenterally.

Short term consequences of early diet

Cow's milk in the first year

Cow's milk is not recommended for children under six months of age, and increasingly the feeling is growing that it is not advisable to give infants cow's milk at all, ie before one year of age. The nutrient composition of cow's milk is not considered to be suitable.[14] Infants who receive cow's milk during the first year appear to be more likely to develop iron-deficient anaemia during the second. As some infants may develop subclinical gastro-intestinal bleeding on cow's milk, this may add to the risk.

Diet of preterm infants during the first extra-uterine month

Since 1983 a prospective multicentre study on the feeding of newborn preterm infants has been run by Dr A. Lucas of the Dunn Nutrition Unit. The results of the study have started to appear over the past few years. The wealth of data which has been generated is going to have an important determinant effect upon many aspects of paediatric practice for some time to come. The study was designed so that varying approaches were used for the feeding of preterm infants during the first month of life. Essentially the infants received one of three supplemental diets: donor breast milk, term formula, or preterm formula. The precise amounts of each feed received are not known, but the preterm formula was nutrient dense, so infants receiving this preparation took increased quantities of energy and most nutrients. Infants receiving the preterm formula gained weight and height at a faster rate than those receiving banked breast milk (18g/kg/d versus 13g/kg/d; 1.38mm/d versus

1.04mm/d) and head circumference increased more rapidly (1.57mm/d versus 1.23mm/d). Of infants weighing less than 1200g at birth, those fed breast milk took an estimated three weeks longer to reach 2000g.[15]

Differences in growth, motor and mental development, have been shown for nine months and 18 months. At nine months of age the infants receiving banked breast milk had a developmental quotient which was significantly behind those receiving preterm formula.[16]

At 18 months, infants fed the nutrient-dense preterm formula were taller and had a larger head circumference than infants given a formula designed for term infants. Those on the preterm formula also showed a significantly better level of performance on a range of tests of psychomotor and mental development with evidence of a more advanced social maturity quotient. The benefits were more evident in males and also in those infants who were small for gestational age.[17]

Put simply, these studies show that if preterm infants receive an adequate intake of nutrients they are more likely to develop normally. It is worth remembering the point so strongly emphasised by Dobbing,[18] that the human brain is at its most sensitive to insult during the last trimester of pregnancy, a period of extra-uterine life for the preterm infant. It is not possible to say from the important series of studies by Lucas whether any particular dietary component is more or less responsible for the beneficial effect, nor how the effect is exerted. Great care needs to be taken in trying to extrapolate these findings to the way in which term infants should be fed, but certainly the results of these studies justify the investigations being extended to an exploration of the effects of diet in early life on the growth and development of term infants.

Phenylketonuria

The phenylketonuria register maintains a national list of all subjects with phenylketonuria (phenylalanine concentration persistently above 480μmol/l) born from 1964 onwards. Prospective follow-up of 808 children who started treatment before four months of age shows that during the early years of the programme the mean intelligence quotient at four years rose with the year of birth, presumably associated with improved standards of dietary care. There has been no further rise since the 1972 cohort, and the mean IQ for the group with optimal care is still eight points below the norms for the population at large. Delay in starting treatment, or a tendency for either high or very low phenylalanine concentrations in blood, were associated with poorer scores. The data suggest that many children who are treated early continue to suffer a mild degree of neurological impairment because of the difficulty with controlling the metabolic abnormality.[19]

However, the potential damage caused by an uncontrolled metabolic state in phenylketonuria is not necessarily restricted to the early period of childhood. Thompson *et al.*[20] have reported a series of seven young adults with phenylketonuria in whom dietary control had deteriorated during childhood. Each individual showed evidence of neurological disability in adolescence or as a young adult. In two of the patients in whom a strict phenylalanine-free diet was introduced, there was a striking improvement in the clinical condition. More objective evidence of improvement was provided in one individual in whom serial magnetic resonance images showed abnormalities after cessation of the dietary treatment, with resolution of the abnormalities once a strict diet was reintroduced. This clinical information suggests that considerations of brain development during childhood cannot simply be restricted to considerations of the sensitive periods around the last trimester of pregnancy and the first two years after birth.

Chronic effects of a single episode of severe malnutrition

For 20 years now the Child Development Group led by Dr Sally Grantham McGregor at the Tropical Metabolism Research Unit in the University of the West Indies in Jamaica have been exploring aspects of child development, with particular emphasis on the effects of a single episode of severe undernutrition upon later development. The greatest single difficulty in studies of this kind is to disentangle the effects of the global environment surrounding malnutrition from the metabolic changes associated with disordered intake of nutrient—substrate and cofactors—itself. Over the years the group has been able to demonstrate the relative contribution to delayed development of the deprivation of food and the deprivation of early stimulation.[10] The evidence would suggest that early undernutrition of itself gives rise to social disadvantage. The more carefully one looks for impairment in function, the more likely it is to manifest itself.

In a recent study the effects of missing breakfast upon the cognitive functions of schoolchildren were explored.[21] The study comprised three groups of children of around 10 years of age, each with 30 subjects. One group had experienced severe malnutrition during the first two years of life; the second group was stunted having experienced chronic undernutrition; and the third group was a control group of normal height. All the children were poor and came from similar social backgrounds. The tests of cognitive function included both measures of fine-grained functions and more global or classroom-type of tasks. Some of the tests were selected because performance would be affected by attention and distractibility, short-term memory, speed and accuracy, or an immediate processing element. The control group was not affected in an adverse way for any of the tests when breakfast was omitted. Indeed, for some of the tests there appeared to be a heightened level of performance, which may be ascribed to an alertness phenomenon. In contrast, children who had been severely malnourished in early childhood, or who were stunted or wasted at the time of the test, were adversely affected in fluency and coding. Relative to the control children they performed less well in arithmetic. Compared with the control children these differences were statistically significant.

These results suggest that a severe insult during the first years of life, or an inadequate intake of food during later periods of childhood, may have an adverse effect upon children's ability to learn, and for these children whether or not they have breakfast before going to school can have a significant effect upon learning ability and performance.

Early growth and long-term health

For many years there has been the feeling among paediatricians that influences early in life might have an important influence upon growth, development, and susceptibility to disease at later ages. The evidence has been of a clinical nature in selected population groups, because long-term epidemiological studies can be impossibly difficult and expensive to carry out. Animal studies have indicated that during development there are sensitive periods during which the ability of the body to function and respond to a range of stimuli might be set. The exact timing and duration of these sensitive periods have never been clear for humans, nor the mechanisms through which metabolic sensitivity might be set; however, the availability of nutrients has implicitly been considered as one variable of importance. Over the past 20 years increased attention has been focused upon the potential for adult obesity to be set in early childhood, with increased emphasis being placed upon ensuring that children should not gain excessive weight during the early years. In consequence the government guidelines on the feeding of children have recommended changes in weaning practice.[22] Associated with this change in recommendation has been a change in the pattern of infant growth. In the recent past children at one year have been significantly shorter and lighter than they were two decades ago.[23] It is time to reassess the possible implications of this policy.

It is now possible to take advantage of the quality of record keeping which was found in some obstetric and paediatric practice in the past. With the refinements that have taken place in the tools of epidemiological investigation, prospective studies have been started and it is increasingly possible to take advantage of the data bases generated in the past.

Questions can be asked in large population groups about the relations of dietary exposure in the past and more recent measures of outcome.

By the use of a retrospective cohort design Barker *et al.*[24] were able to draw relationships between mortality during the first year of life and death from specific diseases later in life in the same population. When the country was divided into 212 local authority areas it was found that there was a strong geographical relationship between infant mortality rates in 1921 to 1925 and mortality rates from ischaemic heart disease in 1968 to 1978. Of 24 other common causes of death there was a relationship between infant mortality and bronchitis, stomach cancer, and rheumatic heart disease. The authors suggested that poor nutrition in early life increased the susceptibility to an affluent diet. In following up the concept and in order to test the hypothesis that environmental influences that impair growth and development in early life might be risk factors for ischaemic heart disease, Barker *et al.*[25] traced 5654 men who were born in six districts in Hertfordshire between 1911 and 1930. Good records had been maintained of the men's weights during infancy, and most of them had been breast fed. The highest rates for ischaemic heart disease were found in those men with the lowest weights at birth and at one year. There was a threefold increase in the standardised mortality rate (SMR) for men who only weighed 18 pounds at one year (SMR 111), compared with men who weighed 27 pounds or more at one year (SMR 42). Thus the men with greater early growth had a reduced risk of heart disease, suggesting that the promotion of infant growth in babies of below average birth-weight might be a priority for health promotion.

One of the known risk factors for heart disease is a high blood pressure. Blood pressure rank in individuals is established at an early age and may in itself be influenced by environmental factors. In a cross-sectional study Whincup *et al.*[26] measured blood pressure in 3591 children aged between five and seven-and-a-half years for whom historical data were available in primary schools in nine British towns. Simple analysis was unable to detect any association between birth-weight and either systolic or diastolic pressure in either sex. However, when an appropriate adjustment was made for current weight a significant relationship emerged. In both sexes birth-weight was inversely related to blood pressure within each grouping for current weight. With multiple regression analysis current weight, birth-weight, maternal age, birth rank, and a maternal history of hypertension remained significant and were little affected by other factors. Thus all of the significant factors were either directly linked to fetal and postnatal growth, or are known to exert a direct influence upon fetal growth. Barker has gone on to explore the relationship further and shown that in national samples of 9921 children aged 10 years and 3259 adults there was an inverse relationship between systolic blood pressure and birth-weight.[27] The results force a consideration of the inter-relationship between birth-weight, attained height, and risk of cardiovascular disease. The association with birth-weight implies that intra-uterine factors may be of importance.

The further demonstration of a complex interaction of placental weight and birth-weight on blood pressure in adulthood suggests that the wellbeing of the mother both before and during pregnancy may be of special importance.[28] The mechanistic basis which underlies these observations is far from clear at this point in time, but the predictive power of the associations is as strong as or stronger than any of the postnatal risk factors which have attracted attention in the past. The message is that a fetus growing well prenatally and an infant growing well postnatally carry the lowest risk for cardiovascular health in later life. This conclusion appears to be substantially at odds with previous recommendations on infant feeding and growth, which sought to limit the weight gained during the first years of life.

Therapeutic options

Nutritional support

The past decade has seen an increase in the range and sophistication of the methods available for providing therapeutic nutritional support of the seriously ill. Most of the changes represent modification of details rather than major advances, and the options have been between oral nutrition, enteral support, and parenteral support. Although parenteral support can be carried out very effectively for long periods of time, there are well-recognised complications associated with its use, especially in inexperienced hands. Nasogastric feeding or nasojejunal feeding is to be preferred where possible, and the importance of providing some enteral input for normal gastro-intestinal development has come to be increasingly appreciated. The introduction of fine-bore nasogastric tubes has substantially reduced both the discomfort and complication rate for this approach. The use of a percutaneous gastrostomy with endoscopically guided placement represents a useful technical advance which offers much promise for the future of individuals with swallowing difficulties or chest problems.[29]

All nutritional support presumes a knowledge of the metabolic demands of the patient and the specific nutrient requirements to satisfy that demand. Intermittent reports of specific nutrient deficiencies or nutrient imbalances, as for example with the correct proportions of phenylalanine and tyrosine, are an inevitable consequence of managing severely ill individuals who are in a brittle metabolic state.

Cystic fibrosis

As a disease entity cystic fibrosis represents all the problems of management for which a clear understanding of nutritional principles is imperative. As children with this condition have maldigestion and malabsorption, it is not possible to make assumptions about the adequacy of their nutrient availability simply from measurements of intake alone.[30] The evidence would suggest that some children have an increased metabolic demand, possibly associated with the underlying disease process itself. The general recommendation has been made that children with cystic fibrosis should have an intake of food which is 120% to 150% of that of normal children. Children with cystic fibrosis do eat more than other children, but not always sufficient to maintain body-weight. It is as important to identify the basis of the limited appetite as to consider the potential benefits of 'forced feeding' régimes. Respiratory infection introduces its own metabolic demand and it is likely that good nutritional support allows for improved respiratory function. The past few years have seen increased attention being given to a more detailed consideration of the nutritional requirements in cystic fibrosis. The results of this work over the next few years will allow for dietary recommendations to be made which will be more specifically tailored to individual requirements as the disease state fluctuates.

Atopic disease

Atopic disorders, such as eczema and asthma, are common causes of childhood illness, and the incidence of both conditions is rising in Britain.[31] There is strong evidence for the role of diet in the management of atopic eczema from a study of children between two and eight years of age.[32] More recent interest has focused upon the possible transference to the offspring of sensitivity to foods in the maternal diet, either prenatally or in the breast milk. In 1988 Ferguson and Watret felt strongly that the best recommendation for the mother of an atopic infant was for her to breast feed the child while taking a healthy mixed diet for herself.[31] This advice might need to be modulated as the results of studies designed to test the propositions concerning maternal diet come through.

For 18 months Chandra *et al.*[33] followed up 221 term infants who were born to mothers with a history of atopy. The infants were either breast fed or not, and the mothers of the breast-fed infants took either a free or a restriction diet. Eczema was less common and milder in infants who were breast fed by mothers on a restricted diet (22% versus 48%). In infants given a formula the development of eczema varied with the formulation; casein hydroylsate 21%; soy milk 63%; cow's milk 70%. In a prospective study of 777 preterm infants Lucas *et al.*[34] found that there was no difference in the development of atopy between infants who received formula or banked donor milk for the group as a whole. However, for those infants whose mothers had a history of atopy, the infants receiving formula had a significantly greater risk of developing eczema than those receiving human milk.

Not all atopic disease can be related directly to the presence of identifiable antigenic stimuli in the environment, and even in those individuals who have asthma or eczema the disease runs an uneven course. Exploration of the basis of atopic disease at a molecular level suggests increasingly that the magnitude of the host inflammatory response may represent an important component of the variability of disease expression. Over the coming years a deeper understanding of the role played by specific nutrients in modulating cytokine responses is likely to play a determinant role in our approach to the dietary management of these disorders.

Conclusion

Twenty years ago concerns in infant feeding were dominated by the concept that fat babies give rise to obese adults. Infant formulae contained a high solute load and a pattern of fat and protein which was considered inappropriate. Early weaning on to cereal-based products was standard. In 1974 the government guidelines on feeding infants promoted breast feeding and the adoption of later weaning.[22] By the mid-1980s the pattern of infant growth appeared to have changed, with breast-fed infants gaining weight along the reference standards during the first six months, but crossing the standards in a downwards direction during the second six months; the result being that by one year of age infants were shorter and lighter with smaller skinfolds than the reference standards. More recent evidence has served to emphasise the importance of fetal growth, infant growth, and achieved weight at one year as predictors of risk for motor and intellectual development and disease in adult life. There is a need in the future for us to be much clearer about the outcome objectives of dietary intervention and management for both the short and the longer term.

The evidence is overwhelming that breast milk confers health benefit in both the short and the long term,[35] and the government's National Breast Feeding Initiative should be vigorously supported by every paediatrician. The mysteries of the unique attributes of breast milk are still a long way from scientific elucidation.

We have very little detailed knowledge of optimal intakes of food and nutrients for normal children between two and 18 years of age. Many recommendations are derived simply by extrapolation between infancy and adulthood. It is impossible to make rational recommendations of food and nutrient requirements in illness without some prior understanding of the requirements for normal growth and development. It is undesirable that dietary guidelines which have been developed for adults should be uncritically extrapolated to children. There is an urgent need to demonstrate that the present dietary guidelines are appropriate for children and do not in themselves carry any risk to health or wellbeing.

The research emphasis over the next decade must focus upon the interaction between diet and genetic expression, including the role played by substrate availability on genetic programming during early life. If we are to be in a position to understand the relationship between diet and disease, it will be necessary to develop a much clearer understanding of the interaction between nutrients and cofactors with the processes of infection and inflammation.

References

1. Jackson, A.A. (1990) Protein requirements for catch-up growth. *Proceedings of the Nutrition Society*, **49**, 507–516.
2. Jackson, A.A., Wootton, S.A. (1990) The energy requirements of growth and catch-up growth. In *Activity, energy expenditure and energy requirements of infants and children* (Eds B. Schürch and N.S. Scrimshaw), 185–214. International Dietary Energy Consultative Group.
3. Gross, R.L., Newberne, P.M. (1980) Role of nutrition in immunological function. *Physiological Reviews*, **60**, 188–302.
4. Tomkins, A., Watson, F. (1989) Malnutrition and infection. ACC/SCN *State of the Art* series, Nutrition Policy Discussion Paper, No. 5, ACC/SCN, Geneva.
5. Grimble, R.F. (1990) Nutrition and cytokine action. *Nutrition Research Reviews*, **3**, 193–210.
6. Howie, P.W., Forsyth, J.S., Ogston, S.A., *et al.* (1990) Protective effect of breast feeding against infection. *British Medical Journal*, **300**, 11–16.
7. Pabst, H.F., Spady, D.W. (1990) Effect of breast feeding on antibody response to conjugate vaccine. *Lancet*, **336**, 269–270.

7A. Department of Health and Social Security (1988) Present-day feeding practice in infant feeding: third report. *Report on health and social subjects series; No 32*. London: HMSO.

8. Avery, M.E., Snyder, J.D. (1990) Oral therapy for acute diarrhoea: the underused simple solution. *New England Journal of Medicine*, **323**, 891–894.
9. Rowland, M.G.M., Cole, T.J., Whitehead, R.G. (1976) A quantitative study into the role of infection in determining nutritional status in Gambian village children. *British Journal of Nutrition*, **37**, 441–450.
10. Grantham-McGregor, S.M. (1990) Malnutrition, mental function and development. In *The malnourished child*, Nestle Nutrition Workshop series, vol 19. Nestec Ltd., Vevey/Raven Press Ltd., New York.
11. Lutter, C.K., Mora, J.O., Habicht, J-P. *et al.* (1989) Nutritional supplementation: effects on child stunting because of diarrhoea. *American Journal of Clinical Nutrition*, **50**, 1–8.
12. Heikens, G.T., Schofield, W.N., Dawson, S., Grantham-McGregor, S. (1989) The Kingston project I: Growth of malnourished children during rehabilitation in the

community, given a high energy supplement. *European Journal of Clinical Nutrition*, **43**, 145–160.
13. Hussey, G. D., Klein, M. (1990) A randomised controlled trial of vitamin A in children with severe measles. *New England Journal of Medicine*, **323**, 160–164.
14. Wharton, B. (1990) Milk for babies and children: no ordinary cow's milk before one year. *British Medical Journal*, **301**, 774–775.
15. Lucas, A., Gore, S.M., Cole, T.J. *et al.* (1984) Multicentre trial on feeding low-birth-weight infants: effects of diet on early growth. *Archives of Disease in Childhood*, **59**, 722–730.
16. Lucas, A., Morley, R., Coles, T.J. *et al.* (1989) Early diet in preterm babies and developmental status in infancy. *Archives of Disease in Childhood*, **64**, 1570–1578.
17. Lucas, A., Morley, R., Cole, T.J. *et al.* (1990) Early diet in preterm babies and developmental status at 18 months. *Lancet*, **335**, 1477–1481.
18. Dobbing, J. (1990) Early nutrition and later achievement. *Proceedings of the Nutrition Society*, **49**, 103–118.
19. Smith, I., Beasley, M.G., Ades, A.E. (1990) Intelligence and quality of dietary treatment in phenylketonuria. *Archives of Disease in Childhood*, **65**, 472–478.
20. Thompson, A.J., Smith, I., Brenton, D. *et al.* (1990) Neurological deterioration in young adults with phenylketonuria. *Lancet*, **336**, 602–605.
21. Simeon, D.T., Grantham-McGregor, S. (1989) Effects of missing breakfast on the cognitive functions of schoolchildren of differing nutritional status. *American Journal of Clinical Nutrition*, **49**, 646–653.
22. Department of Health and Social Security (1974) Present-day practice in infant feeding. *Reports on health and social subjects; No 9*. London: HMSO.
23. Whitehead, R.G., Paul, A.A. (1988) Comparative infant nutrition in man and other animals. In *Comparative nutrition*. London: John Libbey.
24. Barker, D.J.P., Osmond, C. (1986) Infant mortality, childhood nutrition, and ischaemic heart disease in England and Wales. *Lancet*, **i**, 1077–1081.
25. Barker, D.J.P., Winter, P.D., Osmond, C. *et al.* (1989) Weight in infancy and death from ischaemic heart disease. *Lancet*, **ii**, 577–580.
26. Whincup, P.H., Cook, D.G., Shaper, A.G. (1989) Early influences on blood pressure: a study of children aged 5–7 years. *British Medical Journal*, **299**, 587–591.
27. Barker, D.J.P., Osmond, C., Golding, J. *et al.* (1989) Growth *in utero*, blood pressure in childhood and adult life, and mortality from cardiovascular disease. *British Medical Journal*, **298**, 564–567.
28. Barker, D.J., Bull, A.R., Osmond, C., Simmonds, S.J. (1990) Fetal size and risk of hypertension in adult life. *British Medical Journal*, **301**, 259–262.
29. Moran, B.J., Taylor, M.B., Johnson, C.D. (1990) Percutaneous endoscopic gastrostomy. *British Journal of Surgery*, **77**, 858–862.
30. Wootton, S.A. (1991) Energy balance in cystic fibrosis. *Proceedings of the Royal Society of Medicine*. In press.
31. Ferguson, A., Watret, K.C. (1988) Cow's milk intolerance. *Nutrition Research Reviews*, **1**, 1–22.
32. Atherton, D.J., Sewell, M., Soothill, J.F., Wells, R.S. (1978) A double-blind controlled cross-over trial of an antigen avoidance diet in atopic eczema. *Lancet*, **i**, 401–403.
33. Chandra, R.K., Puri, S., Hamed, A. (1989) Influence of maternal diet during lactation and use of formula feeds on development of atopic eczema in high-risk infants. *British Medical Journal*, **299**, 228–230.
34. Lucas, A., Brooke, O.G., Morley, R. *et al.* (1990) Early diet of preterm infants and development of allergic or atopic disease: randomised prospective study. *British Medical Journal*, **300**, 837–840.

4 | The epilepsies

Niall V. O'Donohoe
National Children's Hospital, Dublin

Introduction and epidemiology

The British Paediatric Association, at its Diamond Jubilee meeting in 1988, emphasised the importance of better control of epilepsy among the priorities for child health in the future.[1] Epilepsy is one of the commonest afflictions of humankind worldwide, and it has made a deep and fearful impression on the popular mind. One in 20 of the population have an epileptic seizure at some time in their lives and, at a conservative estimate, 1 in 200 develop epilepsy, the majority during childhood or adolescence.[2] The National Child Development Study established a prevalence rate for epilepsy of 4.1/1000 by the age of 11 years.[3] An American study in Oklahoma found an overall period prevalence of epilepsy of 4.71 per 1000 from birth to the age of 19 years.[4] The incidence of seizures is highest in the first year after birth and some of the most intractable epilepsies begin in infancy and during early childhood. Congenital abnormalities of the brain and more frequent exposure to cerebral insults are responsible, to some extent, for the development of these serious epilepsies.

Experimental evidence suggests that the immature brain is more susceptible to the development of seizures than is its mature counterpart.[5] This is best illustrated by the increased incidence of reactive seizures in response to high fever in the young. However, this susceptibility is coupled with a decreased potential for developing chronic epilepsy as the normal brain matures. We know, for example, that only 4% or less of children having febrile convulsions go on to develop epilepsy in later life.[6] This offers strong support for the presently held view that prophylactic drug therapy is unnecessary except in a small minority of cases.[7]

Pathophysiology

Epileptic seizures result from the sudden, excessive, electrical discharges of large aggregates of neurons, and the clinical components are determined by the site of origin of the discharge and by the pattern of spread. Neurons are rendered susceptible to abnormal electrical behaviour by inherited factors or by disease.

Epileptogenesis is a term which refers to the dynamic process underlying the development of epilepsy. It depends on the predisposition of neuronal aggregates to discharge when stimulated and on synchronisation of firing within the neuronal substrate. The neocortex and the hippocampus are uniquely susceptible to generate abnormal electrical activity of this nature because of their intrinsic organisation and internal connections within the brain. Their excitability is modified both by subcortical and interhemispheric events. Some notable recent research has demonstrated that the substantia nigra, which has strong inhibitory functions through its GABAergic output, functions inadequately in the immature organism.[8]

At the neuronal membrane level Na^+ and Ca^{2+} influx is associated with excitatory depolarisation and K^+ efflux and Cl^- influx with inhibitory hyperpolarisation. Nerve impulses arriving at the terminal bulb of the axon cause release of neurotransmitters which bind to receptors on the post-synaptic membrane and initiate a chain of events within the post-synaptic neuron. For most synapses the transmitter-receptor complex acts as a gate regulating the opening and closing of ion channels on the post-synaptic membrane, with resulting excitation and/or inhibition. Glutamate is the main excitatory neurotransmitter and every neuron has receptors for it. One pharmacologically identified glutamate receptor which binds with a glutamate analogue, N-methyl-D-aspartate, or NMDA, is of particular interest. When activated this receptor opens gated channels permeable to calcium ions. The NMDA receptor has a key role in long-term potentiation, a persistent change in the strength of synaptic connections which is thought to be involved in both the normal reorganisation of neuronal connections which occurs with experience and in the process of epileptogenesis.[9] An exciting recent discovery has been the successful cloning of one of the glutamate receptors in the rat brain.[10] It is expected such research will lead to the identification of the structure of human glutamate receptors. The implications for the subsequent development of glutamate receptor blocking agents which might selectively control epileptic phenomena are clear.

Genetics

Although hereditary factors have long been recognised in the causation of childhood epilepsies, early genetic studies usually considered all forms of epilepsy as a single entity, regardless of age of onset or symptomatology. Metrakos and Metrakos in the early 1960s studied probands of patients with absence attacks and/or grand mal seizures, who had no gross cerebral lesions but a regular 3 Hz. spike-wave abnormality of the EEG.[11]

They proposed that the spike-wave EEG trait was inherited as an autosomal dominant with age-dependent penetrance. Andermann suggested that other genetic, maturational, and environmental factors must interact with the EEG trait before clinical seizures occur.[12] Thus two gene loci may need to interact to produce an appropriate phenotype, and clinically similar disorders, for example atypical absence epilepsy of later onset than classic petit mal, may be due to different genotypes. However, analogy with gene identification in Duchenne and Becker dystrophy[13] and in the spinal muscular atrophies[14] make this unlikely, and it seems probable that different types of the same disease are probably due to an allelic series of mutations at the same gene locus.

In the past 18 months two remarkable advances have been the demonstration of a genetic linkage for benign familial neonatal convulsions with chromosome 20[15] and for juvenile myoclonic epilepsy of Janz with chromosome 6.[16] A gene, once mapped, will sooner or later be isolated and cloned and this will reveal the structure of the gene product.[17] The implications for the greater understanding of the pathophysiology of epilepsy and for more rational therapy are obvious.

Epileptic syndromes

For many years a simplistic, symptom-oriented approach to epilepsy has been used widely. Although it has been taught that seizures may be symptomatic of a wide range of congenital and acquired conditions, if no cause is identified, the label of 'idiopathic epilepsy' has been used. Intense worldwide interest and research in epileptology in the past two decades have gradually begun to solve the mysteries of 'idiopathic epilepsy', and some recent spectacular genetic discoveries have just been mentioned. It has to be admitted, however, that it is much easier to classify epileptic seizures based on symptomatology[18] than it is to classify the epilepsies on an aetiological basis. In recent years, to circumvent this problem, there has been a successful attempt to identify epileptic syndromes of which individual seizures are but one feature, thus drawing attention to the existence of syndromes.[19] The cluster of symptoms and signs which characterise a syndrome include the presence or absence of a family history, the age of onset, the neurological and psychological findings, the features of the interictal and ictal EEG, the natural history of the disorder, the response to medication, and any developmental complications. Some syndromes have also been found to have specific pathological, chromosomal, or biochemical markers.

The epileptic syndromes can be usefully subdivided on the basis of two criteria.[20] Thus, those with generalised seizures (generalised epilepsies) are distinguished from those with partial seizures (partial or localisation-related epilepsies) and those with known aetiology (symptomatic or secondary or lesional) from those with no known aetiology (idiopathic or primary).

Primary epileptic syndromes occur in otherwise normal children, sometimes with a family history of a similar disorder, with no demonstrable underlying pathology and in whom the EEG shows a normal background interictal activity. In these children the response to medication is usually good and remission is likely. In contrast, secondary or symptomatic syndromes are often associated with underlying cerebral disease which may result in developmental abnormality. A positive family history is uncommon and there are abnormal neurological and investigative findings. In these children the response to medication is unpredictable and spontaneous resolution is unlikely. It is important to recognise that similar seizures may occur in different syndromes and that some syndromes are characterised by multiple seizure types. Furthermore, the syndromes vary in specificity from those which represent broad concepts to those which are highly specific. Although not all patients fit into the described syndromes, this approach to the epilepsies has revolutionised the management of these disorders in recent years. It has led to more precise diagnostic, therapeutic, and prognostic attitudes to the individual patient, it has improved communication and exchange of ideas about epilepsy and, inevitably, it will lead to more rational use of the newer and relatively specific anti-epileptic drugs and thereby improve control of seizures.

An alternative neurobiological approach has been advocated by the Montreal School which is complementary to the syndromic method.[21] It is based on the evidence for the multifactorial origin of epilepsy, and on the recognition of a spectrum of clinical and EEG features in patients with both primary and secondary epilepsy. This method attempts to place the individual patient into a biological continuum which exists between the most genetic and the most acquired forms of epilepsy and to use clinical, EEG, radiological, and neuropsychological data to build a profile of the patient, an 'epileptic phenotype'.

The chronology of childhood epilepsies

The chronological approach to the categorisation of childhood epilepsies is particularly attractive to paediatricians. In children, the factors of age, growth, and development are of primary importance in determining whether epilepsy develops or not. Age also determines the type of epileptic syndrome which develops and influences the prognosis.

Aicardi[22] distinguishes four main periods or epochs in childhood epilepsy. These are:

(i) *neonatal period*, which he extends to three months of age, during which seizures are related to structural pathology and the prognosis is poor;

(ii) a period *from three months to four years* in which the seizure threshold of the central nervous system is low and reactive seizures, especially with fever, are common. Serious epileptic syndromes such as West's syndrome and the Lennox-Gastaut syndrome occur in this epoch;

(iii) a period *between four years and nine to ten years* in which there is a predominance of primary or idiopathic generalised and partial epilepsies: for example, childhood absence epilepsy and benign partial epilepsy with rolandic spikes. Complex partial seizures secondary to structural abnormality also become better defined in this epoch;

(iv) from *nine to ten years onward*, primary generalised epilepsies, such as the well-defined juvenile myoclonic epilepsy of Janz, occur while complex partial seizures are more frequently encountered.

This scheme is useful to the paediatrician as a general diagnostic and prognostic framework.

Diagnosis

There are certain facts, critical to the diagnosis of epilepsy, which can only be revealed by interrogation of the patient or his relatives. An eye-witness account is invaluable. History-taking remains the cornerstone of diagnosis[23,24] and is superior to all modern diagnostic aids except perhaps an actual video of an attack together with EEG monitoring. The differential diagnosis of epilepsy from the numerous other paroxysmal, recurrent, non-epileptic events is of crucial importance if unnecessary treatment of children and anxiety for parents are to be avoided. The misdiagnosis of epilepsy is still all too common. Furthermore, history-taking will often define the particular epileptic syndrome: for example, benign partial epilepsy with rolandic spikes and the juvenile myoclonic epilepsy of Janz.

Electro-encephalography

The routine EEG is still the single most valuable test for differentiating epilepsy from non-epileptic conditions.[25] In paediatric practice, however, an EEG is only as good as the skill of the technologist can make it, and correct interpretation requires knowledge of paediatric neurology and epileptology. Because of the relatively short duration of the EEG recording, significant abnormalities may be missed. This has led to the development of ambulatory and intensive monitoring. The techniques available[26,27] consist of:

(i) having the patient wear a set of electrodes connected to a lightweight cassette recorder;
(ii) using FM telemetry in which FM radio signals are sent from a lightweight transmitter worn by the patient and then recorded;
(iii) using simultaneous videotape and EEG monitoring of the patient, with or without a split-screen technique.

Most children do not require any of these procedures but they are useful in:

(a) patients with clinical attacks that by history may be seizures but in whom routine EEGs are normal or equivocal;
(b) patients with suspected pseudoseizures;[28]
(c) patients in whom an exact count of seizures is required;
(d) candidates for epilepsy surgery.

Neuro-imaging

CT scanning is superior to clinical examination and EEG in detecting structural abnormalities of the central nervous system. It does, however, involve radiation, the patients may need sedation, and allergic reactions to contrast media can occur. The frequency of abnormal CT scans in children with epilepsy is of the order of 33% and these are more frequently found in patients with abnormal neurological signs, in those with partial seizures (excluding benign rolandic epilepsy), and where there is focal slowing in the EEG.[27,29,30] Although one of the usual reasons for doing a CT scan is to rule out a neoplasm or other treatable lesion, it has to be said that abnormalities of therapeutic significance are found in only a small proportion of cases. However, the CT may help to throw light on the aetiology of the epilepsy, and should at least be considered in all patients with epilepsy except those with childhood absence seizures, benign partial epilepsy with rolandic spikes, and febrile seizures. A CT scan should always be done where there is any change in the neurological examination or in the seizure pattern, especially during adolescence.

The MRI scan has significant advantages over CT because of its higher sensitivity, superior image quality, lack of radiation exposure, and capacity for multiplanar display. MRI scan is increasingly used to attempt to locate lesions in the temporal lobes or elsewhere which may be responsible for causing complex partial seizures in children. Such seizures occur in up to 25% of children with epilepsy and can begin as early as under two years of age.[31]. Cerebral lesions which may be responsible include arterio-venous malformations, subarachnoid cysts, hamartomas, areas of old infarction, mesial temporal sclerosis, and slow-growing gliomas. Remission rates in childhood have been reported to be as low as 10% and 18% in two recent series,[31,32] although Lindsay *et al.* found a remission rate off drugs of 33% in their 1966–1979 series.[33] Increasingly, surgical treatment is considered and used earlier for refractory cases.[34]

In their 1987 retrospective study, the Montreal group detected abnormalities with MRI in all their patients with temporal lobe epilepsy due to the presence of structural brain lesions and in 70 per cent of those where mesial temporal sclerosis was responsible.[35] In both respects it was superior to CT and they recommend that patients with intractable complex partial seizures should have this investigation since a number of structural epileptogenic lesions are not visualised by other imaging techniques.

Evaluation of the patient with seizures and recurrence risks

Before prescribing anti-epileptic drugs for a child with suspected epilepsy, one should establish a firm diagnosis, categorise the seizure type or types,
attempt to identify the epileptic syndrome present, and try to make an aetiological diagnosis. The initiation of treatment needs to be considered on a risk-versus-benefit basis.[36] The nature of the epileptic syndrome will influence the decision. For example, in the common benign partial epilepsy with rolandic spikes, up to one-quarter of the patients may have only one seizure, and approximately half have fewer than five seizures.[37]

Single seizures, which occur in response to transient toxic and metabolic disturbances or to trauma, are often referred to as reactive seizures. Febrile convulsions constitute the only well-defined reactive seizure disorder which can be considered a syndrome. Non-recurrent seizures are not epilepsy.

In recent years many studies have investigated the recurrence risks following the first unprovoked seizure in a child. Children with epileptic syndromes usually or invariably associated with recurrence, such as infantile spasms, the myoclonic epilepsies, and childhood absence epilepsy, were excluded as were those with febrile convulsions. Hirtz *et al.*,[38] following children to seven years, found a recurrence risk of 57%. Camfield *et al.*[39], following children to 16 years, found a recurrence rate of 52%. Shinnar *et al.*[40] in a prospective study, found that subsequent seizures were experienced by 36% of children in a mean period of 30 months after the first unprovoked seizure. The majority of children in the latter study were not treated. All three studies found that the key risk factors for recurrence are the aetiology of the seizures (idiopathic versus symptomatic) and the EEG. Idiopathic grand mal seizures with a normal EEG indicate a low risk, whereas partial seizures with a remote symptomatic cause, a previous history of neonatal seizures, and an abnormal neurodevelopmental examination indicate a high risk. It is important to note that when recurrences take place 70% do so within six months and nearly all within two years. After a second attack, further recurrences are likely in 80–90% of children.

Anti-epileptic drugs and their effects

Anti-epileptic drugs are potent substances which may cause side-effects, including idiosyncratic side-effects and acute and chronic toxicity. Camfield *et al.*[41] found that 15% of newly treated patients required a change of medication due to allergic or behavioural side-effects, and Abu-Arafeh and Wallace[42] had the same experience in 20% of their patients. Long-term side-effects include cosmetic changes, altered bone metabolism, haematological changes, and subtle cognitive and behavioural changes. The great majority of children who develop epilepsy after infancy are of normal intelligence and attend ordinary schools. No drug is free of risk although modern drugs are superior, especially where cognition and behaviour are concerned. The benign nature of much of childhood epilepsy is insufficiently appreciated. Emerson *et al.*[43] found that 70–75% of children who were seizure free for four years remained so when medication was stopped. Shinnar *et al.*[44] noted the same outcome when treatment was stopped after only two years. Putting this in the context of 50%–65% of children who remain seizure free with or without medication after the first seizure should make us pause and consider before embarking on long-term therapy. If we do use anti-epileptic drugs, we should give as much as is needed but as little as is necessary to control the seizures, we should avoid polytherapy, and we should use drug-level monitoring wisely,[45] remembering that it is the clinical response of the patient which is of paramount importance and not an arbitrarily defined 'therapeutic window' determined by serum levels.

Established drugs have come in for much critical appraisal recently. The behavioural side-effects of phenobarbitone are well known. In

February 1990 Farwell *et al.*[46] in a study of children taking phenobarbitone prophylaxis for febrile convulsions, concluded that phenobarbitone depressed cognitive performance and that this disadvantage, which may outlast the administration of the drug by several months, was not offset by the benefit of seizure prevention. Although this study has been criticised,[47] there is no doubt that, for these and other reasons, the therapeutic pendulum has swung strongly against the pharmacological prophylaxis of febrile convulsions during the past decade. Intermittent forms of prophylactic therapy, using diazepam rectally or even orally, are now preferred.[48,49]

Sodium valproate prophylaxis for febrile convulsions is not really an option under two years of age because the danger of fatal hepatotoxicity is greatest then.[50] The good news, however, is that Dreifuss *et al.*[51] have reported that, despite increased use of the drug, fatal hepatotoxicity from sodium valproate in the USA is declining. In the period 1978–1984, the risk was 1/10,000; in 1985–1986 it had fallen to 0.2/10,000; in that period, no hepatic fatalities were reported over the age of ten years. They ascribed the fall to the fact that more patients were receiving sodium valproate as monotherapy, that more low-risk patients were being treated with sodium valproate, and that fewer high-risk patients (0–2 years) were receiving sodium valproate. Sodium valproate should not be given in a polytherapy regime under the age of three years, it should be avoided in patients with pre-existing liver disease or a family history of such disease, and salicylates should not be given to a patient on sodium valproate. Fasting should be avoided in patients on sodium valproate with an intercurrent illness, and immediate withdrawal of the drug is mandatory if hepatotoxicity is suspected. Although it is prudent to monitor liver enzyme levels during the first three months of treatment when the risk is greatest, withdrawal of medication is necessary only if substantial rises occur. One-stage prothrombin time and fibrinogen levels are more sensitive than other tests of liver function in detecting hepatic compromise. Although valproate hepatotoxicity is rare, it may occur at any age and vigilance is required to detect its early onset.

New anti-epileptic drugs

There are several new anti-epileptic drugs undergoing trials at present, and there is an excellent short review of these by Porter in the *Lancet* of August 18, 1990.[52] They include vigabatrin, oxcarbazepine, lamotrigine, gabapentin, zonisamide, flunarizine and felbamate. Of these agents, vigabatrin (Sabril) is now available commercially in the UK. This substance is a specific irreversible inhibitor of gamma aminobutyric acid (GABA) aminotransferase.[53] As an adjuvant or add-on drug, it is reported to reduce seizure frequency in about half the patients treated, mainly adults. There is some concern about its long-term safety because it has been reported to produce reversible, non-inflammatory changes in the myelin of white matter in some experimental animals. There is no evidence that these lesions can occur in man. Very recently, lamotrigine (Lamictal) which may act by inhibiting the release of excitatory amino acids such as glutamate, has also been marketed.

Prospects for the future

There is intense interest worldwide in the neurosciences and in the epilepsies. The United States Congress designated the 1990s 'The Decade of the Brain', and this was endorsed by the Council of Delegates at the 14th World Congress of Neurology in New Delhi in October 1989. The following research objectives have been proposed.[54]

1. Determine the basic cellular mechanisms of epilepsy.
2. Characterise the genetic susceptibility to epilepsy.
3. Develop new anti-epileptic drugs.[55]
4. Study further the efficacy of surgery for seizures.
5. Identify types of behavioural abnormalities associated with epilepsy and develop specific therapies for these abnormalities.
6. Devise technical innovations including development of new light-weight ambulatory monitoring devices to warn patients of impending seizures, self-regulatory drug delivery systems, and more sophisticated imaging methods to measure brain function.

Epilepsy in childhood is different from the condition in adults in its causes, in the various syndromes which occur and how they present clinically, and in the response to treatment. Medication itself has far-reaching effects on the developing brain and on cognition. The psychological and social consequences of epilepsy are also different in childhood. It behoves all paediatricians, not only paediatric neurologists, to interest themselves in the child with seizures so that the objective of the British Paediatric Association[1] in bringing about better treatment and control of epilepsy in the future may be achieved.

References

1. Court, D., Alberman, E. (1988) Worlds apart. In: *Child Health in a Changing Society* (ed. J.O. Forfar), pp 1–30. British Paediatric Association, Oxford University Press.
2. Shorvon, S.D. (1990) Epidemiology, classification, natural history, and genetics of epilepsy. *Lancet*, **336**, 93–96.
3. Ross, E.M., Peckham, C.S. (1983) Seizure disorder in the National Child Development

Study. In: *Research Progress in Epilepsy* (ed. F.C. Rose) pp 46–59. London: Pitman.
4. Cowan, L.B., Bodensteiner, J.B., Leviton, A., Doherty, L. (1989) Prevalence of the epilepsies in childhood and adolescence. *Epilepsia*, **30**, 94–106.
5. Moshé, S.L. (1987) Epileptogenesis and the immature brain. *Epilepsia*, **28**, Supplement I, S3–S15.
6. Annegers, J.F., Hauser, W. A., Shirts, S.B., Kurland, L.T. (1987) Factors prognostic of unprovoked seizures after febrile convulsions. *New England Journal of Medicine*, **316**, 493–498.
7. Addy, D.P. (1990) Phenobarbitone and febrile convulsions. *Archives of Disease in Childhood*, **65**, 921.
8. Moshé, S.L., Sperber, E.F., Brown, L.L. *et al.* (1989) Experimental epilepsy: developmental aspects. *Cleveland Clinic Journal of Medicine*, **56**, Supplement, Part I, S92–S99.
9. Kalil, R.E. (1989) Synapse formation in the developing brain. *Scientific American*, **261**, 38–45.
10. Hollman, M., O'Shea-Greenfield, A., Rodgers, S.W., Heinemann, S. (1989) Cloning by functional expression of a member of the glutamate receptor family. *Nature*, **342**, 643–648.
11. Metrakos, K., Metrakos, J.D. (1961) Genetics of convulsive disorders. II. Genetic and electroencephalographic studies in centrencephalic epilepsy. *Neurology*, **11**, 474–483.
12. Andermann, E. (1982) Multifactorial inheritance of generalised and focal epilepsy. In: *Genetic Basis of the Epilepsies* (eds V.E. Anderson, W.A. Hauser, J.K. Penry, C.F. Sing) pp 355–374. New York: Raven Press.
13. Rowland, L.P. (1988). Clinical concepts of Duchenne muscular dystrophy. The impact of molecular genetics. *Brain*, **111**, 479–495.
14. Melki, J., Sheth, P., Abdelhak, S. *et al.* and French Spinal Muscular Atrophy Investigators (1990) Mapping of acute (type 1) spinal muscular atrophy to chromosome 5q12–q14. *Lancet*, **336**, 271–273.
15. Leppert, M., Anderson, V.E., Quattlebaum, T. *et al.* (1989) Benign familial neonatal convulsions linked to genetic markers on chromosome 20. *Nature*, **337**, 647–648.
16. Delgado-Escueta, A.V., Greenberg, D.A., Treiman, L. *et al.* (1989) Mapping the gene for juvenile myoclonic epilepsy. *Epilepsia*, **30**, Supplement 4, S8–S18.
17. Editorial (1987) Mapping the human genome. *Lancet*, **329**, 1121–1122.
18. Commission on Classification and Terminology of the International League Against Epilepsy. Proposal for revised clinical and electroencephalographic classification of epileptic seizures. (1981) *Epilepsia*, **22**, 489–501.
19. Roger, J., Dravet, C., Bureau, M. *et al.* (eds) (1985) *Epileptic Syndromes in Infancy, Childhood and Adolescence*. London: John Libbey.
20. Dreifuss, F.E. (1989) Classification of epileptic seizures and the epilepsies. In: *Seizure Disorders* (ed. J.M. Pellock). *Pediatric Clinics of North America*, **36**, 265–279. Philadelphia, London: W.B. Saunders.
21. Berkovic, S.F., Andermann, F., Andermann, E., Gloor, P. (1987) Concepts of absence epilepsies. Discrete syndromes or biological continuum? *Neurology*, **37**, 993–1000.
22. Aicardi, J. (1986) *Epilepsy in Children*. New York: Raven Press.
23. O'Donohoe, N.V. (1985) *Epilepsies of Childhood* (2nd edn). London: Butterworths.
24. Brett, E.M. (1990) 'It isn't epilepsy is it, doctor?'. Editorial, *British Medical Journal*, **300**, 1604–1606.
25. Drury, I. (1989) Epileptiform patterns of children. *Journal of Clinical Neurophysiology*, **6**, 1–39.
26. Stores, G. (1984) Intensive EEG monitoring in paediatrics. *Developmental Medicine and Child Neurology*, **26**, 231–234.
27. Holmes, G.L. (1989) Electro-encephalographic and neuroradiologic evaluation of

children with epilepsy. In: *Seizure Disorders* (ed. J.M. Pellock). *Pediatric Clinics of North America*, **36**, 395–420. Philadelphia, London: W.B. Saunders.
28. Wyllie, E., Friedmann, R.N., Rothner, A.D. *et al.* (1990) Psychogenic seizures in children and adolescents. Outcome after diagnosis by ictal video and electroencephalographic recording. *Pediatrics*, **85**, 480–484.
29. Yang, P.J., Berger, P.E., Cohen, M.E., Duffner, P.K. (1979). Computed tomography and childhood seizure disorders. *Neurology*, **29**, 1084–1088.
30. Shorvon, S. (1987) Imaging in the investigation of epilepsy. In: *Epilepsy*. (Ed. A. Hopkins) pp 201–228. London: Chapman and Hall.
31. Harbord, M.G., Manson, J.L. (1987) Temporal lobe epilepsy in childhood. Reappraisal of aetiology and outcome. *Pediatric Neurology*, **3**, 263–268.
32. Kotagal, P., Rothner, A.D., Erenberg, G. *et al.* (1987) Complex partial seizures of childhood onset. A five-year follow-up study. *Archives of Neurology*, **44**, 1177–1180.
33. Lindsay, J., Ounsted, C., Richards, P. (1980) Long-term outcome in children with temporal lobe seizures. IV. Genetic factors, febrile convulsions and remission of seizures. *Developmental Medicine and Child Neurology*, **22**, 429–439.
34. Mizrahi, E.M., Kellaway, P., Grossman, R.G. *et al.* (1990) Anterior temporal lobectomy and medically refractory temporal lobe epilepsy of childhood. *Epilepsia*, **31**, 302–313.
35. Kuzniecky, R., de la Sayette, V., Ethnier, R. *et al.* (1987) Magnetic resonance imaging in temporal lobe epilepsy. Pathological correlations. *Annals of Neurology*, **22**, 341–347.
36. Freeman, J.M. (1987) A clinical approach to the child with seizures and epilepsy. *Epilepsia*, **22**, Supplement I, S103–S109.
37. Beaussart, M., Faou, R. (1978) Evolution of epilepsy with rolandic paroxysmal foci. A study of 324 cases. *Epilepsia*, **19**, 337–342.
38. Hirtz, D.G., Ellenberg, J.H., Nelson, K.B. (1984) The risk of recurrence of nonfebrile seizures in children. *Neurology*, **34**, 637–641.
39. Camfield, P., Camfield, C., Dooley, J. *et al.* (1985) Epilepsy after a first unprovoked seizure in childhood. *Neurology*, **35**, 1657–1660.
40. Shinnar, S., Berg, A.T., Moshé, S.L. *et al.* (1990) Risk of seizure recurrence following a first unprovoked seizure in childhood. A prospective study. *Pediatrics*, **85**, 1076–1085.
41. Camfield, P.R., Camfield, C.S., Smith, E.C., Tibbles, J.A.R. (1985) Newly treated childhood epilepsy: A prospective study of recurrence and side-effects. *Neurology*, **35**, 722–725.
42. Abu-Arafeh, I.A., Wallace, S.J. (1988) Unwanted effects of anti-epileptic drugs. *Developmental Medicine and Child Neurology*, **30**, 117–121.
43. Emerson, E., D'Souza, B.J., Vining, E.P. *et al.* (1981) Stopping medication in children with epilepsy: predictors of outcome. *New England Journal of Medicine*, **304**, 1125–1129.
44. Shinnar, S., Vining, E.P.G., Mellits, E.M. *et al.* (1985) Discontinuing anti-epileptic medication in children with epilepsy after two years without seizures. *New England Journal of Medicine*, **313**, 976–980.
45. Wallace, S.J. (1990) Anti-epileptic drug monitoring: an overview. *Developmental Medicine and Child Neurology*, **32**, 923–926.
46. Farwell, J.R., Lee, Y.J., Hirtz, D.G. *et al.* (1990) Phenobarbital for febrile seizures – effects on intelligence and on seizure recurrence. *New England Journal of Medicine*, **332**, 364–369.
47. Hirsch, R.P., Painter, M.J. (1990) Phenobarbital for febrile seizures (Letter). *New England Journal of Medicine*, **333**, 484.
48. Knudsen, F.U. (1985) Recurrence risk after first febrile seizure and the effect of short-term diazepam prophylaxis. *Archives of Disease in Childhood*, **60**, 1045–1049.
49. Rylance, G.W. (1990) Treatment of epilepsy and febrile convulsions in children. *Lancet*, **336**, 488–491.

50. Brown, J.K. (1988) Valproate toxicity. *Developmental Medicine and Child Neurology*, **30**, 121–125.
51. Dreifuss, F.E., Langer, D.H., Moline, K.A., Maxwell, J.E. (1989) Valproic acid hepatic fatalities. II. U.S. experience since 1984. *Neurology*, **39**, 201–207.
52. Porter, R.J. (1990) New anti-epileptic agents: strategies for drug development. *Lancet*, **336**, 423–424.
53. Dreifuss, F.E. (ed.) (1989) Gamma Vinyl GABA (Vigabatrin) in epilepsy. The international experience. *Epilepsia*, **30**, Supplement 3, S1–S35.
54. Editorial (1990) *Epilepsy Advances in Clinical and Experimental Research*. **5**, No. 4, 1. Epilepsy Foundation of America.
55. Leppik, I.E. (ed.) (1989) Research in epileptogenesis. The search for tomorrow's anti-epileptic drugs. *Epilepsia*, **30**, Supplement 1, S1–S68.

5 | Cerebral palsy

Richard O. Robinson
Department of Paediatrics, Guy's Hospital, London

Reviewing the published work in cerebral palsy in the past five years, one is tempted to organise it into 'Epidemiology' and 'The Rest'. While it may be true to say that the enormous amount of work done in the epidemiological field has not as yet benefited directly a single child with cerebral palsy, it would be wrong, for reasons which I shall come to, not to wish for further developments in this field.

Epidemiology

Much of the epidemiological work has been fuelled by the need to know to what extent birth asphyxia contributes to cerebral palsy. Not only are there cogent medico-legal reasons for attempting to define this, but also this question has underlain much of the development of interventional obstetrics with fetal monitoring over the past 20 years. We all know that birth asphyxia causes some cerebral palsy. We are all too familiar with the unequivocally severely asphyxiated term infant who, surviving a stormy neonatal period with fits and either hypo- or hypertonia, goes on to develop a spastic quadriplegia with progressing microcephaly and severe mental handicap. We also see other children developing cerebral palsy rather insidiously at 4–6 months after an apparently blameless pregnancy, labour, and birth.

It was of course Freud who nearly 100 years ago made an apparently simple subject more complex by suggesting: 'One has to consider the anomaly of the birth process, rather than being the central aetiological factor, may itself be the consequence of the real perinatal aetiology'.[1] Having dropped this bombshell to counter William Little who found it difficult to conceive of any aetiology other than birth asphyxia,[2] he concluded that paediatric neurology was too complicated and went on to other things.

As far as this question as to 'How much cerebral palsy is caused by birth asphyxia?' is concerned, the epidemiologists are generally agreed that the answer is: 'Not as much as we had thought'. The most influential studies coming to this conclusion have been based on the data from the approximately 54,000 pregnancies recruited to the National Collaborative Perinatal Project in America.[3,4,5] They found that only 6% of children with complicated term deliveries, with 5-minute Apgar scores of less than 6 and neonatal signs of hypoxic, ischaemic encephalopathy will develop cerebral palsy. Conversely, although 21% of children with cerebral palsy had at least one marker of severe intra-partum asphyxia, about one-third of these had a major malformation outside the central nervous system. Similarly, one-half of those with cerebral palsy and an intra-partum asphyxia factor also had additional abnormal features present before labour. Indeed, full-term infants with low 10-minute Apgar scores, neonatal fits, hypotonia, meconium in the liquor, neonatal apnoeic spells, neonatal neurological abnormalities, and slow head-growth after birth were all more often associated with congenital disorders than with birth asphyxia. Depending on the criteria employed it was concluded that somewhere between 3–13% of cerebral palsy was associated with intra-partum asphyxia. It should be noted, however, that the first children recruited to this study are now over 30 years old. Mortality following birth asphyxia was high and continued during the first few years. How justified would their conclusions be today that birth asphyxia bad enough to damage the brain usually kills?

The more recent 1975–1980 cohort from Stanley's Western Australia study supports this conclusion.[6] She estimated that even taken across all birth-weights—ie including the pre-term—14.1% of cases of cerebral palsy were thought to be caused by (or at any rate associated with) birth asphyxia. She estimated that 8.2% of cases of spastic cerebral palsy were probably or definitely caused by birth asphyxia or trauma—figures very similar to those of the National Collaborative Perinatal Project.

The implication of this is that, at least as far as term infants are concerned, there are for the majority no identifiable preceding factors, ie we do not know what causes at least two-thirds of cases. A corollary is that further refining obstetric practice is unlikely to make much difference to the overall cerebral-palsy rate. Intra-partum monitoring, for example, does not appear to affect the incidence of cerebral palsy[7] although it may affect the incidence of neonatal fits. This implication is borne out by the comparison of the results obtained by the 1958 British Perinatal Mortality Survey and the 1970 British Births Survey.[8] During that period obstetric practice became more interventional. Some of the changes are detailed in Table 1. Despite all these changes in practice and survival, the congenital cerebral palsy prevalence rate remained precisely the same at 2.5/1,000. A cautionary note has been sounded elsewhere. In the latter half of the 1960–1975 period there was in the North-East of England a rise in the cerebral-palsy rate among babies of

Table 1. Changes in obstetric practice between 1958 and 1978.

Year	BPMS† 1958	BBS* 1970
Births in consultant units	48%	66%
Caesarean section rate	3%	5%
Induction rate	13%	26%
Forceps rate	5%	9%
Prop. with labour > 24 hours	8%	4%
Prop. with 2nd stage > 1 hour	21%	12%
Mortality from cerebral trauma	0.3%	0.04%
Stillbirth rate	2.2%	1.3%
Neonatal mortality rate	1.6%	1.2%

*BBS (British Births Survey):
Chamberlain, R., Chamberlain, G., Howlett, B., Claireaux, A. (1975) *The first week of life. British births 1970* (vol. 1). London: Heinemann Medical Books.
Chamberlain, G.V.P., Philipp, E., Howlett, B., Masters, K. (1978) *Obstetric care. British births 1970* (vol. 2). London: Heinemann Medical Books.
†BPMS (British Perinatal Mortality Survey):
Butter, N.R., Bonham, D.G. (1963) *Perinatal mortality: the first reports of the 1958 British perinatal mortality survey*. Edinburgh: E. & S. Livingstone.
Butler, N.R., Alberman, E.D. (1969) *Perinatal problems. The second report of the 1958 British perinatal mortality survey*. Edinburgh: E. & S. Livingstone.

birth-weight more than 2.5kg—particularly in the more severely handicapping forms of cerebral palsy.[10] Similar changes have been seen in Hagberg's series of studies from Southern Sweden.[11] These changes were not seen in Merseyside.[12] It would be premature to conclude much from this. It may be that social and medical changes are allowing women to carry handicapped fetuses to term who would otherwise have been born pre-term or still-born. On the other hand, we must always bear in mind that interventional obstetrics carries its own risks.

The other question which has motivated epidemiological studies has been the role of neonatal intensive care units. Are they generating increasing numbers of handicapped, often pre-term, infants? This is in effect the Little/Freud controversy moved to a modern arena. No one disputes the exponential rise in the cerebral-palsy rate in infants less than 2,000g birth-weight. Are the processes leading to pre-term birth also causing cerebral palsy, or is the brain being damaged directly as a consequence of the complications of prematurity?

Stewart and her co-workers surveyed the world literature up to 1977, concluding that for infants of very low birth-weight (less than 1500G), although the mortality rate had steadily fallen, the morbidity rate was largely unchanged.[13] That the morbidity rate had not by and large actually increased was in itself a remarkable achievement. Indeed, it is possible to quote studies to 1983 from Tübingen[14] and to 1984 from Alberta[15] which show a decreased morbidity rate in very low birth-weight infants. However, more recently a cautionary note has once again been sounded. It first should be pointed out that as the perinatal mortality rate among low birth-weight infants falls, even if morbidity rates stay the same, the actual numbers of handicapped survivors increase. This is indisputable. In order to obtain some sort of perspective we need figures such as those once again from Western Australia which suggest that, between 1968 and 1981, for every 1,000 babies born less than 1500g, 375 additional normal survivors were gained at the 'cost' of 13 children with cerebral palsy.[9] This question of survival is also crucial in trying to compare studies in different countries. We can envisage the situation where the perinatal mortality figures fall so low that one sees the start of an exponential rise in rates of cerebral palsy overall. The lowest perinatal mortality figures come from Sweden with rates of 7.4/1,000 live births for the period 1979–1982[11] (see Table 2). They now also have the highest proportion of children with cerebral palsy born pre-term (ie less than 37 weeks' gestation)—45%.[16] Their rate of cerebral palsy in the less than 1500g birth-weight group at 89/1,000 is now the highest quoted and is reflected in their increasing overall cerebral-palsy rate, particularly in the pre-term diplegic children, which has been consistently rising for the past 20 years. Figures showing similar trends are also available from Finland[17] and Ireland.[18] The Hagbergs suggest that the Scandinavian fall in perinatal mortality rates is about 10 years ahead of the United Kingdom and Western Australia. They predict that we will find similar changes here in due course. I would

Table 2. Children born before term as a proportion of the total of children with cerebral palsy (CP).

		Pre-term proportion of total with CP	Perinatal mortality rate
BBS[8]	1970	2.5%	2.5%
BPMS[8]	1958	5%	3.8%
Merseyside[12]	1966–77	29%	?
W. Australia[9]	1975–80	39%	1.1%
Sweden[11]	1979–82	43%	0.7%

Note: See Table 1 for full references for BBS and BPMS.

suggest, therefore, that a suitable subject for audit in this country is continuing morbidity rates in population-based studies of very low birth-weight infants.

Where has all this led us to? There is no doubt that this work has altered the way that the Courts deal with individual cases of questionable birth asphyxia. However, more importantly, we remain as ignorant now about the causes of most cerebral palsy as we did a hundred years ago when these matters were first discussed by Little and Freud. We have, however, been given two clues which need following up. The first is the hint about congenital defects which comes from the National Collaborative Perinatal Project and elsewhere. Perhaps more detailed architectural and functional brain imaging in these children will give us better defined categories for study. Computed tomography (CT) abnormalities are not always present in children with cerebral palsy and, when they are, the patterns do not relate predictably to the type of motor abnormality found. Cerebral blood-flow abnormalities may be found on SPECT when the CT scan is normal, but again are not always predictably related to the type of motor handicap.[19] There are considerable problems in deriving absolute values for regional glucose metabolism by positron emission tomography (PET) in infants and children. A study of relative values in normal and asphyxiated term infants showed loss of 'metabolic architecture' in those with hypoxic ischaemic encephalopathy.[20] We need detailed information about patterns of congenital anomalies together with accompanying cytogenetic studies. The other hint comes from Bundey's and Gustavson's empirical recurrent risk studies of the outcome of subsequent pregnancies in families where a child with non-perinatal cerebral palsy has already been born.[21,22] A figure of 1 : 200 for congenital hemiplegia and other lateralised forms of cerebral palsy suggests that these are arbitrary non-recurrent events. Conversely, a figure of 1 :8–9 following symmetrical cerebral palsy—whether spastic or dyskinetic —suggests that half of these are autosomal recessive. These familial cases, otherwise clinically indistinguishable from the rest, may be a fruitful area for genetic linkage studies as well as intensive antenatal monitoring.

I have thus far managed to avoid defining what kinds of cerebral palsy I am referring to. The antecedents of cerebral palsy will differ not only between types but also probably between the pre-term and term, between the fetally malnourished (and types and timing of fetal malnutrition) and appropriately grown infants, and between populations with different perinatal mortality rates (which again must be birth weight/gestational age related). The Liverpool team have made a start on defining antecedents of diplegia[23] and hemiplegia[24] in low birth-weight infants. Hagberg has described the antecedents of spastic tetraplegia in a defined population.[25] We need to continue population-defined cohort studies of cerebral palsy. We might be able to use the need for audit to persuade regions to establish paediatric epidemiologists. We may now, by getting the question more focused, be able to look at clues which lead us to prevention.

Two final thoughts. Factors associated with prematurity are well known. There is one French study which describes the fall in prematurity rate coinciding with an improved antenatal care system.[26] I know of no controlled interventional studies aimed at reducing the prematurity rate, but clearly the more recent cerebral palsy data from Sweden and elsewhere makes this more pertinent.

Secondly, the increasingly brain-orientated management approach of neonatologists must continue to be further refined. The epidemiology suggests that only stabilisation of infants following carefully monitored and controlled deliveries will continue to give us an advantageous cost-to-benefit ratio with a declining perinatal mortality rate.

Acquired cerebral palsy is no less important for being less mysterious. Depending on age limits within the definition, it constitutes some 5–15% of the total. The most recent data again come from Merseyside.[27] About half of the total are caused by central nervous system infections and a substantial proportion of the rest by injury. Many are potentially preventable either by the development of effective vaccines or by properly safeguarding our children on roads, in cars, around swimming pools, and the like.

Management

I have selected various areas for consideration by confining myself only to those changes which have influenced my own practice in the past five years. I should perhaps first say that stereotactic thalamotomy for the relief of dystonia has been largely abandoned, mainly because of the unacceptably high risk of impairing speech but also because improving dystonia was by no means synonymous with improving ability.[28] Galvanic stimulation of the cerebellum or spinal cord has not been proved effective.

Physiotherapy

I believe the main effect of physiotherapy is giving parents confidence in handling their children, providing suitable aids, and preventing secondary deformity. Perhaps no sentence starting 'I believe' should have a place in a scientific presentation, but one only has to visit Third World countries which lack physiotherapists for belief to shade into factually based certainty. Physiotherapists are forced into a counselling role also, for which they are completely untrained. They are a tremendous psychotherapeutic resource—a function which perhaps should be recognised and formalised in their training.

Contractures are the result of abnormal periods of muscle shortening, leading to secondary shortening of connective tissue as well as reduction of sarcomere numbers. Tardieu and colleagues studied the time the soleus muscle gets stretched dynamically during a normal day's activity (mean 7 hours 10 minutes). They showed in 10 walking diplegic children that no contractures occurred when stretching time was more than 4 hours 50 minutes but did when it was less than 3 hours 30 minutes.[29] Most non-ambulant children with cerebral palsy might get two 10-minute periods of passive stretching per day if their parents are not too busy. On this data the effect of this practice is questionable. Perhaps the role of the physiotherapist in treating the partially active is to provide motivation for adequate periods and ranges of movement. This approach finds echoes in the work of Peto in Budapest. Comparison of the effect of physiotherapy with a cognition stimulation programme in diplegic infants without contractures, showed earlier acquisition of walking and higher overall developmental scores in those in the cognition stimulation group.[30]

An attempt to show the effect of so-called 'inhibitive' casting as an adjunct to physiotherapy on walking performance in partially ambulant diplegic children without contractures was similarly unsuccessful.[31] Here the feet were immobilised in the neutral position with the toes dorsiflexed for 10–14 days, followed by use of light polypropylene ankle/foot orthoses during the day. The changes which occurred of a greater range of foot dorsiflexion and greater foot–floor contact were accompanied neither by a decrease in static muscle tone nor by improvement in developmental skills. What changes there were had worn off five months later. Perhaps the lesson is to let the more able get on with life in whatever way they find easiest, but to monitor closely for any deterioration in function or any increasing effort to maintain function, together with any accompanying deformities.

If secondary deformity in the less active is the result of immobility in abnormal postures, prevention should be achieved by correct positioning which for much of the time implies an appropriate seating system. Here Nwaobi from Memphis, Tennessee, has introduced some science into what was previously an art form. He has shown that children with spastic and dyskinetic cerebral palsy feel unbalanced in any position other than a vertical trunk-and-head position with the hips at a right-angle. If the child is tipped back—reclined—or forward out of this position, the spinal muscles tense. Opening out the hip angle has the same effect.[32]

He has shown that deviation from this position impairs upper-limb function—presumably by increasing arm muscle-tone.[33] Green at Chailey has shown that similar displacements from the vertical, while not impairing simple perceptual tasks in vision and hearing, do impair more complex cognitive tasks involving auditory or visual memory or visual matching.[34] While the educational implications of this work require further exploration, one immediate lesson is that it is no good sending children for evaluation of sophisticated word processor and communication aid systems until their seating system is appropriate. In general, seating is usually found to be most effective when orthogonal. Other features which may need to be included are a ramped cushion in order to keep the femur–pelvis angle (as opposed to the leg–trunk angle) at a right angle, and a sacral pad in order to accommodate the normal spinal curvature above (see Fig. 1).

Surgery

The detection of secondary deformities has already been mentioned as an important part of the paediatrician's job. It involves listening to what parents, therapists, and children say, together with informed liaison,

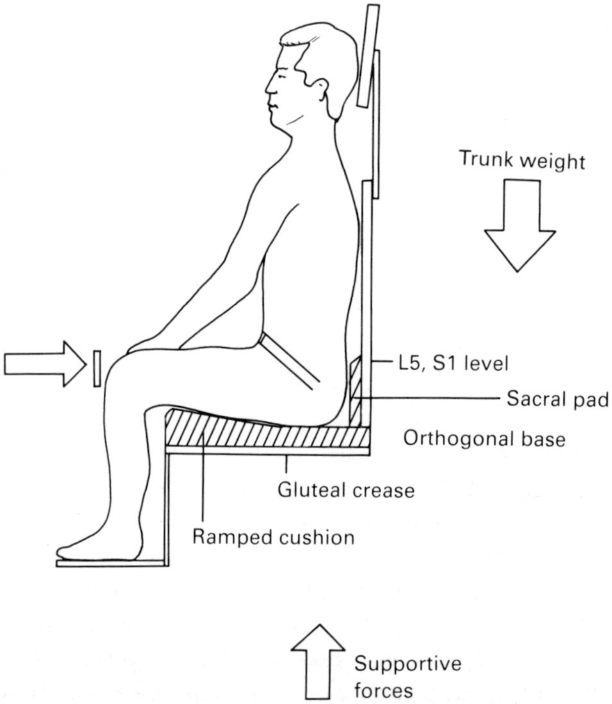

Fig. 1. *Cross-section through the Chailey Adaptaseat*

preferably through combined clinics with an interested orthopaedic colleague. I shall mention just two important areas where a consensus has emerged in the past five years.

The first concerns the prevention of secondary hip deformity.[35,36] Performed early, ie pre-school, soft tissue surgery can prevent most hip dislocations. Hips particularly at risk are those where there is little weight bearing with excessive adductor tone and posturing.[37] Progression of subluxation in hips such as these is undetectable clinically. They should be X-rayed every six months. Dislocation without acetabular dysplasia is rare. That proportion of the femoral head uncovered should be measured at each X-ray. Dislocation is rapidly progressive when more than half the femoral head is uncovered, and some surgeons will proceed when one-third is uncovered. Surgery should be considered on clinical grounds alone; however, if there is a fixed contracture limiting abduction to 30° or a fixed flexion contracture of more than 45°, dislocation is probable in due course. Conversely Scrutton and Baird have shown that hips are unlikely to be a problem in children who can learn to pull to stand. The effect of passive weight-bearing in standing frames is unknown but needs to be tested.

The other major deformity for consideration is scoliosis.[38] This can develop with a subluxing hip (cause and effect, if any, here is controversial) or independently. When it occurs with a hip deformity, the spine deformity must be corrected first. If the curve extends to the pelvis, fusion should involve the pelvis, particularly if the child is skeletally immature. Progression of postural, ie unfixed, curves might be prevented or deferred if of less than 30° by a well-made brace, known as a 'thoraco-lumbar spinal orthosis'. Curves of more than 40° will need surgery. In some hands extensive and frequently two-stage fusions have been successfully abandoned in favour of para-spinal rods with segmental fixation. These allow sitting up the day after surgery and subsequent early mobilisation. This implies that paediatricians should learn how to measure Cobb angles, on thoraco-lumbar spine films obtained in sitting and suspension (in order to evaluate what is fixed and what is not).

We may get further and better particulars on the management of progressive deformity from *longitudinal* studies of cohorts of children with cerebral palsy. Most of our knowledge is based on cross-sectional data which may be somewhat misleading in various areas. We have seen, for example, femoral head uncovering decrease when walking is achieved.

A developing area is in surgery aimed at improving the stability and ease of walking. Much surgery has been recommended on clinical data alone. Bad and unpredictable results still occur following apparently well-based clinical decisions. It is to be hoped that this situation will be improved by gait laboratory studies. For example, in-toeing in walking is usually due to over-active medial hamstrings, and can be corrected by lateral transfer of the semitendinosus. If femoral ante-version is present, a de-rotation osteotomy will also be considered.[39] However, the over activity may be coming from the ileopsoas or other hip internal rotators. Only analysis of the electromyogram (EMG) during the walking cycle will detect which is the offending muscle. The different EMG patterns in the affected leg in hemiplegic cerebral palsy have been described.[40] Similarly analysis of the function of muscles which cross two joints, such as the rectus femoris, can assist operative decisions.[41] Normally the rectus is active in early swing to help hip flexion as well as to prevent excessive knee flexion. If the rectus is active in stance also, and the problem is excessive hip flexion in standing, proximal release is logical. If, however, there is activity after early swing and the problem is excessive extension leading to a stiff gait, distal release or transfer is a better option. I think the function of paediatricians will be to encourage orthopaedic surgeons to take an intelligent interest in this work. It is likely that the pattern of practice that will develop is for patients to be referred for gait analysis and consequent surgical recommendations. The decision for surgery will remain with the referring doctor. In the United States, where this pattern of work is well established, there has been a tendency to recommend, if appropriate, several procedures at once, in contrast to the 'let's do this and then see' approach that prevails in the UK. Perhaps a good way to persuade our orthopaedic colleagues to take an interest is to ask slightly searching questions about common patients which give the impression that we are well informed.

A final exciting development in this area has been that of selective dorsal rhizotomy.[42,43] This entails collaboration with neurosurgeons. It is based on the following principle. Each dorsal root has up to 20 macroscopically definable rootlets. Each rootlet is stimulated at surgery while recording from the muscles of its own and nearby segments. If there is an abnormal excitatory pool in the spinal cord at that point, only a low threshold of stimulation will be required to evoke a muscle response; or at normal levels of stimuli a sustained contraction or even spread of contractions to other muscle segments will be evoked. If any of these happens the offending rootlet is divided. In practice about half the rootlets from L2 to S1 are so involved. This is thus a peripheral afferent attack on lower limb spasticity.[44] The most extensive experience comes from Peacock's group of 60 children with cerebral palsy. Forty of those with diplegia have now been followed up for 3–7 years. The criteria for inclusion were an ability to side sit (with or without arm support), four-point kneeling, to rise from squatting, and some form of forward locomotion. Of the 60, 44 could crawl and 22 could walk with or without aids. All but three had an IQ of more than 70. Any form of dystonia was a contra-indication, as were significant fixed contractures. The results of Peacock's series appear impressive. In all 40 diplegics, side sitting, crawling, and standing improved. Of 14 independent walkers, 12 had a much improved walking pattern. Of eight children walking with aids, five could afterwards manage without. Of 13 who could only walk with assistance beforehand, one became independent, eight walked with aids, and four still needed assistance. In all, numbers of community walkers rose from four to 15. Interestingly, he also claimed improvement in *upper* function in 19 of the 38 who had arm involvement, as well as in speech in five of nine with articulation defects. Immediately post operatively some children were weaker—probably from exposure of pre-existing weakness in an antagonist to a powerfully spastic muscle—but persisting weakness was only a problem in one. Sensory loss was not detectable, nor were cortical somato sensory evoked potentials affected.[44] Poor foot postures persisted, and 24 children have had subsequent foot and leg surgery. No progression of hip subluxation has been seen. Thirty-two of 35 sets of parents thought the procedure worthwhile. This is clearly important work. However, it needs re-duplication ideally with gait laboratory evaluation, careful measurement of post-operative hypotonia and weakness, documentation of any change in bladder or bowel function, and—most crucially—a control group receiving equal amounts of physiotherapy.

Oro-motor function

Another area where there has been significant improvement in management in the past five years has been that of dribble control. One-quarter to one-third of all children with cerebral palsy drool; for some this is a major social handicap. Drooling is caused by a number of factors[45] (see Table 3). The actual rate of salivary secretion is normal. The problem lies in the co-ordination of the oral phase of swallowing, as the pharyngeal and oesophageal phases are usually normal. As with most aspects of cerebral palsy, the assessment and management of these various factors requires a multi-disciplinary team approach involving physiotherapist,

Table 3. Drooling in cerebral palsy.

Poor head control
Open mouth
Poor lip closure
Disordered tongue mobility
Disordered gag reflex

speech therapist, doctors, and ENT surgeons. If an upright posture and lip seal can be achieved with physiotherapy and speech therapy training alone, perhaps using auditory cues and bio-feedback techniques to initiate and monitor swallowing frequency, there will be significant reduction in drooling,[46] which can be aided by the gradual introduction of an anticholinergic such as benztropine.[47] Where this is not possible, translocation of the submandibular ducts (which are responsible for half the saliva drooled) to the anterior fauces—thereby bypassing the oral phase of swallowing—achieves excellent results in about three-quarters of patients.[48] Not all surgeons carry out routine tonsillectomy beforehand. Therapy and drugs may still have a part to play post operatively.

A neglected area of oro-motor function is that of dysphagia. Croft, at Chailey Heritage, has recently shown that nutritional status is related to poor oro-motor function. Feeding ability is influenced by the textures of food offered and, as usual in severely handicapped children, by appropriate seating systems. We need to be aware that aspiration, particularly in dystonic children, is clinically undetectable in 40% and may be a regular cause of chest infections. Feeding may be a trial for all concerned. These children should be investigated by barium swallow.[49] The role for gastrostomy, perhaps as an adjunct to oral feeding, needs to be defined now that gastrostomy using an endoscopic technique is almost a bedside procedure.

Urinary continence

A further neglected area in cerebral palsy is that of bladder control. Urinary symptoms not appropriate to the child's mental development may be present in up to one-third of children with cerebral palsy. Diurnal enuresis is not uncommon, as are urgency and frequency. Forty-two of 49 cerebral-palsied children with urinary symptoms had abnormal urodynamic studies—usually uninhibited contractions from an overactive detrusor muscle.[50] Incomplete emptying due to inappropriate internal sphincter contraction, at the same time as detrusor contraction (known as dyssynergia), carries the usual risks of infection and vesicoureteric reflux. The treatment prescribed was based on the videourodynamic findings—anticholinergic agents for abnormal bladder contractions or intermittent catheterisation for incomplete emptying. Adequate follow-up was available in 27. Of these, worthwhile improvement was gained in 18 and a further three became totally dry. This work bears repetition further to define not only symptomatic management in a substantial number but also preservation of renal function in a minority.

One final thought. It is in the nature of things that we can never know the morbidity or life expectancy of children we are treating now. We should, however, pause at the thought that not only are there no actuarial statistics for people with cerebral palsy born at any time, but also we do not know what proportion have jobs, live independently, get married, or have children. It will come as no surprise that in a recent short-term follow-up study, IQ at school was not a predictive factor in achieving employment—but degree of disability was.[51]

References

1. Freud, S. (1968) *Infantile Cerebral Paralysis* (trans. L.A. Russin). Coral Gables, Florida: University of Miami Press, p. 142.
2. Little, W.J. (1862) On the influence of abnormal parturition, difficult labours, premature birth and asphyxia neonatorum on the mental and physical condition of the child, especially in relation to deformities. (Transactions of the Obstetrical Society London), **3**, 293–344.
3. Nelson, K.B., Ellenberg, J.H. (1986) Antecedents of cerebral palsy; multivariant analysis of risk. *New England Journal of Medicine*, **31**, 581–586.
4. Nelson, K.B. (1988) What proportion of cerebral palsy is related to birth asphyxia? *Journal of Pediatrics*, **112**, 572–574.
5. Naeye, R., Peters, E.C., Bartholomew, M., Landis, J.R. (1989) Origins of cerebral palsy. *Am J Dis Chi*, **143**, 1154–1161.
6. Blair, E., Stanley, F.J. (1988) Intrapartum asphyxia: a rare cause of cerebral palsy. *Journal of Pediatrics*, **112**, 515–519.
7. Grant, A., O'Brien, N., Joy, M-T. *et al.* (1989) Cerebral palsy among children born during the Dublin randomised trial of intrapartum monitoring. *Lancet*, **1**, 1233–1235.
8. Emond, A., Golding, J., Peckham, C. (1989) Cerebral palsy in two national cohort studies. *Archives of Disease in Childhood*, **64**, 848–852.
9. Stanley, F.J., Watson, L. (1988) The cerebral palsies in Western Australia: trends 1968–1981. *American Journal of Obstetrics and Gynecology*, **15**, 889–893.
10. Jarvis, S.N., Holloway, J.S., Hey, E.N. (1985) Increase in cerebral palsy in normal birth-weight babies. *Archives of Disease in Childhood*, **60**, 1113–1121.
11. Hagberg, B., Hagberg, G., Olow, I., van Wendt, L. (1989) The changing panorama of cerebral palsy in Sweden. V: The birth year period 1979–82. *Acta Paediatrica Scandinavica*, **78**, 283–290.
12. Pharoah, P.O.D., Cooke, T., Rosenbloom, L., Cooke, R.W.I. (1977) Trends in birth prevalence of cerebral palsy. *Archives of Disease in Childhood*, **62**, 379–384.
13. Stewart, A.L., Reynolds, E.O.R., Lipscomb, A.P. (1981) Outcome for infants of very low birth-weight: survey of the world literature. *Lancet*, **ii**, 1038–1040.
14. Haas, G., Buchwald-Saal, M., Leidig, E., Mentzel, H. (1986) Improved outcome in very low birth-weight infants from 1977 to 1983. *European Journal of Paediatrics*, **145**, 337–340.
15. Robertson, C.M.T., Etches, P.C. (1988) Decreased incidence of neurologic disability among neonates at high risk born between 1975–1984 in Alberta. *Canadian Medical Association Journal*, **139**, 225–229.
16. Hagberg, B., Hagberg, G., Zetterstrom, R. (1989) Decreasing perinatal mortality —increase in cerebral palsy morbidity? *Acta Paediatrica Scandinavica*, **78**, 664–670.
17. Riikonen, R., Raumavirta, S., Sinivuori, E., Seppala, T. (1989) Changing pattern of cerebral palsy in a south-west region of Finland. *Acta Paediatrica Scandinavica*, **78**, 981–987.
18. Dowding, V.M., Berry, C. (1988) Cerebral palsy: changing patterns of birth-weight and gestational age. *Irish Medical Journal*, **81**, 25–29.

19. Taudorf, K., Vorstrup, S. (1989) Cerebral blood-flow abnormalities in cerebral palsy children with a normal CT scan. *Neuropediatrics*, **20**, 33–40.
20. Thorp, P.S., Levin, S.D., Garnett, E.S. *et al.* (1988) Patterns of cerebral glucose metabolism using ^{18}FDG and positron tomography in the neurological investigation of the full-term newborn infant. *Neuro Paediatr*, **19**, 146–153.
21. Bundey, S., Griffiths, M. (1977) Recurrence risks in families of children with symmetrical spasticity. *Developmental Medicine and Child Neurology*, **19**, 179–191.
22. Gustavson, K.H., Hagberg, B., Sanner, G. (1969) Identical syndromes of cerebral palsy in the same family. *Acta Paediatrica Scandinavica*, **58**, 330–340.
23. Powell, T.G., Pharoah, P.O.D., Cooke, R.W.I., Rosenbloom, L. (1988) Cerebral palsy and low birth-weight infants—II. Spastic diplegia; associations with fetal immaturity. *Developmental Medicine and Child Neurology*, **30**, 19–25.
24. Powell, T.G., Pharoah, P.O.D., Cooke, R.W.I., Rosenbloom, L. (1988) Cerebral palsy and low birth-weight infants—I. Spastic hemiplegia: association with intrapartum stress. *Developmental Medicine and Child Neurology*, **30**, 11–18.
25. Edebol-Tysk, K., Hagberg, B., Hagberg, G. (1989) Epidemiology of spastic tetraplegic cerebral palsy in Sweden—II. Prevalence, birth data, and origin. *Neuropediatrics*, **20**, 46–52.
26. Papiernick, E., Bouyer, J., Dreyfus, J. *et al.* (1985) Prevention of preterm births; a perinatal study in Haguenan, France. *Paediatrics*, **76**, 154–158.
27. Pharoah, T.O.D., Cooke, T., Rosenbloom, L. (1989) Acquired cerebral palsy. *Archives of Disease in Childhood*, **64**, 103–106.
28. Speelman, J.D., Van Maren, J. (1989) Cerebral palsy and stereotactic neurosurgery: long-term results. *Journal of Neurology, Neurosurgery and Psychiatry*, **52**, 23–30.
29. Tardieu, C., Lepagot, A., Tabary, C., Bret, M.D. (1988) For how long must the soleus muscle be stretched each day to prevent contracture? *Developmental Medicine and Child Neurology*, **30**, 3–10.
30. Palmer, F.B., Shapiro, B.K., Wachtel, R.C. *et al.* (1988) The effects of physical therapy on cerebral palsy. A controlled trial in infants with spastic diplegia. *New England Journal of Medicine*, **318**, 803–808.
31. Watt, J., Sims, D., Harckham, F. *et al.* (1986) A prospective study of inhibitive casting as an adjunct to physiotherapy for cerebral-palsied children. *Developmental Medicine and Child Neurology*, **28**, 480–488.
32. Nwaobi, O.M. (1986) Effect of body orientation in space on tonic muscle activity of patients with cerebral palsy. *Developmental Medicine and Child Neurology*, **28**, 41–44.
33. Nwaobi, O.M. (1987) Seating orientation and upper extremity function in children with cerebral palsy. *Physical Therapy*, **67**, 1209–1212.
34. Green, E. (1990) Personal communication.
35. Scrutton, D. (1989) The early management of hips in cerebral palsy. *Developmental Medicine and Child Neurology*, **31**, 108–116.
36. Hoffer, M.M. (1986) Management of the hip in cerebral palsy. *Journal of Bone and Joint Surgery*, **68A**, 629–631.
37. Cooke, P.H., Cole, W.G., Carey, R.P.L. (1989) Dislocation of the hip in cerebral palsy. Natural History and Predictability. *Journal of Bone and Joint Surgery*, **71B**, 441–446.
38. Ferguson, R.L., Allen, B.L. (1988) Considerations in treatment of cerebral palsy patients with spinal deformities. *Orthopedic Clinics of North America*, **19**, 419–425.
39. Hoffer, M.M., Stein, G.A., Koffman, M., Prietto, N. (1985) Femoral varus derotation osteotomy in spastic cerebral palsy. *Journal of Bone and Joint Surgery*, **67A**, 1229–1235.
40. Winters, T.F., Gage, J.R., Hicks, R. (1987) Gait patterns in spastic hemiplegia in children and young adults. *Journal of Bone and Joint Surgery*, **69A**, 437–441.
41. Perry, J. (1987) Distal rectus femoris transfer. *Developmental Medicine and Child Neurology*, **29**, 153–158.
42. Peacock, W.J., Arens, L.J., Berman, B. (1987) Cerebral palsy spasticity. Selective posterior rhizotomy. *Pediatric Neuroscience*, **13**, 61–66.

43. Arens, L.J., Peacock, W.J., Peter, J. (1989) Selective posterior rhizotomy: A long-term follow-up study. *Child's Nervous System*, **5**, 148–152.
44. Kundi, M., Cahan, L., Starr, A. (1989) Somato-sensory evoked potentials in cerebral palsy after partial dorsal root rhizotomy. *Archives of Neurology*, **46**, 524–527.
45. O'Dwyer, T.P., Timon, C., Walsh, M.A. (1989) Surgical management of drooling in the neurologically damaged child. *Journal of Laryngology and Otology*, **103**, 750–752.
46. Koheil, R., Sochaniwskij, A.E., Bablick, K. *et al.* (1987) Biofeedback techniques and behavioural modification in the conservative remediation of drooling by children with cerebral palsy. *Developmental Medicine and Child Neurology*, **29**, 19–26.
47. Camp-Bruno, J.A., Winsberg, B.J., Green-Parsons, A.R., Abrams, J.P. (1989) Efficacy of benztropine therapy for drooling. *Developmental Medicine and Child Neurology*, **31**, 309–319.
48. Harris, S.R., Purdy, A.H. (1987) Drooling and its management in cerebral palsy. *Developmental Medicine and Child Neurology*, **29**, 807–811.
49. Helfrich-Miller, K.R., Rector, K.L., Straka, J.A. (1986) Dysphagia: its treatment in the profoundly retarded patient with cerebral palsy. *Archives of Physical Medicine and Rehabilitation*, **67**, 520–525.
50. Dector, R.M., Bauer, S.B., Khoshbin, S. *et al.* (1987) Urodynamic assessment of children with cerebral palsy. *Journal of Urology*, **138**, 110–112.
51. O'Grady, R.S., Nishimura, D.M., Kohn, J.G., Bruweld, W.A. (1985) Vocational predictions compared with present vocational status of 60 young adults with cerebral palsy. *Developmental Medicine and Child Neurology*, **27**, 775–778.

6 | Genetics

Dian Donnai
Department of Clinical Genetics, St Mary's Hospital, Manchester

The core activity of clinical genetics is genetic counselling; this aims to establish a genetic diagnosis and to assess risks for family members. The process of genetic counselling involves a team which offers information about the condition and the risks and about available options, and helps families adjust to their genetic situation. The specialty of clinical genetics is concerned with individuals of all ages with disorders of all body systems, and there needs to be collaboration with many different medical disciplines.

Clinical genetic practice has been revolutionised in the past 10 years by our ability to manipulate deoxyribonucleic acid (DNA); this has allowed more precise genetic counselling and increased the range of options for families with single gene disorders. Improved cytogenetic techniques coupled with molecular studies have led to the recognition of many microdeletion syndromes, and counselling in families, for example, with fragile-X mental retardation is dependent on a combination of cytogenetic and molecular techniques.

The interface between clinical genetic and paediatric practice involves families with single gene disorders, but it also involves the investigation and care of children with birth defects and malformation syndromes where the aetiology of the problem is not clear, and counselling cannot be so precise. This paper will discuss areas of genetic practice which have significantly changed due to the introduction of DNA technology; it will also discuss newly recognised mechanisms which may explain many malformations and syndromes and improve genetic counselling for families of children with birth defects.

The application of DNA technology to clinical practice

DNA can be extracted from nucleated cells, most commonly white blood cells, but any tissue can be used. The extracted DNA is treated with restriction enzymes derived from bacteria, which cut double-stranded DNA only at certain specific sequences (restriction sites). The DNA is denatured to the single-stranded state and the pieces separated by gel electrophoresis. There are inherited differences between the DNA of normal healthy people in their restriction sites, giving rise to restriction fragment length polymorphisms (RFLPs). If the DNA pieces in the gel are transferred to a filter which binds them (Southern blot) the RFLPs can be revealed by radio-active probes, often cloned fragments of natural DNA, which recognise and hybridise to their complementary DNA sequence on the filter.[1]

Gene tracking

Gene tracking involves the use of a gene probe which identifies an RFLP from an area of the chromosome very near to the gene being studied—a linked marker—in order to follow the transmission of a disease gene in a family. Depending on the inheritance pattern of the condition, this allows for carrier detection, pre-symptomatic diagnosis, or prenatal diagnosis. Several markers are needed, so that if one marker is uninformative (ie does not clearly distinguish one of a pair of chromosomes from the other at the specific area of interest) another can be used. Gene tracking can only be done in families with a suitable pedigree structure and with DNA samples from key individuals. During meiosis exchange of DNA occurs between a chromosome pair and the risk of recombination between an RFLP and the disease gene increases the further they are apart. This limits the accuracy of gene tracking and for this reason, to limit errors, markers on either side of the disease gene location are used.

Intragenic probes

For some genes, intragenic RFLPs have been recognised and therefore recombination errors in risk prediction are negligible. Similarly, if the specific mutation within the gene is a deletion of a DNA sequence, for some conditions probes can recognise the presence or absence of the sequence allowing precise prenatal diagnosis or carrier prediction.

Reverse genetics

When a gene is cloned and its DNA code sequenced, by what is now called reverse genetics, it is possible to work out what the gene does, and hence determine the underlying cause of a particular disease. Analysis of the protein product of the gene which is faulty in Duchenne dystrophy has already been helpful in diagnosis, and in the future it may be possible to design more rational treatments using this knowledge, or even to consider gene therapy.

Prenatal diagnosis

Couples at high genetic risk may request prenatal diagnosis, and if the fetus is shown to be affected, elect to have termination of the pregnancy. DNA can be extracted from a chorionic villus biopsy performed nine weeks after the last menstrual period. If the preliminary laboratory work has been done prior to pregnancy on key family members, it is possible to have a result in a few days. New techniques, such as polymerase chain reaction (PCR),[2] mean that for some conditions results are available within 24 hours. The scope of prenatal diagnosis for genetic disorders formed part of the report of a recent working party on prenatal diagnosis and genetic screening.[3]

DNA analysis in specific genetic disorders

(a) Duchenne muscular dystrophy (DMD)

DMD is a serious muscle disorder resulting in death of affected individuals in the second or third decade. The X-linked pattern of inheritance has been recognised for years, but many boys are the only affected individual in their families, suggesting a high mutation rate. Ten years ago all that could be offered to female relatives who wished to know their carrier status was creatinine kinase measurement, pedigree analysis, and calculation of a risk using Bayesian analysis. For some women the risk obtained was very high, indicating they were likely to be carriers. For those with intermediate or low-risk figures, however, their status was less certain, and many such women still elected to have pre-natal diagnosis of fetal sex by amniocentesis, and to abort all males.

The first clue to the specific location on the X chromosome of the DMD gene came from study of the few girls with the disease who had one X chromosome disrupted by a translocation between it and an autosome. The normal X would be preferentially inactivated. The break point in all the girls on the X chromosome was in the band Xp21 and DNA probes from this region were shown to be linked to DMD in family studies.[4] The gene for the milder Becker type of muscular dystrophy, previously thought to be a separate entity, was also proved to be at the same site.[5]

Soon probes detecting RFLPs within the large dystrophin gene were developed, giving greater accuracy in carrier prediction and prenatal diagnosis, and using complementary DNA probes about 60–70% of males were shown to have deletions in coding sequences.

Now many Regional Genetic Services have genetic registers,[6] so that families can be fully investigated and counselled. The register staff ensure that long-term contact is maintained with the family, that young women at risk of being carriers can be offered tests at the appropriate time, and that new technologies are applied as soon as they become available. Further possibilities for diagnosis, and perhaps eventually treatment, have resulted from the characterisation of the large protein, dystrophin, which is coded for by the gene disrupted in DMD.[7]

(b) Cystic fibrosis (CF)

The mode of inheritance has been known for CF for some time, but unlike DMD the chromosomal location was not known. Until 1985 all that the genetic services could offer to families who had an affected child was to inform them of the one-in-four risk of a further affected child, and the possibility of a late prenatal test which had significant false negative and false positive rates.[8] The discovery of RFLPs linked to the CF locus on chromosome 7[9,10,11] allowed prenatal diagnosis to be performed earlier in pregnancy using chorionic villus biopsy with a low error rate. The new tests also allowed carrier testing within a family, providing the markers were informative.

It also became possible to extract tiny DNA samples from stored Guthrie blood spot cards, or histological specimens of CF children who had died, and amplify the DNA using the polymerase chain reaction (PCR).[2]

The gene in which a mutation can lead to CF has recently been identified[12] and it codes for a protein which has been called the cystic fibrosis transmembrane conductance regulator (CFTR). Of CF mutations in the UK population, 70–80% are accounted for by a deletion of 3 DNA base pairs, in position 508 of the protein, now termed the 'delta F508 mutation'. This can be detected with relatively simple DNA analysis and allows screening of the unrelated spouses of individuals known to be carriers. It also opens up the possibility of population carrier screening for CF, the commonest serious recessively inherited disorder of Caucasians.[13]

DNA technology is applicable to many other genetic disorders where the gene location is known and probes available. These include Huntington's chorea, adult polycystic kidney disease, haemophilia, haemoglobinopathies, fragile X, spinal muscular atrophies, neurofibromatosis, and many more. The paediatrician can ensure that families receive the most up-to-date genetic services by referring early for genetic investigation and counselling, that is before a further pregnancy occurs. It is important that samples from individuals with single-gene disorders are collected for DNA analysis or storage, even from those with disorders not yet mapped to a chromosome location. It is likely that before long all of the human genome will have been sequenced.[14]

Mechanisms in dysmorphology

Dysmorphology is the clinical activity concerned with the diagnosis and study of congenital anomalies. At one time this was largely concerned with description and recognition of syndromes, but the speciality has now moved into an era where the molecular, cytogenetic, biochemical, and embryological mechanisms involved in the causation of birth defects can be explored and elucidated. Three approaches recently employed in dysmorphology research will be further discussed.

Mouse–human homology

One successful strategy has been to study possible homologies between mouse and human congenital anomaly syndromes.[15] Comparative gene mapping can be carried out allowing more detailed investigation at the molecular level. This approach has been successful in mapping the gene location of Greig's syndrome,[16] X-linked vitamin D resistant rickets,[17] Waardenberg's syndrome,[18] and several more. Once the gene location is known it should be possible to work out the exact sequence of the gene itself and by recognition of the protein product maybe find the mechanisms behind the abnormal morphology.

Mosaicism

It is generally assumed that all cells in the body have an identical genetic constitution, but with wider investigations using cytogenetic and molecular techniques it is becoming apparent that mosaicism at a chromosomal or single-gene level is more common than previously thought, and may account for examples of anomalous inheritance patterns and for certain patterns of birth defects.

Chromosomal mosaicism may be fairly common in placental tissue, while the fetus has a normal karyotype. The ACC collaborative study of chorionic villus biopsy[19] indicates that there is an aneuploid cell line in the tiny sample taken in 1% of pregnancies. It would be reasonable to speculate that if more areas of the placenta were analysed, mosaicism would be detected even more frequently. In the majority of cases, the resulting baby was cytogenetically normal with no clinical abnormalities and no evidence on cord blood analysis of the mosaicism. There are anecdotal reports of infants with intra-uterine growth retardation who were cytogenetically normal but where the placentae had a large proportion of trisomic cells.[20]

A converse situation may also apply, and a recent publication[21] reported cytogenetic analysis of blood and placentae from liveborn infants or from terminated fetuses with trisomy 13 and 18, and revealed that all were mosaic, the mosaicism consisting of trisomic and normal cells confined to the cytotrophoblast. The percentage of cells with normal karyotype in each placenta varied from 12% to 100%, the average being 70%. The authors interpreted these findings as suggesting that a post-zygotic loss of a trisomic chromosome in a progenitor cell of tropho-ectoderm facilitated the intra-uterine survival of trisomy 13 and 18 conceptuses. It also suggests that there may be a mechanism for 'self-correction' of trisomies, which will be discussed further in the section on uniparental disomy.

The main clinical syndromes reported in the past as being associated with mosaicism have been trisomy 21 mosaicism, where the phenotype on the whole is milder than full Down's syndrome, and trisomy 8 mosaicism where the child characteristically has unusual creases on the palms and soles, a congenital heart defect, and joint contractures worsening with increasing age. A syndrome described by Pallister and Killian[22] with a characteristic facial appearance, extra nipples, short fingers, and joint contractures has more recently been shown to be due to mosaicism, the abnormal cell line having an extra chromosome consisting of two short arms of 12, so-called '12p tetrasomy'. In most cases the lymphocyte chromosome analysis was absolutely normal and the abnormal cell line only detected on cultured skin fibroblasts.

As skin biopsy has been increasingly employed more and more children with puzzling constellations of anomalies have been shown to be chromosomal mosaics. Features common to many such children are mental retardation, joint contractures, asymmetry, and skin pigmentary abnormalities.

We studied a number of patients with the cutaneous manifestations of hypomelanosis of Ito. Previously the cause of the disorder was not known, and 74% of reported patients had one or more abnormalities of the central nervous system, eyes, hair, teeth, or musculo-skeletal system, in addition to the depigmented markings which followed Blaschko's lines. Because our patients, in addition to the skin pigmentary anomalies, had asymmetry and joint contractures, we felt chromosomal or single-gene mosaicism was a distinct possibility. Skin biopsy with chromosome analysis of cultured fibroblasts revealed that two out of three of our patients had a mixture of diploid and triploid cells in their skin.[23] Many reports of chromosomal mosaicism in hypomelanosis of Ito have subsequently been reported and we concluded that the skin anomalies are nonspecific manifestations of mosaicism. The distribution of the skin markings may well indicate that the mosaicism arose before neural crest cell migration.

Recent publications[24,25] have discussed the likelihood that many cases of apparent genetic heterogeneity or anomalous inheritance could be due to mosaicism involving single-gene mutations. Indeed, there are a number of reports in the literature now of a parent having several children affected with a gene mutation detectable with DNA probes, where they themselves do not apparently carry the mutation in their somatic tissue. This indicates that germline mosaicism is likely. A person may also have an apparently 'mild' manifestation of a disorder because the mutation is present in only a proportion of cells, whereas if their offspring inherits the mutation, it will be present in each cell and the child will be severely affected.

It is possible that mosaicism could account for other sporadic conditions such as Sturge-Weber syndrome, neurocutaneous melanosis, Proteus syndrome, Klippel-Trenauny-Weber syndrome, and McCune-Albright syndrome, and it has been suggested[26] that in this type of disorder, fetal survival is only possible when the mutation is present in mosaic state and has therefore arisen during development. If the mutation is lethal in the non-mosaic state, then of course 'fully affected' individuals would not be seen, since they would be likely to miscarry.

Differential imprinting and uniparental disomy

During the formation of sperm or eggs, chromosomes are somehow labelled (imprinted) with their parental origin, and for some chromosomal regions correct function requires the presence of both a paternally and maternally imprinted genome. Evidence that there are functional differences between the maternal and paternal genome is provided by hydatidiform moles and triploid conceptuses. A conceptus with a 46,XX karyotype entirely of paternal origin develops as a hydatidiform mole, instead of a normal female. Triploid conceptuses with two paternal chromosome sets have a molar placenta, whereas those with two maternal genomes have a more normal placenta. At the single chromosome level it has been demonstrated in mice that the paternally derived X chromosome is preferentially inactivated in placental tissue, indicating that there is some imprint which confers functional difference.

Differential imprinting may explain the different expression of the same mutation within a family depending on the sex of the transmitting parent. In families with myotonic dystrophy the severe congenital form of the disease only occurs in babies who inherit the abnormal gene from their mothers; within the same family, the affected offspring of a male transmitting the mutation may not develop signs or symptoms until the third or fourth decade. In the rare cases of juvenile onset of Huntington's disease, the transmitting parent is usually the father.[27]

Further evidence of imprinting in humans comes from studies of Prader-Willi and Angelman's syndromes. Both syndromes are associated with mental retardation, but with physical phenotypes which in some respects are very different and in some complementary. Individuals with Prader-Willi syndrome are hypotonic and develop severe obesity due to insatiable appetite. They have small hands and feet, small genitalia, and a characteristic face. Patients with Angelman's syndrome have seizures, ataxic movements, sudden outbursts of inappropriate laughter, microcephaly, and rather large jaws. Some, but not all, patients with both syndromes have a deletion of the chromosomal region 15q11–13. When there is a deletion, it affects the paternally derived chromosome 15 in Prader-Willi syndrome but the maternally derived chromosome 15 in Angelman's syndrome.[28]

Differential imprinting may still be responsible for an abnormal phenotype, even if there is no single-gene mutation (such as in myotonic dystrophy) or chromosome deletions (such as the cytogenetically abnormal Prader-Willi and Angelman syndrome children). This is through the mechanism of uniparental disomy (UPD). UPD describes the situation where an individual has the correct number of chromosomes, but both chromosomes of one particular pair are derived from one parent and none from the other. Although the chromosome number is correct, in some cases UPD is associated with pathological effects. Experimental manipulations have been used to produce mice with UPD for various chromosomal regions.[29] For some regions there are no ill effects, while for others there are pathological consequences, usually including severe general growth retardation or excess.

In 1988 Spence *et al.*[30] showed that a girl with cystic fibrosis and severe growth retardation had inherited two copies of the same chromosome 7 from her mother and none from her father. Subsequently, two other similar cases have been described, and in fact uniparental disomy may not be so excessively rare in man. Monosomy and trisomy are very common in early embryos, but are usually incompatible with continued development. Thus monosomic or trisomic conceptuses are under strong selection to duplicate or lose one chromosome. Perhaps Spence's patient had trisomy 7 at conception due to non-disjunction in maternal meiosis II. The trisomy might then have 'self-corrected' to disomy by eliminating the paternal homologue. Had the maternal 7 not carried the CF mutation, the situation would have remained undetected, since karyotypic investigation of her short stature would have been 'normal'. It is interesting that human chromosome 7 is homologous to mouse chromosome 11; Cattanach and Kirk[29] have shown that mice are growth retarded when both homologues of chromosome 11 are derived from the mother.

Further support that uniparental disomy is associated with recognisable human phenotypes has been shown by recent reports of patients with Prader-Willi syndrome and Angelman syndrome who have no visible chromosome deletion. These patients with Prader-Willi syndrome have been demonstrated to lack a paternal chromosome 15, and they have either both maternal homologues (maternal heterodisomy) or two copies of one of the mother's chromosome 15 (maternal isodisomy)[31]. The fact that heterodisomy is seen argues against the phenotype being due to the homozygous expression of recessive genes. The unifying conclusion from the deletion and uniparental disomy evidence is that Prader-Willi syndrome is due to the lack of a paternal imprint in the chromosomal region 15q11–13. Recent work with Angelman's syndrome has revealed paternal disomy in some non-deletion cases.[32]

Uniparental disomy for other chromosomal regions is very probably associated with recognisable clinical phenotypes. Extrapolating from the work with mice, suitable candidate disorders would be recurrent pattern syndromes, which are usually sporadic, and are associated with under- or overgrowth. These include Russell-Silver, Rubinstein Taybi, Sotos and Williams syndromes. For most of these disorders, there are few, if any, reports in siblings or parents, but there are well documented cases in identical twins. Thus the cause is almost certainly genetic, but argues against a simple genetic mechanism.

If the cause of these recurrent pattern syndromes could be shown to be uniparental disomy, this would aid genetic counselling and allow low recurrence risk to be confidently given. The study of abnormal mechanisms of development may paradoxically also lead to progress in the study of normal mechanisms of morphogenesis.

References

1. Weatherall, D.J. (1985) *The new genetics and clinical practice* (2nd edn) Oxford: Oxford University Press.
2. Lynch, J.R., Brown, J.M. (1990) The polymerase chain reaction: current and future clinical applications. *Journal of Medical Genetics*, **27**, 2–7.
3. Report of the Royal College of Physicians (1989) *Prenatal diagnosis and genetic screening: community and service implications*. Royal College of Physicians of London.
4. Davies, K.E., Pearson, P.L., Harper, P.S. (1983) Linkage analysis of two cloned DNA sequences flanking the Duchenne muscular dystrophy locus on the short arm of human X chromosomes. *Nucleic Acids Research*, **11**, 2302–2312.
5. Kingston, H.M., Safarazi, M., Thomas, N.S.T., Harper, P.S. (1984) Localisation of the Becker muscular dystrophy gene on the short arm of the X-chromosome by linkage to cloned DNA sequences. *Human Genetics*, **67**, 6–17.
6. Read, A.P., Kerzin-Storrar, L., Mountford, R.C. *et al.* (1986) A register-based system for gene tracking in Duchenne muscular dystrophy. *Journal of Medical Genetics*, **23**, 581–586.
7. Monaco, A.P., Kunkel, L.M. (1988) Cloning of the Duchenne/Becker muscular dystrophy locus. In *Advances in human genetics*, Harris, H., Hirschhorn, K. (eds) Plenum, New York, vol. 17, pp 61–98.

8. Brock, D.J.H., Bedgood, D., Barron, L., Hayward, C. (1985) Prospective prenatal diagnosis of cystic fibrosis. *Lancet*, **i**, 1175–1178.
9. Knowlton, R.G., Cohen-Hagenaver, O., Cong, N.V. *et al.* (1985) A polymorphic DNA marker linked to cystic fibrosis is located on chromosome 7. *Nature*, **318**, 380–382.
10. White, R., Woodward, S., Leppert, M. *et al.* (1985) A closely linked genetic marker for cystic fibrosis. *Nature*, **318**, 382–384.
11. Wainwright, B.J., Scambler, P.J., Schmidtke, J. *et al.* Localisation of cystic fibrosis locus to human chromosome 7cen-7q22. *Nature*, **318**, 384–385.
12. Riordan, J.R., Rommens, J.M., Kerem, B.S. *et al.* (1989) Identification of the cystic fibrosis gene: cloning and characterisation of complementary DNA. *Science*, **245**, 1066–1073.
13. Modell, B. (1990) Cystic fibrosis screening and community genetics. *Journal of Medical Genetics*, **27**, 475–479.
14. Stephens, J.C., Cavanaugh, M.L., Gradie, M.I. *et al.* (1990) Mapping the human genome: current status. *Science*, **250**, 237–244.
15. Winter, R.M. (1988) Malformation syndromes: a review of mouse/human homology. *Journal of Medical Genetics*, **25**, 480–487.
16. Huson, S.M., Brueton, L., Williamson, R., Winter, R.M. (1988) Greig cephalopolysyndactyly: a clinical survey, identification of a mouse model, and molecular genetic studies. *Journal of Medical Genetics*, **25**, 638A.
17. Read, A.P., Thakker, R.V., Davies, K.E. *et al.* (1986) Mapping of human X-linked hypophosphataemic rickets by multilocus linkage analysis. *Human Genetics*, **73**, 267–270.
18. Foy, C., Newton, V., Wellesley, D. *et al.* (1990) Assignment of the locus for Waardenburg Syndrome Type I to human chromosome 2q37 and possible homology to the Splotch mouse. *American Journal of Medical Genetics*, **46**, 1017–1023.
19. ACC Collaborative Study (1989) *Chorionic Villi 1987 and 1988.* Chorionic Villi Working Party, Association of Clinical Cytogeneticists.
20. Stioui, S., De Silvestris, M., Molinari, A. *et al.* (1989) Trisomic 22 placenta in a case of severe intra-uterine growth retardation. *Prenatal Diagnosis*, **9**, 673–670.
21. Kalousek, D.K., Barrett, I.J., McGillivray, B.C. (1989) Placental mosaicism and intra-uterine survival of trisomies 13 and 18. *American Journal of Human Genetics*, **44**, 338–343.
22. Hunter, A.G.W., Clifford, B., Cox, D.M. (1985) The characteristic physiognomy and tissue specific karyotype distribution in the Pallister-Killian syndrome. *Clinical Genetics*, **28**, 47–53.
23. Donnai, D., Read, A.P., McKeown, C., Andrews, T. (1988) Hypomelanosis of Ito: a manifestation of mosaicism or chimerism. *Journal of Medical Genetics*, **25**, 809–818.
24. Edwards, J.H. (1989) Familiarity, recessivity and germline mosaicism. *Annals of Human Genetics*, **53**, 33–47.
25. Hall, J.G. (1988) Review and hypotheses: somatic mosaicism: observations related to clinical genetics. *American Journal of Medical Genetics*, **43**, 355–363.
26. Happle, R. (1986) The McCune-Albright syndrome: a lethal gene surviving by mosaicism. *Clinical Genetics*, **29**, 321–324.
27. Reik, W. (1988) Genomic imprinting: a possible mechanism for the parental origin effect in Huntington's chorea. *Journal of Medical Genetics*, **25**, 805–808.
28. Knoll, J.H.M., Nicholls, R.D., Magenis, R.E. *et al.* (1989) Angelman and Prader-Willi syndromes share a common chromosome 15 deletion but differ in parental origin of the deletion. *American Journal of Medical Genetics*, **32**, 285–290.
29. Cattanach, B.M., Kirk, M. (1985) Differential activity of maternally and paternally derived chromosome regions in mice. *Nature*, **315**, 496–498.
30. Spence, J.E., Perciaccante, R.G., Greig, G.M. *et al.* (1988) Uniparental disomy as a mechanism for human genetic disease. *American Journal of Human Genetics*, **42**, 217–226.

31. Nicholls, R.D., Knoll, J.H.M., Butler, M.G. *et al.* (1989) Genetic imprinting suggested by maternal heterodisomy in non-deletion Prader Willi syndrome. *Nature*, **342**, 281–285.
32. Malcolm, S., Nichols, M., Clayton-Smith, J. *et al.* (1990) Angelman syndrome can result from uniparental disomy. *American Journal of Human Genetics*; **47**, 227A.

7 | Paediatric rheumatology

Barbara M. Ansell
Northwick Park Hospital, London

Rheumatic diseases of childhood

There are still no clues as to the initiating stimulus or stimuli in the majority of disorders coming under the umbrella term of rheumatic diseases of childhood. It is, however, important to recognise what pattern of illness is present so as to be alert for possible complications and to institute appropriate management.

It is pertinent to start with *Lyme disease*, named after the small town of Lyme in Connecticut, where it was first recognised. This develops after a bite by a tick, the *Ixodes damminus* or *ricinus*, which implants the *Spirochaete burgdoferi*. It is usually a mono- or pauci-articular arthritis, which may have been preceded by a general illness with fever for a few days, and approximately half the children afflicted will have, or have had, the characteristic skin lesion of erythema migrans chronicum; these symptoms may have occurred up to several months before those affecting the joints. Other features include neurological abnormalities and carditis. Although recognised as a worldwide problem, in Europe more emphasis has been placed on the neurological aspects of the disease than on the arthritis.[1] However, Lyme arthritis can occur in Britain, and in patients who travel to countries where it is more common. Early recognition is important so that early treatment with antibiotics can be initiated, the patient then being more likely to recover completely.

Erythema infectiosum, first described in 1889, was shown in the 1980s to be due to infection with parvovirus B19. In 1985 cases of acute arthritis in children and adults were described associated with serological evidence of recent B19 infections, even in the absence of typical rash. A school outbreak of erythema infectiosum affected more than half the children; some 5% complained of joint pain, but less than half had noticeable swelling.[2] In general, joint symptoms in children are mild, but occasionally a marked arthropathy or even an appearance suggesting systemic juvenile arthritis can develop. The rash is classically a 'slapped cheek erythema' which affects the face but can appear on the limbs. It may disappear and reappear over several months, sometimes lasting only a few hours. The arthritis has an excellent prognosis even in those few cases in which it is prolonged for some months, and only requires supportive measures.

While *rheumatic fever* has continued to be a major problem in developing countries, there has been a resurgence in the United States involving not only Hispanics, Puerto Ricans, Polynesians, and American Indians, who tend to have more frequent and severe disease, but also Caucasians.[3] To a lesser extent this has also happened in Europe. The age of incidence has increased so that the first attack can occur in the teens. The most common manifestations are an acute migratory polyarthritis and carditis. Erythema marginatum, which used to be considered the characteristic rash, as well as nodules and chorea, appears to be rare. The cause of this is not certain: it could be that the streptococcus itself has changed. The importance of effective prophylaxis, either by monthly injections of penicillin or by daily oral administration of penicillin or a similar antibiotic, in preventing recurrences cannot be overstated; it is probably wise to continue it indefinitely if there has been any carditis.

Reactive arthritis can follow dysenteric infections, the most common organisms being salmonella, shigella, or yersinia. While occasionally a typical Reiter's syndrome occurs some two or three weeks after the bowel infection, more commonly the syndrome is incomplete, and frequently the symptoms of transient red eye or dysuria are not considered by parents important enough to report when bringing the child up with an acute arthritis; the majority of such children will carry HLA B27. The arthritis is self-limiting, but if it persists the early use of sulphasalazine may be helpful.

Juvenile chronic arthritis

It is generally agreed that chronic arthritis of childhood comprises a heterogeneous group of conditions of unknown aetiology, although immunoregulatory imbalances are thought to be involved in pathogenesis. The majority are different from adult seropositive rheumatoid arthritis, but nomenclature and classification criteria are far from satisfactory.[4] In the USA Cassidy *et al.*[5] suggested the term 'juvenile arthritis' should cover all disorders which have a peripheral or axial arthritis, reserving the term 'juvenile rheumatoid arthritis' for idiopathic peripheral arthritis, with seronegative spondyloarthropathy and reactive arthritis separated out.

Whatever overall name is adopted, there is agreement that chronic childhood arthritis usually starts in one of three ways: with systemic illness; as a polyarthritis which is further divided by the presence or absence of IgM rheumatoid factor; or in pauci-articular form in which four or fewer joints are involved in the first three to six months. This last group is subdivided by age of onset, without precise definition as to what the ages should be, young children aged six years and under who carry antinuclear antibodies and are at risk for iridocyclitis forming one group, and older children, particularly boys aged nine and over, who frequently carry HLA B27, forming another. These subgroupings are supported by tissue-typing studies, as young-onset pauci-articular disease is associated with HLA A2 DR5 and DRw8, while the older onset is characterised by the presence of HLA B27. Young-onset polyarthritis is associated with DRw8, while IgM rheumatoid factor polyarthritic onset is associated with DR4 (see Table 1).[6] Polyarthritis remains a heterogeneous group and within the pauci-articular onset group there are probably further subgroups; these include older girls aged seven, eight, or nine, whose disease is confined to a single joint and who have no rise in ESR or positive serology, as well as those with several joints affected who ultimately develop psoriatic arthritis. As yet, diagnostic criteria for juvenile psoriatic arthritis have not been validated.[7]

Management begins with the recognition of which pattern of illness is present. The importance of maintaining the position and function of joints from the moment they become involved cannot be overstated. This requires the use of rest splints, particularly for the hands and wrists, knees, ankles, and feet, which will have to be made for each child. Appropriate physiotherapy will also be necessary to keep the joints mobile and prevent muscle wasting and joint deformity. The worry about Reye's syndrome being associated with aspirin has led to an increased use of other non-steroidal anti-inflammatory drugs, and a number are now available for children aged five years and over (see Table 2). However, diclofenac sodium (Voltarol) and, particularly, ibuprofen are the only ones that are generally accepted for the young child. The ibuprofen suspension allows easy administration, but it should be given in four divided doses. In the older schoolchild, the twice-daily administration of naproxen suspension is particularly appreciated by parents. All these drugs are potent, with no particular one being more effective than another, but there is individual preference.[8] Such drugs will be required until the joint inflammation settles. In our original naproxen tolerance study, 10 of 30 patients had stopped within two years because the disease had gone into remission.

The indications for corticosteroid therapy include serious systemic disease, failure to maintain position and function in joints in disease with polyarthritic onset, particularly in the young, or serious polyarthritis after a pauci-articular onset; very occasionally it may be required for severe uveitis. Every attempt should be made to use an alternate day

Table 1. Onset patterns of juvenile chronic arthritis

Systemic	Polyarthritic		Pauci-articular		
Boys = girls	IgM rheumatoid factor negative	IgM rheumatoid factor positive	Early (under 6)	Late (6 years +)	Others including
Young	Girls > boys often young	Girls > boys late childhood	Girls > boys	Boys > girls	Juvenile psoriatic arthritis
Majority develop polyarthritis	Symmetrical	Symmetrical, particularly hands, feet, knees	Lower limb joints particularly		Arthritis and inflammatory bowel disease
	Large joints initially		Chronic uveitis Acute iritis	Enthesopathy	
Tendency to relapsing course		Nodules Latex RAHA+	ANA frequently present		
	Under 6 carry HLA DRw8	HLA DR4 often present	HLA A2 DR5 DRw8	HLA B27 often present	

Table 2. Non-steroidal anti-inflammatory drugs for juvenile chronic arthritis

		mg/kg/d
Propionic acid derivatives:	Ibuprofen	20–40
	Naproxen	10–15
Indoles	Tolmetin	15–30
	Indomethacin	2–5
Phenyl alkanoic acid derivative	Voltarol	3
Piroxicam	Feldene	0.5

régime except in systemic onset disease, when it is difficult to do so. It is then usual to suggest 1mg/kg/day given as a single daily dose, but at times this will have to be divided to achieve adequate control. The possible use of pulses of intravenous methylprednisone at approximately five-day intervals has also been considered in systemic disease, as it will maintain hypothalamic pituitary adrenal function. However, it is not a satisfactory régime for young children. The effect of intravenous methylprednisone in the young child with systemic disease appears to last only about 48 hours, after which severe illness recurs. Thus the infusions either have to be increased in frequency, rendering the child cushingoid and therefore obviating the rationale behind this treatment, or there are wide swings in disease activity. A combination of non-steroidals and corticosteroids is safe and helpful in allowing a minimum dose of corticosteroids to be used. The possible use of deflazacort (an oxazolone derivative of prednisone), when it becomes available, will need consideration as there is little doubt that this produces less cushingoid appearance and maintains bone density better than ordinary prednisone.[9,10]

Failure of growth in height occurs both in serious illness and as a result of daily corticosteroid therapy. This can be improved by human growth hormone. In our study it was found that improvement occurred on both 12 and 24 units per week given on six out of seven days over a one-year period. Normal growth was not resumed and when the growth hormone was stopped the height velocity fell again.[11] The role of human growth hormone in improving ultimate height still needs further investigation and, by the very nature of this relatively rare disorder, a multicentre study will be required.

Intravenous gammaglobulin has been suggested as valuable in the management of systemic juvenile rheumatoid arthritis.[12] In our hands it was ineffective in those children with a low IgG at outset of therapy, but in those with a high IgG it was of some help in controlling the systemic features.

The use of long-acting local corticosteroid injections, particularly in the management of pauci-articular disease, is proving to be beneficial, with the knee the most studied joint.[13] It is also valuable in the wrist, foot, and elbow. However, injection of local steroid into a child's joint is not always easy, and should not be performed as a one-off procedure, particularly in an adult clinic, as there are complications which include subcutaneous tissue atrophy (recorded in as many as 8.3% of patients),[14] and intra-articular calcification, to say nothing of the fear caused to the child who has been subjected to this procedure under local anaesthetic while being held down.

Slow-acting anti-rheumatic drugs have relatively little place in the management of childhood arthritis. Indeed, in systemic onset disease gold, penicillamine, and sulphasalazine have all been shown to have a high incidence of serious side effects, including a modified disseminated intravascular coagulation syndrome after the second injection of gold, thrombocytopenia of severe degree with pencillamine, and leucopenia with high fever on day nine with sulphasalazine; none of these should be used in the presence of systemic features. The US/USSR co-operative study of hydroxychloroquine and penicillamine against placebo in seronegative polyarthritis showed no significant increased improvement in children on either hydroxychloroquine or penicillamine compared with placebo.[15] A study on auranofin (an oral gold preparation) gave similar results.[16] Intramuscular gold has never actually been put to the test, although we did a small study comparing placebo with auranofin with intramuscular gold. The only four children who improved markedly were two on auranofin and two on myocrisin (intramuscular gold) who had had an onset of seronegative polyarthritis around the age of eight or nine. My own feeling is that myocrisin may have a place in such patients, but this needs to be substantiated. This would suggest that we have to look more critically at the type of patient included in such studies. There is certainly need for further work on seronegative polyarticular onset at the age of eight and upwards. The only other long-acting drug which has been shown to cause significant improvement in polyarthritis is methotrexate.[17] However, not every child with polyarthritis warrants treatment with methotrexate. We have had a relatively limited success with this drug in systemic onset disease, but there have been no serious side-effects.[18] Multicentre studies will be required to establish the place of methotrexate in systemic-onset disease, and also to look at its role in the management of pauci-articular disease extending to polyarthritis.

Amyloidosis, which is the one potentially fatal complication of juvenile arthritis and occurs particularly in those children with a systemic onset of disease, but also in other groups with persistently high C-reactive protein concentrations (CRPs), can now be recognised early and monitored by a new imaging technique.[19] This consists of labelling serum amyloid P with iodine^{123} which, when injected into patients with amyloidosis, rapidly leaves the circulation and localises in the amyloid, in contrast to normal subjects in whom it remains in circulation. Its distribution can be imaged by scintigraphy, usually performed after 24 hours.

In a recent review,[20] the risk of amyloidosis appeared to be approximately 7% at the 15-year follow-up; if disease activity can be controlled by chlorambucil, mortality is greatly reduced. Hawkins's technique[19] will allow better monitoring of the progress of amyloidosis during cytotoxic therapy.

In the juvenile spondylo-arthropathies it is important to try and get better criteria,[21] as sacro-iliitis is not usually present early in the course of the disease, and presently one relies on the age of onset, presence of enthesopathy, a lower-limb arthropathy, affecting particularly boys, as well as acute iridocyclitis and a history of bowel inflammation. That differences in management may be required is suggested by the fact that flurbiprofen proved to be the most effective of the non-steroidal anti-inflammatory drugs.[22] Sulphasalazine also appears to be particularly effective in controlling the peripheral arthritis in this group.[23]

Rarer connective tissue disorders

Systemic lupus erythematosus

The incidence of systemic lupus erythematosus (SLE) in children is low. Thus in southern Sweden it has been estimated as 0.4 per 100,000 compared with 1.2 per 100,000 in the 15-to-24 decade,[24] but it remains a serious multisystem disease. There is still no agreement as to the best management of serious renal involvement, but reliance on corticosteroids alone is no longer justified. In the USA pulses of cyclophosphamide are favoured, while in the UK a régime similar to that for nephrotic syndrome—ie induction with cyclophosphamide followed by azathioprine—may well prove to be as effective and less toxic to the gonads. Central nervous system (CNS) involvement is causing an increased morbidity in paediatric SLE with neuropsychiatric manifestations occurring in 15–45% of patients.[25] Psychological testing has shown that some 35% of children may have impairment of function, in addition to overt problems such as a stroke or chorea. As in adults, anti-cardiolipin antibodies are frequently present in the blood of children with CNS lupus. Magnetic resonance imaging is showing up areas of involvement in the cerebrum in cases with minor symptoms.[26] Mortality is from infection and atherosclerotic heart disease, the cause of the latter being uncertain, but the possibility of dyslipoproteinaemia needs further consideration, as does the role of steroids.[27] Another cause of morbidity in children is aseptic necrosis. This does not appear to correlate with the total dose or duration of corticosteroid therapy.[28]

Neonatal lupus has been reported in children born to mothers carrying anti-Ro antibodies and consists of either congenital heart block or rashes, with or without haematological problems. It is of particular interest that these children may be born to mothers with no definitive history of lupus and who are subsequently found to have anti-Ro antibodies. The exact risk for those mothers who are known to carry anti-Ro is not certain, but it appears relatively low.[29]

Overlap syndrome (or 'mixed connective tissue disease')

This syndrome is characterised by the presence of anti-RNP antibodies. Such children usually present with polyarthritis associated with odd rashes, Raynaud's phenomenon, and sometimes fever, serositis, and nodules. Renal involvement is rare.[30] The majority of these children will develop other features of scleroderma over a prolonged period, while an occasional one will develop systemic lupus erythematosus.[31]

Dermatomyositis

The possible role of Coxsackie-B infection requires further elucidation, as does the role of the immune system.[32,33] In the management of such children intravenous pulses of methylprednisone are considered a quick way of bringing them into remission, and they may not necessarily require subsequent corticosteroid therapy,[34] although most rheumatologists continue with oral corticosteroids, with the hope of getting the child onto an alternate day régime fairly quickly. If there is failure to improve or deterioration as the corticosteroid dose is reduced, the question of second-line therapy will arise, and here cyclosporin A appears to be the drug of choice.[35] Methotrexate and alkylating agents should be reserved for those children who do not improve.

Factor-VIII-related antigen is raised in active dermatomyositis—as it is in other vasculitides—and may be a useful monitoring tool.[36]

Scleroderma in childhood

Scleroderma is much more likely to be localised than generalised when it occurs in childhood. However, its classification is becoming more

Table 3. Vasculitic syndromes in childhood

Polyarteritis	microscopic
	macroscopic
Kawasaki disease	
(muco-cutaneous lymph node syndrome)	
Granulomatous vasculitis	
Wegeners granulomatosis	
Churg Strauss syndrome	
Leucocytoclastic	
Henoch Schonlein purpura	
Hypersensitivity angiitis	
Vasculitis in connective tissue disorders	
Dermatomyositis	
SLE	
MCTD/overlap	
Scleroderma	
Sero+ JRA	
Behçets	

difficult as we see more cases, and appreciate that some children have both morphea and linear scleroderma and an associated synovitis.[37] The latter will usually be accompanied by a raised erythrocyte sedimentation rate (ESR), but not necessarily so. A high proportion of children with localised scleroderma do have antinuclear antibodies. Another variant of scleroderma sometimes seen in childhood is fasciitis with eosinophilia.[38] This is associated with a marked peripheral eosinophilia, often a high ESR, and general stiffness. There may be associated patches of multiple morphea. It is reputed to respond to corticosteroids.

Vasculitis

Many different types of vasculitic syndromes are recorded in childhood (Table 3).[39] Two warrant comment: first and notably, Kawasaki's syndrome, which usually begins below the age of five and is associated with high fever, conjunctival injection, odd rashes, massive cervical lymphadenopathy, arthralgia and arthritis, and eventually peeling skin. The major problem, however, is cardiac involvement. A high ESR and very high platelet count will lend support to the diagnosis. It appears that those children treated with intravenous gammaglobulin do better than those without (see chapter 8).[40]

The second form of vasculitis is that associated with streptococcal infections. The importance of recognising this is twofold; while usually cutaneous it can affect viscera, and relapse is common after further streptococcal infections, therefore prophylactic antibiotics are desirable after the acute phase is over.

References

1. Sigal, L.H. (1988) Lyme disease: a worldwide borreliosis. *Clinical & Experimental Rheumatology*, **6**, 411–421.
2. Smith, C.A., Woolfe, A., Lenci, M. (1987) Parvoviruses: infections and arthropathies. *Rheumatic Diseases Clinics of North America*, **13**, 249–263.
3. Pope, R.M. (1989) Rheumatic fever in the 1980s. *Bulletin of Rheumatic Diseases*, **38**, 1–8.
4. Ansell, B.M. (1990) Classification and nomenclature. In: *Paediatric Rheumatology Update.* Woo, P., White, P., Ansell, B.M. (eds). Oxford: Oxford University Press, pp 3–6.
5. Cassidy, J.T., Levinson, J.E., Brewer, E.J. (1989) The development of classification criteria for children with juvenile rheumatoid arthritis. *Bulletin of Rheumatic Diseases*, **38**: 1–7.
6. Hall, P.J., Burman, S.J., Barash, J. *et al* (1989) HLA and complement C4 antigens in polyarticular onset seronegative juvenile chronic arthritis: association of early onset with HLA DRw8. *Journal of Rheumatology*, **16**, 55–59.
7. Southwood, T.R., Petty, R.E., Malleson, P.N. *et al.* (1989) Psoriatic arthritis in children. *Arthritis & Rheumatism*, **32**, 1007–1013.
8. Leak, A.M., Richter, M.R., Clemens, L.E. *et al.* (1988) A crossover study of naproxen, diclofenac, and tolmetin in seronegative juvenile chronic arthritis. *Clinical & Experimental Rheumatology*, **6**, 157–160.
9. Loftus, J.K., Allen, R., Hesp, R. *et al.* (1989). A comparative trial of diflazacort and prednisone in juvenile chronic arthritis. *Clinical & Experimental Rheumatology*, **7**, 458.
10. Loftus, J., Allen, R., Hesp, R. *et al.* (1991) A randomised double blind trial of deflazacort vs. prednisone in juvenile chronic (or rheumatoid) arthritis. A relatively bone-sparing effect of deflazacort. *Paediatrics* (in press).
11. Davies, U.M., Ansell, B.M., Woo, P. (1990). Growth retardation in juvenile chronic arthritis: effect of treatment with biosynthetic human growth hormone. *Arthritis and Rheumatism*, **33**, Supplement Abstract No. 29 S. 14.
12. Silverman, E.D., Laxer, R.M., Greenwald, M. *et al.* (1990) Intravenous gammaglobulin therapy in systemic juvenile rheumatoid arthritis. *Arthritis & Rheumatism*, **33**, 1015–1022.
13. Earley, A., Cuttica, R., McCullough, C. *et al.* (1988) Triamcinolone into the knee-joint in juvenile chronic arthritis. *Clinical & Experimental Rheumatology*, **6**, 153–155.
14. Job-Deslandre, C., Menkes, C.J. (1990) Complications of intra-articular injections of triamcinolone hexacetonide in chronic arthritis of childhood. *Clinical & Experimental Rheumatology*, **8**, 413–416.
15. Brewer, E.J., Giannini, E.H., Kuzmina, N. *et al.* (1980) Penicillamine and hydroxychloroquine in the treatment of severe juvenile rheumatoid arthritis: results of the USA/USSR double-blind placebo controlled trial. *New England Journal of Medicine*, **23**, 404–411.
16. Giannini, E.H., Brewer, E.J., Kuzmina, N. *et al.* (1990) Auranofin in the treatment of juvenile rheumatoid arthritis. *Arthritis & Rheumatism*, **33**, 466–476.
17. Giannini, E.H., Brewer, E.J. (1989) Methotrexate in the treatment of recalcitrant JRA—results of the double-blind placebo controlled randomised trial. *Arthritis & Rheumatism*, **32**, S82.

18. Speckmaier, M., Findeisen, J., Woo, P. *et al.* (1989) Low-dose methotrexate in systemic onset juvenile chronic arthritis. *Clinical & Experimental Rheumatology*, **7**, 647–650.
19. Hawkins, P. (1989) Imaging amyloidosis in Still's disease. *British Medical Journal*, **299**, 848–850.
20. Vouyiouka, O., David, J., Ansell, B.M. *et al.* (1990) Mortality and morbidity of a cohort of juvenile arthritis patients with amyloidosis. *Arthritis and Rheumatism*, **33**, Supplement and abstract D61 S. 144.
21. Hussein, A., Abdul-Khaliq, H., Von der Hardt, H. (1989) Atypical spondyloarthritis in children: proposed diagnostic criteria. *European Journal of Paediatrics*, **148**, 513–517.
22. Leak, A.M., Richter, M.R., St-Cyr, C.H. *et al.* (1986) Flurbriprofen is as effective as naproxen in juvenile spondylitis. *Journal of Rheumatology*, **13**, 664–665.
23. Ansell, B.M. (1991) Sulphasalazine. *Clinical & Experimental Rheumatology* (In press).
24. Jonsson, H., Nived, O., Sturfelt, G., Silman, A. (1990) Estimating the incidence of systemic lupus erythematosus in a defined population using multiple sources of retrieval. *British Journal of Rheumatology*, **29**, 185–188.
25. Papero, P.H., Bluestein, H.G., White, P. *et al.* (1990) Neuropsychologic deficits and antineural antibodies in pediatric systemic lupus erythematosus. *Clinical & Experimental Rheumatology*, **8**, 417–424.
26. Jacobs, L., Kinkel, P.R., Costello, P.B. *et al.* (1988) Central nervous system lupus erythematosus: the value of magnetic resonance imaging. *Journal of Rheumatology*, **15**, 601–606.
27. Ilowite, N.T., Samuel, P., Ginzler, E. *et al.* (1988) Dyslipoproteinaemia in paediatric systemic lupus erythematosus. *Arthritis & Rheumatism*, **31**, 859–863.
28. White, P. (1990) Morbidity of childhood SLE. In: *Paediatric Rheumatology Update*. Woo, P., White, P., Ansell, B.M. (eds). Oxford: Oxford University Press, pp 217–226.
29. Lockshin, M.D., Bonfa, E., Elkon, K. *et al.* (1988) Neonatal lupus risk to newborns of mothers with systemic lupus erythematosus. *Arthritis & Rheumatism*, **31**, 697–701.
30. Singsen, B.H. (1985) Mixed connective tissue disease in childhood. *Pediatric Review*, **7**, 309–314.
31. Allen, R.C., St-Cyr, C., Maddison, P.J. *et al.* (1986) Overlap connective tissue syndromes. *Archives of Diseases in Childhood*, **61**, 284–288.
32. Christensen, M.L., Pachman, L.M., Scherderman, R. *et al.* (1986) Prevalence of Coxsackie B virus antibodies in patients with juvenile dermatomyositis. *Arthritis & Rheumatism*, **29**, 1365–1370.
33. Cambridge, G. (1990) What is the role of the immune system in juvenile dermatomyositis? In: *Paediatric Rheumatology Update*. Woo, P., White, P., Ansell, B.M. (eds). Oxford: Oxford University Press, pp 182–193.
34. Malleson, P.N. (1990) Controversies in juvenile dermatomyositis. *Perspectives in Pediatric Rheumatology*, **17**: 1–2.
35. Heckmatt, J., Sanders, C., Peter, A.M. (1989) Cyclosporine in juvenile dermatomyositis. *Lancet*, **i**, 1063–1066.
36. Bowyer, S.L., Ragsdale, C.G., Sullivan, D.B. (1989) Factor-VIII-related antigen and childhood rheumatic diseases. *Journal of Rheumatology*, **16**, 1093–1097.
37. Allen, R.C., Waller, R., Williamson, S. *et al.* (1987) Localised scleroderma treatment response measured by infra-red thermography. *Thermography*, **2**, 550–553.
38. Grisanti, M.W., Moore, T.L., Osborn, T.G. *et al.* (1989) Eosinophilic fasciitis in children. *Seminars of Arthritis & Rheumatism*, **19**, 151–157.
39. Dillon, M.J. (1990) Vasculitic syndromes. In: *Paediatric Rheumatology Update*. Woo, P., White, P., Ansell, B.M. (eds). Oxford: Oxford University Press, pp 227–242.
40. Bissenden, J.G., Hall, S. (1990) Kawasaki syndrome: lessons for Britain. *British Medical Journal*, **300**, 1025–1026.

8 | Advances in paediatric immunology

Roland J. Levinsky
Institute of Child Health, London

Introduction

The 1980s have seen an exponential growth in knowledge about immunological mechanisms and disease. Whereas prior to this decade much of immunological knowledge had come from study of the mouse, and little of it seemed relevant to human immunology other than by extrapolation, research in the 1980s has seen the growth of human immunology as a major topic. The major reasons for this have been the exceptional rapidity in which monoclonal antibody and molecular biological techniques have been used to dissect the human immune system. The major advances which have clinical application to paediatric immunology are in five main areas. These are:

1. the genetics of immunodeficiency diseases;
2. the use of intravenous immunoglobulin in different diseases;
3. the therapeutic use of cytokines;
4. the use of monoclonal antibodies;
5. advances in bone-marrow transplantation, in particular crossing HLA barriers.

Genetics of immunodeficiency diseases

Prior to 1980 very few of the inherited immunodeficiency diseases could be defined in terms of their molecular aetiology. The only ones understood at that level were the purine enzyme deficiency diseases of adenosine deaminase deficiency and purine nucleoside phosphorylase deficiency. These two enzymes are involved in the purine degradation pathways, and in both diseases the affected children have severe cell-mediated immunodeficiency. In the early 1980s antenatal diagnoses for a wider range of inherited immunodeficiency diseases were described, many based on the functional analysis of the affected cell series, for instance the failure to generate superoxide in polymorphs or monocytes in chronic granulomatous disease (CGD) or the lack of a specific T-cell subpopulation in other forms of severe combined immunodeficiency. However, in the past five years many of these diseases have been defined in terms of their genetic defect; in some the genes have in fact been cloned and the precise defect, either a point mutation or a gene deletion, defined.

Family linkage studies using restriction fragment length polymorphisms (RFLP) have now identified the gross genetic loci of all the immunodeficiency diseases coding on the X chromosome. For instance, if one moves down the X chromosome then the gene for X-linked properdin deficiency is located in the Xp11.23–21.1 region, the gene for X-linked chronic granulomatous disease, which has now been cloned, is located in the Xp21.1 region, the gene for Wiskott-Aldridge syndrome is located at Xp11 just above the centromere, the gene for X-linked severe combined immunodeficiency (SCID) is in the region of Xq13, that for X-linked agammaglobulinaemia (XLA) in the Xq22 region, X-linked hyper IgM in the Xq24 region, and X-linked lymphoproliferative disease (XLP) at the Xq26–27 region. This is illustrated in Figure 1.

In the autosomal recessive diseases the genes for the autosomal recessive forms of CGD have all been cloned and these code for three different proteins, a 47kd phospho-protein (coded on chromosome 10), and 67kd phospho-protein (chromosome 1), and a 22kd α subunit of the cytochrome b245 complex (chromosome 16). The X-linked CGD gene codes for the β subunit of that complex. All these proteins are involved

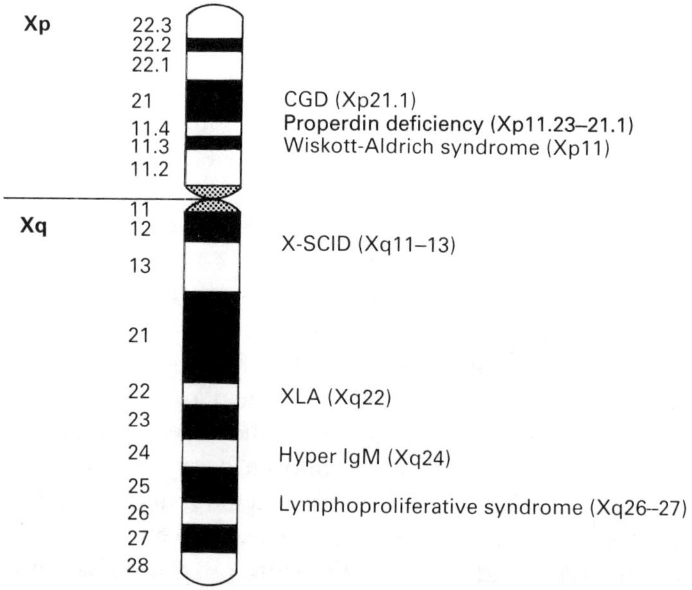

Fig 1. *Genetic loci of the X-linked immunodeficiency diseases*

in superoxide generation by the NADPH system. Similarly, the genetic defect underlying the leucocyte adhesion deficiency has now been well defined. In this syndrome, in which affected children present with delayed umbilical cord separation, purulent pyogenic abscesses, and in severe cases develop pyoderma gangrenosum type lesions leading ultimately to death in early childhood, the gene defect has now been defined as one of several point mutations in the β subunit (CD18 coded at 21q22.3) of the LFA1 complex, a molecule involved in cell adhesion. More recently, the gene coding for the majority of cases of ataxia telangectasia has been mapped to a region of chromosome 11 (11q23).

All these diseases are now amenable to antenatal diagnosis before 12 weeks of pregnancy by analysing the DNA obtained from chorionic villus biopsy material by restriction fragment length polymorphisms and Southern blotting. For most of these diseases a range of probes is informative, and although not all carrier women can be offered this service it is certainly available for the majority.

Another disease which has been defined at the molecular level is the HLA class II deficiency (bare lymphocyte syndrome) in which affected children lack the HLA class II molecules on their lymphocyte cell surfaces. This has now been defined as a functional abnormality of a DNA binding protein regulating the promoter region of the HLA class II gene complex. The exact molecular defect in the family of DNA binding proteins has not yet been defined. Antenatal diagnosis in this disease, as in other forms of severe immunodeficiency, may be performed by analysis of 18- to 20-week gestation foetal blood, and in the former case looking for the HLA class II molecules on the cell surface and in the latter case the presence or absence of T-cell subpopulations.[1]

Use of intravenous immunoglobulin in different diseases

The 1971 Medical Research Council (MRC) clinical trial established the use of intramuscular immunoglobulin as a therapeutic modality for hypogammaglobulinaemia whatever the cause. Since that time patients continued to receive immunoglobulin in the intramuscular form in a schedule of 25 to 50mg/kg weekly. In the mid-1980s intravenous immunoglobulin preparations became available and these are now in widespread use. Most preparations are very safe, having been screened for HIV, hepatitis A and B viruses, and, more recently, with the addition of liver function tests to exclude the possibility of subjects conveying hepatitis C. Most of the preparations contain the normal distribution of the four IgG subclasses and contain a wide spectrum of antibody repertoire. Certain preparations have been selected for increased antibody activity to particular viral antigens such as those containing anti-measles antibody, anti-CMV antibody, and anti-varicellar zoster antibody. In this country, as in the United States and Europe, most patients with severe forms of hypogammaglobulinaemia now receive intravenous immunogobulin infusions.[2] In paediatric practice the dose is titrated to maintain the trough levels above the normal range for age, and this results in the infusion being given in doses between 200–600mg/kg administered every three to four weeks.[3] As a result of this form of treatment the quality of life of all subjects has improved dramatically, there is a greatly reduced incidence of severe infections, and—most pleasing of all—the late sequelae of hypogammaglobulinaemia, namely the chronic chest infections with resultant bronchiectasis and permanent lung damage, are now totally avoidable. The growth of these children is also now normal. Most adults on long-term maintenance therapy lead totally normal lives, and a recent trend to improve the quality of life of both adults and children has been the introduction of home administration of intravenous immunoglobulin by patients themselves, if they are old enough, or by their parents in the case of younger children. After a suitable course of training such home administration may be given quite safely.

In addition to its use in the major forms of immunodeficiency diseases, intravenous immunoglobulin has been tried and found to be effective as a form of treatment for acute and chronic idiopathic thrombocytic purpura,[2] and in the prevention of coronary artery disease in Kawasaki syndrome.[4] Furthermore, controlled trials have shown that severe neonatal sepsis may be significantly reduced in premature-baby wards if intravenous immunoglobulin is administered prophylactically to premature infants of less than 32 weeks' gestation, ie prior to the maternal transfer of IgG across the placenta.

There have also been anecdotal reports of the effect of intravenous immunoglobulin in a wide variety of auto-immune diseases including systemic lupus erythematosis (SLE), Behçet's syndrome, various forms of vasculitis, rheumatoid arthritis, and even in asthma and idiopathic epilepsy. None of these has been subjected to careful controlled clinical trials, and before this has been done one cannot recommend this form of therapy in these diseases. Furthermore, the mechanisms of action of intravenous immunoglobulin in such diseases are at least controversial. It is possible that the antibodies within the preparation interact with antigen excess immune complexes and in so modifying the immune complexes lead to enhanced clearance, but there is no clear evidence for such activity. Another possible mode of action in auto-immune disorders with profound auto-antibody synthesis is anti-idiotype down-regulation of the auto-antibody production. There is animal experimental evidence in support of such activity, but the use of multi-donor immunoglobulin preparations would be a very hit-and-miss affair in order to achieve such a specific effect.

A use of intravenous immunoglobulin for which there is clear evidence of efficacy is in the support therapy given during the aplastic phase of bone-marrow transplantation where sepsis may be greatly reduced by such treatment. However, the use of cytokines, particularly those which affect the granulocyte series and so ameliorate the pancytopaenia following marrow ablation therapy prior to the bone-marrow transplant, will in time reduce the need for intravenous immunoglobulin therapy. It must be remembered that intravenous immunoglobulin preparations are very expensive and there is always the potential of transmitting an unknown virus with such preparations. For these reasons they should not be used lightly.

Use of cytokines

Cytokines are soluble proteins which act in much the same way as hormones. Some, such as γ interferon, may be produced by several cell types, but others are produced exclusively by one cell type, eg interleukin 3 (IL3) by T cells. A list of cytokines is given in Table 1.

The various cytokines which fall into the group known as interleukins have diverse effects on a variety of cell types and function. Some act as growth factors in their own right, others act as differentiating factors or initiators of first or second cell signals, etc. It is likely that specific events in a cell cycle are triggered by a local interaction of one or more cytokines with their specific receptors at the cell surface, and that the concentration of a cytokine at the cell in question is the important event rather than its specific concentration in the circulation. Many of these cytokines are now entering clinical trial for a variety of conditions. For instance, γ interferon has been known to be effective in a form of leukaemia found in adults, ie hairy-cell leukaemia, and remission is rapidly induced with this agent. Trials of other cytokines in a variety of cancers are in progress but the three more specifically used for cancer therapy, albeit still in the initial trial stage, are interleukin 2 (IL2), γ interferon, and tumor necrosis factor (TNF), either singly or in combination.

In the immunodeficiency disorders cytokines have also found a clinical use and there are established indications for the use of two separate cytokines. There is now clear evidence via a randomised double-blind study in the USA and Europe for the use of γ interferon in chronic granulomatous disease. The cytokine, given subcutaneously in a three-times-a-week schedule, significantly reduced the number and severity of severe infections in the treated group.[5] The mode of action is

Table 1. The use of cytokines

Cytokine	Cell source	Major activity
IL1	Macrophages, T and B cells	Stimulates T and B cells proliferation, induces fever
IL2	T/NK cells	Activates and is mitogenic for many cells (T, B, macrophage NK)
IL3	T cells	Stimulates early haemopoiesis
IL4	T cells/most cells	B and T cell mitogen. B cell differentiation. Isotype selection
IL5	T cells	Stimulates eosinophil activity. Isotype selection
IL6	T, B, macrophages, endothelium	Stimulates B cell differentiation
IL7	Bone-marrow stroma	Pre B cell differentiation
IL8	Macrophages	Granulocyte activating factor
GM-CSF	T cells, macrophages, fibroblasts	Stimulates haemopoiesis granulocyte/monocyte lines
G-CSF	Macrophages, fibroblasts	Stimulates granulocyte production and activity
M-CSF	Macrophages, fibroblasts	Stimulates monocyte production and activity
Erythropoietin	Kidney medulla	Stimulates red cell production
α interferon	Granulocytes	Induces cellular antiviral state. Enhances MHC class I
β interferon	Fibroblasts	Stimulates NK activity
γ interferon	T cells	Multifunctional regulatory protein stimulates some activities, inhibits others
TNF	Macrophages, T and B cells	Activates macrophages, induces acute phase response and fever
TGFβ	Macrophages, T cells	Inhibits many cytokine activities

not known, and whereas it was initially thought that γ interferon up-regulated cytochrome b expression via its effect on the promotor region of the gene, the evidence for this is no longer convincing. It certainly increases microbiocidal activity possibly via an increase in superoxide production, but there is also evidence that other cytokines such as interleukin 3 (IL3), granulocyte-macrophage colony stimulating factor (GM-CSF) and granulocyte colony stimulating factor (G-CSF) may have similar activity. None of these has yet been tried clinically in this condition.

The growth factors for haemopoietic cell lineages have also found clinical use especially in congenital agranulocytosis (Kostmann's syndrome) where the defect appears to cause granulocyte maturation arrest in the bone marrow at the promyelocyte stage. Regular injections of G-CSF, but not GM-CSF, restore the neutrophil count to the normal range and cessation of treatment leads to relapse.[6] There is clear evidence of decreased response to this growth factor as pharmacological amounts need to be given to achieve the therapeutic effect. There is no evidence of a G-CSF receptor deficiency in this disease.

It is likely that other diseases will respond to treatment with different cytokines; for instance IL2 coupled to polyethylene glycol (IL2-PEG) is being tried in combined immunodeficiency due to IL2 deficiency, and also in common variable immunodeficiency. Furthermore, as one of the mouse models of osteopetrosis has been shown to be due to a defect in the macrophage colony stimulating factor (M-CSF) gene, it is likely that a similar defect exists within the human forms which may respond to injections of the cytokine.

Therapeutic use of monoclonal antibodies

The discovery of monoclonal antibodies in the 1970s is one of the more fundamental breakthroughs in medical science of this century. Since that time it has been shown that monoclonal antibodies can be raised to almost any antigen and such antibodies, once defined, become invaluable tools for both diagnosis and therapy. The exponential growth in knowledge about the human immune system is partly because of the ability to analyse cell surface molecules initially at glycoprotein level and then ultimately at genetic level, and this has invariably come about by virtue of there being a monoclonal antibody reacting with the molecule in the first instance. In terms of paediatric immunology, monoclonal antibodies have major use as diagnostic tools in cell surface molecule analysis, detection of malignant cells in pathological sections, or as anti-viral and anti-bacterial detection agents in simple diagnostic assays. In therapeutic terms, their use both *in vitro* and *in vivo*, as tools either to get rid of unwanted cells or to create transplantation tolerance, is invaluable. In the field of bone-marrow transplantation, which will be dealt with in the next section, monoclonal antibodies are now widely used in purging malignant cells from the bone marrow prior to re-introduction of bone marrow at autologous transplantation, for T-cell removal to prevent graft versus host disease (GVHD) in allogeneic blood-marrow transplantation, and more recently for isolation of human stem cell enriched populations using anti-CD34 monoclonal antibodies in order to promote positive selection for stem cells for both autologous transplantation for malignancy and also for gene therapy in the future.

Monoclonal antibodies are also now being used *in vivo* as specific mechanisms for immunosuppression, for the treatment of severe GVHD following bone-marrow transplantation, and to prevent the rejection crises occurring following organ transplantation. The most widely used of these are anti-T-cell monoclonal antibodies. The problems with *in vivo* use of such monoclonal antibodies is that there is the likelihood of subsequently creating anti-species antibody responses, ie against the mouse proteins, and subsequent courses of these monoclonal antibodies would therefore be rendered ineffective. This problem is now in the process of being circumvented by genetic engineering techniques in which the human heavy and light chain parts of the immunoglobulin molecule of any isotype can be spliced onto the mouse hyper-variable antigen binding site of the molecule. This hybrid molecule retains the specificity of the original mouse monoclonal antibody but is no longer immunogenic. A further development from the genetic engineering experiments is the development of monovalent Fv fragments of antibodies which again can be humanised, and these much smaller fragments of antibodies still retain the binding specificity, albeit with lower affinity. These molecules presumably could cross into compartments where other molecules may be excluded by virtue of their size. Such molecules, if combined with either toxins or a potent radiolabel such as I^{125}, could be useful for *in vivo* targeting of cells such as malignant clones or the removal of other unwanted cells. There is also the possibility of creating bivalent antibodies where one arm of the antibody molecule recognises, say, a T cell, and the other arm recognises a particular cell for which there is a need to eliminate. The cross linking of these two cell types by this bivalent antibody would activate the T cell to kill the target cell. All these approaches are still in the developmental stage.

Advances in bone-marrow transplantation, in particular crossing HLA barriers

Bone-marrow transplantation is now widely available for a wide range of diseases, from immunodeficiency diseases to most leukaemias and many metabolic diseases. However, due to the small family sizes in Western Europe and the USA, the chances of obtaining an HLA-compatible sibling donor is no greater than 33%. This means that for bone-marrow transplantation to be an effective treatment for all patients with such diseases, techniques have to evolve to transplant effectively across histocompatibility barriers without the development of lethal GVHD. Animal experiments in the 1970s showed that by effective removal of T lymphocytes from the bone-marrow inoculum, GVHD could be substantially reduced and possibly even prevented. Since 1980, with the development of more sophisticated forms of T-cell removal, initially by soy bean lectin agglutination and E rosetting and subsequently by the use of monoclonal antibodies which bind more specifically, it has now become possible to perform bone-marrow transplantation across HLA barriers. One of the problems encountered, however, is that with effective T-cell removal, ie greater than 2 logs and sometimes 3 logs depletion, if the graft takes, although there is no GVHD, there is a much higher rate of graft rejection. The major research in the past five years has been to overcome the innate graft rejection capabilities of the host. Again in animal experiments it has been shown that if one increases the conditioning, ie radio or chemotherapy of the recipient, such graft rejection can be prevented. However, the levels of radiation are virtually at unacceptable levels of toxicity and other techniques need to be applied.

Recently the use of monoclonal antibodies such as those blocking adhesion, ie leucocyte function antigen 1 (anti-LFA1), and those blocking effector function, but not destroying the cells, ie anti-CD4 and CD8 antibodies, have been shown in animal experimental models and even in human studies to be effective at blocking graft rejection. It is likely that once these monoclonal antibodies have been humanised they will go into clinical trial in order to perfect these techniques. For the immunodeficiency diseases at least, and in particular for severe combined immunodeficiency, the results of haplo-identical HLA bone-marrow transplantation are rapidly approaching those of HLA-matched sibling transplants. For the latter one now expects greater than 90% full cure in good centres, whereas for HLA mismatched bone-marrow transplants many of the centres are achieving greater than 60% full cure,[7] and the Memorial Sloane Kettering Hospital in New York, in particular, is leading the way at over 70% full cure. These results no doubt will be matched for other forms of bone-marrow transplantation and in particular for leukaemia, a disease in which, at present, it is more difficult to cross HLA barriers effectively.

The future

Many of the techniques discussed in the last two sections are relevant to the future treatment of a wide range of diseases. The ability to isolate bone-marrow stem cells and to manipulate bone marrow *in vitro* should allow the treatment of a wide range of genetic diseases by somatic gene therapy. In such therapy it is not envisaged at present that the defective gene in question be replaced *in situ*, but that the good gene be inserted randomly within the human genome. Although there are potential risks with such a manoeuvre, for many of the diseases which are fatal without effective treatment the benefits would quite clearly outweigh the risks. The research at present involves insertion of the functioning gene via a retroviral non-replicating vector into bone-marrow stem cells in the hope that the progeny cells derived from these stem cells will continue to express the gene product. To date, it has proved exceptionally difficult to obtain stable expression, and so far such expression has only been obtained in cell lines or for short duration in the SCID mouse model. Experiments in monkeys have not shown long-term stable expression as yet. Ultimately, better vectors will be developed and this technique should become feasible for treatment of all the genetic diseases which are currently treated by bone-marrow transplantation (Table 2).

Somatic gene therapy, however, has much wider implications as there is the possibility of modulating the immune system by the insertion of different genes. It may be possible to target a particular cytokine, ie tumour necrosis factor or γ interferon, to malignant cells and so kill the cells locally. Similarly, it may be possible to provide somatic gene therapy as a form of drug delivery system for deficiencies of hormones, for instance in insulin-dependent diabetes or growth-hormone deficiency.

Table 2. Genetic diseases currently treated by bone-marrow transplantation

Immunodeficiency:	Diseases such as severe combined immunodeficiency and other forms of combined immunodeficiences, HLA class 2 deficiency, and leucocyte adhesion deficiency
Haemoglobinopathies:	Thalassaemia
Metabolic diseases:	Lysosomal storage disorders such as Hurlers, Hunters, Fabry, Gaucher, etc.
Miscellaneous:	Osteopetrosis

Note: This table is by no means comprehensive and merely indicates examples within the different groupings. Cells derived from the bone-marrow pluripotential stem cell may provide the missing cell series, protein, enzyme, or other unknown factor.

In this type of disease it would not be necessary to insert the gene in question into the bone-marrow stem cells, but other cells, such as the endothelium or kerotinocytes, could provide the correct environment and become the substitute endocrine organ. Haemophilia may ultimately be treated in similar ways.

In summary, therefore, these new techniques which have been developed in the 1980–1990 decade will ensure a particularly exciting future for medicine in the 21st century. Human immunology has come of age and has finally become a useful discipline in terms of both diagnosis and therapy.

References

1. Kinnon, C., Pelham, A., Levinsky, R.J. Antenatal diagnosis of immunodeficiency disorders. In *Prenatal Diagnosis and Screening* (eds. Brock, M.H., Rodeck, C.A., Ferguson-Smith, M.). Churchill-Livingstone: Edinburgh.
2. Waters, A.H., Webster, A.D.B. (eds) Intravenous immunoglobulins in immunodeficiency syndromes and idiopathic thrombocytopaenic purpura. *The Royal Society of Medicine International Congress and Symposium series*, 1985, No. 84.
3. Roifman, C.M., Levison, H., Gelfant, E.W. High-dose versus low-dose intravenous immunoglobulin in hypogammaglobulinaemia and chronic lung disease, 1987, *Lancet*, **2**, 1075–1077.
4, Rowley, A.H., Shulman, S.T. What is the status of intravenous gamma-globulin for Kawasaki syndrome in the United States and Canada? *Journal of Paediatric Infectious Diseases*, 1988, **7**, 463–466.
5. Segers, R. The use of γ interferon in chronic granulomatous disease. In *Progress in Immunodeficiency III* (eds. Chapel, H., Levinsky, R.J., Webster, A.D.B), 1991. Royal Society of Medicine Publications: London/New York.
6. Welte, K. Colony stimulating factor for granulocyte deficiency. In *Progress in Immunodeficiency III* (eds. Chapel, H., Levinsky, R.J., Webster, A.D.B.), 1991. Royal Society of Medicine Publications: London/New York.
7. Fischer, A., Landais, P., Friedrich, W., *et al.* European experience of bone marrow transplantation for severe combined immunodeficiency. *Lancet*, 1990, **ii**, 850–854.

9 | Advances in diabetes therapy in childhood

Fotini-Heleni Karachaliou and J. David Baum
Institute of Child Health, University of Bristol

Introduction

Seventy years ago diabetes was a life-threatening, incurable, progressive, wasting disease of childhood. The development of injectible insulin therapy changed diabetes to a life-limiting, incurable, chronic disorder—insulin-dependent diabetes mellitus (IDDM). Despite enormous effort, little practical progress was made in the clinical management of childhood diabetes over the next 50 years. Over the past two decades, and especially in the past few years, we have witnessed a picture of accelerating change in the details of therapy but diabetes remains a lifelong and life-limiting disease.

The aim of this review is to look back over the past five years at advances in diabetes therapy and to speculate on advances we can reasonably expect during the 1990s. However, it would be appropriate to set out the aims of therapy before detailing the instruments involved. These aims are:

1. to provide children with diabetes and their families lives free from the effects of extremes of blood-glucose concentration, aiming for the ideal of stable and physiological blood-glucose regulation;
2. to secure for children with diabetes a normal life-expectancy coupled with a near-normal life style;
3. to reduce to a minimum the interference with normal living and normal health caused by the instruments of therapy;
4. to empower the child and family to be autonomous in their health care;
5. to identify early and reliable pointers to the long-term complications of diabetes and introduce the appropriate therapies, as and when the value of such treatment is clarified;
6. to identify those free from the risk of long-term complications and liberate them from the rigours of current therapeutic regimens;

7. to identify early and reliable markers of the diabetogenic process and introduce the appropriate interventions, as and when such are clarified, with the aim of suppressing or reversing the process;
8. to identify those genetically predisposed to the development of diabetes and implement appropriate interventions, as and when such are identified, to avoid or counteract those environmental factors (if any) shown to be involved in the initiation of the diabetogenic process;
9. to identify factors that protect against the diabetogenic process, as and when such are identified, whether they be genetic or environmental, and enhance them by appropriate interventions.

Insulins

Human insulin

Over the past five years we have witnessed a massive changeover from animal insulin to formulations of human insulin manufactured by either recombinant DNA technology or semisynthesis (enzymatic conversion from porcine insulin). At least 75% of diabetic patients taking insulin in Britain are now using human insulin, while five years ago only about 6% of insulin sold in Britain was of human type.[1]

Apart from the avoidance of lipo-atrophy and the rarity of allergic reactions, the advantages of human insulin are largely theoretical or philosophical. There have been a few reports of a small number of adult patients in whom the transfer to human insulin was associated with an increased frequency of hypoglycaemia or loss of premonitory symptoms or both.[2] It is advised that the dose of human insulin should be reduced by 10% if the initial dose of beef insulin was 40–100U daily, and by 25% if the previous dose was more than 100U.[3] Transfer from porcine to human insulin seems to require no dosage reduction. Transfer to human insulin should take place in the home environment under medical or nursing supervision with frequent home blood-glucose determination in the first few days. On balance the use of human insulin for children with decades of insulin therapy ahead of them seems justified, perhaps especially for newly diagnosed children being initiated on treatment.

Analogues of human insulin

An important pharmacological goal in diabetes management has been to achieve a rapid increment of plasma-free insulin to coincide with the time of meal consumption. The subcutaneous injection of currently available soluble insulin produces peak plasma concentrations some 90–120 min later; to be optimally effective soluble insulin should therefore be injected 30–60 mins before the meal.[4] In the real world such a long interval is at best inconvenient and usually impossible. The delay in the absorption of human insulin is thought to be due to the predominance of insulin dimers and hexamers rather than monomers. It has been recently reported that a single amino-acid substitution yields monomeric insulin analogues with largely preserved biological activity but which are absorbed 2–3 times faster after subcutaneous injection than conventional soluble human insulin.[5] The first study in human subjects recording a much faster absorption of a monomeric insulin analogue compared with soluble human insulin was published in 1988.[6] The place for such preparations in the care of children with diabetes will need to be clarified by clinical trials over the next quinquennium.

The field of insulin analogues will inevitably expand over the next decade. The development of insulin analogues with quicker and more consistent subcutaneous absorption rates, as well as longer-acting insulin preparations with chemical stability and predictable patterns of absorption, will be the target. The early results are encouraging, but clinical trials of appropriate size and design are required to evaluate the efficacy of the analogues under field conditions.

Different insulin regimens

A multitude of different insulin regimens are used in current clinical practice, ranging from single injections to mixtures of insulins in the syringe, to three or four injections daily. Little real progress has been made over the past five years towards an agreed optimal regimen for children. Clinical investigations, studies of pharmacokinetics and miscibility of different kinds of insulin continue. We can hope that the next five years will yield a consensus since it profits neither patient nor physician to continue in the current muddle.

Pumps, or continuous subcutaneous insulin infusion

Continuous subcutaneous insulin infusion (CSII) has been confirmed to produce near-normal glycaemic control only within supervised research protocols.[7] With a few exceptions, long-term results of CSII on large non-research population groups have not confirmed the early encouraging metabolic results from pilot studies.[8,9] CSII requires continuing available care by skilled professionals in well-organised diabetes clinics with a 24-hour telephone service, continuing education, and meticulous home blood-glucose monitoring.[10] Children have in fact voted that pump therapy, at least as currently practised, is not acceptable under the normal free-range conditions of everyday life.

Pens

The introduction of the insulin pen (NovoPen I) in 1984/85 undoubtedly represented a great advance in the practical delivery of insulin. It took the form of a simple device beautifully engineered in chromium-plated brass, shaped like a pen and holding cartridges containing short-acting insulin. In 1987 NovoPen II was introduced in plastic, lighter in weight but perhaps less attractive, designed to deliver more easily larger doses of insulin with cartridges containing either intermediate-acting or a premixed insulin.[11]

The use of a Pen has led to no general improvement in blood-glucose control itself, but has permitted a more flexible lifestyle, in particular freedom in planning meals, in exchange for multiple injections.[12] Additionally a Pen is easily portable, more socially acceptable, and injections can be given simply and quickly. Mechanical problems seldom occur and the cost is comparable to conventional injections using disposable syringes and needles. For highly motivated and well-educated children and teenagers, with a good understanding of dose adjustment, the Pen represents a substantial advance in diabetes management, as proven by its popularity.

No doubt the next five years will see further developments of Pen devices and insulins for cartridge use. The appropriate clinical trials should then clarify the best regimens for children and not leave us with more choice and clinical chaos.

Other insulin delivery systems

There is a case for standardising conventional subcutaneous injection technique, since it has been reported that random intramuscular injection may occur particularly with injections in the thigh.[13] This may in itself result in unexpected variations in absorption rate.

A new device called the 'sprinkler needle' has been introduced with a sealed end-hole and fine small holes in the side walls which, it is claimed, allows a better distribution of insulin in the subcutaneous tissue and a better absorption.[14]

The jet injector is a device designed to force an ultra-thin liquid stream of insulin through the skin under high pressure, which aims to decrease the pain of injection. Jet injection is mechanically reliable and is claimed to produce a 10–20% greater decrease in blood glucose and a more rapid rise in free-insulin levels than conventional insulin delivery.[15,16] However, problems associated with jet injectors include after-pain, bruising, and leakage of insulin from the jet site.

Nasal insulin administration is needle-free, though not strictly non-invasive. It permits a rapid insulin absorption (plasma insulin peaks 15–30 min after nasal application) followed by a rapid decline in plasma insulin concentrations. However, the problem of poor insulin absorption (only 10% of the administered dose is absorbed) needs to be resolved.[17]

The appropriate clinical trials are now required to clarify the proper place in routine care of the sprinkler needle, jet injectors, nasal insulin, and other innovations in insulin delivery.

Implants

Since the subcutaneous route for insulin administration is almost invariably associated with peripheral hyperinsulinaemia and under-insulinisation of the liver, the intraperitoneal (IP) or intravenous (IV) routes for insulin delivery have been considered. The use of an external pump for IP or IV insulin infusion has been limited by patient discomfort, significant infections, and biomechanical problems of material and pump failure.[18,19]

In the early 1980s the first implantable externally programmable pumps for insulin administration became available for clinical evaluation. Both in Europe and USA these were associated initially with great optimism but subsequently and inevitably with many problems.[20] By May 1989, according to the Human Implantable Pump International Registry, 280 pumps had been implanted in 215 diabetic patients, 73% of whom had IDDM, and 70% aged between 20 and 50 years.[21,22]

Although many technical problems have been overcome, the most important unresolved problem is the biocompatibility of catheters. The most common reasons reported for pump failure have been flow slow-down and catheter obstructions due to tissue reactions. Reports from the two most recent programmable pump clinical trials, the European POINT study[23] and the US PIMS study,[24] show that generally pumps function safely and satisfactorily; most problems encountered have been catheter related.

Artificial endocrine pancreas

From the beginning of the 1980s there has been a quest for a portable or, even better, a wearable artificial endocrine pancreas, incorporating a durable implantable glucose sensor, a computer calculating infusion rates of insulin based on specific glucose-insulin algorithms, and an infusion pump. Without doubt the development of some kind of implantable glucose sensor device (even without connection to a pump) would represent an extremely welcome and important advance in the care of children with diabetes.

Advances in technology can reasonably be expected to resolve the problems of biocompatibility in catheters, leading to better pump function and longevity. Methods for early detection of catheter malformation as well as efficient techniques for catheter repair can be anticipated. However, it is generally accepted that the major advance in implantable or portable insulin pump progress will be to 'close the loop' by means of an implantable sensor which will continuously monitor blood-glucose concentrations. Unfortunately the bio-engineering problems for producing sensors stable in the tissues for more than a few hours and with a consistent response remain unsolved. Polarography, infrared, and electrochemical needle-type sensors[25,26,27] are among the devices currently under investigation.

Today, only the large closed-loop system exists in the form of the bedside artificial pancreas, or Biostator.[28] This has great research value but no place in normal clinical management. Over the next decade we can hope for an implantable IV or IP pump, adjusting doses in response to tissue glucose readings provided by a needle-type glucose sensor. The major advance will be a long-term stable and reliable sensor enabling the device to be implanted and the loop to be closed at last.

Transplantation

Islet transplantation

Over the past five years attempts to transplant pancreatic islet tissue, derived from either human fetal pancreas or from dispersed adult human pancreas, have continued. Impressive progress has been reported in islet-cell isolation techniques, understanding the immunological mechanisms underlying islet-cell rejection, and the development of methods for immunomodulation to overcome rejection-related problems.[29,30] However, successful islet transplantation in human diabetic subjects currently remains elusive.

The most important requirements for successful islet transplantation lie in the quality and the quantity of the islet tissue (at least six fetal pancreata are required for each adult recipient). Over the next few years we can expect improvements in culturing methods to reduce the amount of fetal tissue needed, effective prevention of immune rejection of islet allografts by reducing the immunogenicity of fetal islet tissue, and advances in the understanding and application of immunomodulation.

Alternative strategies may derive from developments in molecular biological techniques. Manipulations of the insulin gene are expected to enable the creation of artificial β-cells by transfection of genes for synthesis and processing of insulin into the patient's own skin fibroblasts.[31]

Pancreatic transplantation

Data from the International Pancreas Transplant Registry report 856 transplants in 796 patients in 73 institutions since July 1977.[32,33] In most instances they were kidney and pancreas transplants in end-stage renal disease. Results show that with technically successful dual transplantation the one-year patient survival is about 80% and one-year graft survival about 50%.[33] The results are similar for all commonly used surgical techniques. However, to further improve the results and prevent the complications of diabetes it would be logical to perform transplantation much earlier in the course of the disease. The reported pancreatic graft survival rate is low in non-uraemic patients, with one-year survival rate of only 32% in specialised centres.[33] This is hardly an encouraging prospect when contemplating transplantation in an otherwise healthy child with diabetes.

Recipient selection

Transplantation, whether of islet cells or of the whole pancreas in non-uraemic patients, will be justified only when the secondary complications of diabetes in an individual subject are predictably more serious than the side-effects of the transplantation process. Renal transplantation can exemplify the clinical hazards of immunosuppression. Reliable predictors of diabetic complications in adults and in children will be priority developments in the 1990s.

Diet

Food is one of the fundamental therapeutic modalities in the treatment of IDDM. The general recommendations concerning diet for children with diabetes have changed little over the past five years:

(i) meal plan rather than 'diet' based on good eating habits for the whole family;

(ii) flexible meal plans to allow for hugely variable activity, growth and development;
(iii) the meal plan to include food appropriate to the patient's ethnic, cultural, and social background.

In the 1980s the emphasis was on certain food types,[34,35,36] as follows:

(a) Whole carbohydrate food *rich in dietary fibre* in which the cell walls are slow to be disrupted and the viscous fibre content is high, thus delaying carbohydrate digestion, was advocated. Foods provoking the smallest rise in blood-glucose include leguminous vegetables, some whole fruit, and oats.
(b) *A reduction in total fat intake*, and particularly animal fat, was advised. For saturated fats a partial substitution with mono- and poly-unsaturated fats was recommended.
(c) *Mineral absorption* can be affected by high-fibre foods, and adequate intake of calcium, iron, and zinc was suggested.

Over the next five years it seems unlikely that major new foods will be introduced to this dietary regimen. The emphasis will be on healthy eating for the whole family with the details of the dietary prescription and meal plan following, rather than leading, changes in the practice of insulin delivery.

Education, support and empowerment

The extensive and continuous educational needs of the family and the child, together with lifetime reinforcement and maintenance of motivation, are now well recognised. What is less clearly established is: who are the educators, how effective is their methodology, and how are they updated and motivated?[37] There is, moreover, challenging work to be done to evaluate to what extent such educational efforts succeed. What are the outcome measures: the child's knowledge of diabetes, his or her attitude to diabetes, the daily details of the child's personal practice, or blood-glucose control?

It is generally agreed as good practice that the child's care is best supervised by a multidisciplinary team including physician, dietician, specialist nurse, psychologist, and social worker.[38] This allows the proper flexible emphasis to range between blood-glucose surveillance, psychological best-buy, family stability, school, jobs, independence, and so forth. In the years to come, in this country at least, an equilibrium will be established between the demands for best practice from the professional and consumer groups on the one hand and the constraints of the health authority purchasers on the other. It is likely that the role of the British Diabetic Association will be further developed along the lines of organising parent weekends, youth courses and summer camps, in support of the families' educational and psychological needs.

Complications

Over the past five years the need to focus on early pointers to the long-term complications of diabetes has been recognised.[39,40] Micro-albuminuria (elevated urinary albumin excretion not detectable by standard clinical tests) constitutes the clearest indicator of risk for renal failure and premature cardiovascular mortality. The predictive value of micro-albuminuria for adults with diabetes has been derived from relevant prospective studies.[41,42] Limited joint mobility[43] has been shown to precede the development of microvascular complications. Recently, studies on early abnormalities in diabetic children of autonomic[44] and peripheral neural function[45] have been reported, which may prove to be markers of neuropathy in the future. However, whether it be micro-albuminuria, limited joint mobility or autonomic nervous dysfunction, the published observations are limited and will require very long-term follow-up to clarify their predictive value, especially in the case of children.

If the value of early markers of latent complications of diabetes is to be enhanced, and certainly if such tests are to be introduced into routine clinical practice, there is an urgent need for standardising the details of the methodology prior to long-term studies of their predictive value when they can serve as the baseline for intervention studies.

Intervention studies in adults have included strict blood-glucose control, intensified insulin treatment, antihypertensive therapy, and restricted protein diet.[46] However, such studies need to be extended in duration, to recruit larger numbers of subjects using as outcome variables such clear end-points as end-stage renal failure or cardiovascular morbidity/mortality. For children the studies will need to be longer in duration and larger in size, if for example the value of blood-pressure monitoring and selective blood-pressure reduction is to be justified and open to evaluation.

Epidemiology

National surveys and family studies will contribute towards establishing the incidence of the disease[47] and the identification of genetic predisposition, environmental triggers, and markers of the early diabetogenic process.[48,49] Additionally, priorities for the 1990s will include prospective cohort studies, case-control studies, family studies with cell lines established for genomic analyses. Co-ordinated research in epidemiology and genetics will offer the best chance of identifying genetic predisposition and resilience, environmental trigger factors and protective factors, and protection against or avoidance or reversal of the diabetogenic process.

Immunotherapy

Recent studies suggest that IDDM is (a) the consequence of an autoimmune process leading to the destruction of islet β-cells; (b) not a disease of acute onset but a disease with a prolonged preclinical phase.[50] This period of latency, during which several immunological abnormalities have been reported, is regarded as the most auspicious for an immune therapeutic intervention. The most frequent abnormalities described are islet-cell antibodies (ICA), insulin antibodies, circulating activated T-lymphocytes, and impaired suppressor cell function. Of these, high persistent ICA levels, especially when they are complement fixing (CF-ICA), seem to have the highest positive predictive value for the development of IDDM.[51] Investigators have now begun to explore the possibility of intervention therapy (immunomodulation, nicotinamide, dietary restriction, or even insulin administration before the onset of clinical disease) to halt or reverse the disease process.[52,53]

In April 1990, there was a consensus from the National Institute of Health (NIH) that there is a methodology that can identify with near certainty, among first-degree relatives of diabetic patients with IDDM, those who will develop diabetes, and that immuno-intervention therapy before the onset of symptoms may prevent the disease.[54]

In June 1990, the expert committee of the American Diabetes Association on the prevention of IDDM published a position statement. According to this, screening of the population is discouraged outside the context of defined research studies, while screening of high-risk individuals is encouraged, provided that individuals who are found positive are referred to centres participating in co-operative intervention studies. Also, intervention studies must use standardised methods, assays, entry criteria, and end-point definitions.[54]

There have been clinical trials on immunosuppression or immunomodulation on the basis of diabetogenic hypotheses, in both children and adults.[55,56,57] Immunosuppression with cyclosporin associated with immunomodulators and nicotinamide should be conducted only in patients enrolled in clinical trials,[58] as soon as possible after presentation, in highly organised centres, according to protocols including control groups and strict evaluation of side-effects, within the guidelines issued by the International Diabetes Immunotherapy Group.[59] Such an exclusive approach is justified given the grave side-effects associated with the use of potentially oncogenic and nephrotoxic drugs for long periods, if not for the child's lifetime.

The clinic scene in the 1990s

There is a potential conflict between simplification of regimens for diabetic children and their families and the increased armoury for potential impositions on the children's lifestyles with measures of latent microvascular disease, enrolment in immunosuppression, and other clinical trials.

Whether or not the incidence of IDDM is increasing, and whether or not attempts to simplify the basis of the daily insulin prescription is achieved, it seems likely for the clinic and for the children and families that the load of work and responsibility will increase over the next five years. This will demand increased training of medical and nursing staff, additional members of staff for regional and district clinics, and inevitably an increased financial commitment by the Health Service. It is to be hoped that the ten-year view might be different, with the harvest from molecular biological research yielding simple and safe islet-cell transplantation, reliable markers of the diabetogenic process with the capacity to reverse it, identification of environmental risk factors to be avoided, and perhaps identification of protective factors to be enhanced. At least we might work towards identifying the majority of children with diabetes who may be destined *not* to develop the complications of the disease, and who might be allowed the autonomy of a minimalist regimen, freedom from the dictatorship of diet, and a much more distant dependency on clinics and doctors and the other multidisciplinarians.

References

1. Pickup, J.C. (1989) Human insulin. *British Medical Journal*, **299**, 991–993.
2. Turner, T.A., O'Mullane, M.M., Sinver, A. *et al.* (1988) Switching to human insulin. *Lancet*, **ii**, 1150.
3. Gill, G.V., Jones, K.E. (1988) Beef to human insulin: dose for dose? *Lancet*, **ii**, 1305.
4. Kinmonth, A.L., Baum, J.D. (1980) Timing of pre-breakfast insulin injection and postprandial metabolic control in diabetic children. *British Medical Journal*, **280**, 604–606.
5. Brange, J., Ribel, U., Hansen, J.F. *et al.* (1988) Monomeric insulins obtained by protein engineering and their medical implications. *Nature*, **333**, 679–682.
6. Vora, J.P., Owens, D.R., Dolben, J. *et al.* (1988) Recombinant DNA derived

monomeric insulin analogue: comparison with soluble human insulin in normal subjects. *British Medical Journal*, **297**, 1236–1239.
7. Shiffrin, A.D., Desroisiers, M., Alegassine, H., Belmonte, M.M. (1984) Intensified insulin therapy in the type 1 diabetic adolescent: a controlled trial. *Diabetes Care*, **7**, 107–113.
8. Brink, S.J., Stewart, C. (1986) Insulin pump treatment in children, adolescents, and young adults with insulin dependent diabetes mellitus. *Journal of the American Medical Association*, **255**, 617–621.
9. Knight, G., Boulton, A.J.M., Ward, J.D. (1986) Experience of continuous subcutaneous insulin infusion in the outpatient management of diabetic teenagers. *Diabetic Medicine*, **3**, 82–84.
10. American Diabetes Association (1982) Indications for use of continuous insulin delivery systems and self-measurement of blood glucose. *Diabetes Care*, **5**, 140–141.
11. Kolendorf, K., Beck-Nielsen, H., Oxenboll, B. (1988) Clinical experience with NovoPen II and insulin Protaphane HM Penfill. *Postgraduate Medical Journal*, **64** (suppl 3), 14–16.
12. Jefferson, G., Marteau, T.M., Smith, M.A. (1985) A multiple injection regimen using an insulin pen and prefilled cartridged soluble human insulin in adolescents with diabetes. *Diabetic Medicine*, **2**, 493–495.
13. Vaag, A., Damgaard Pedersen, K., Lauritzen, M. *et al.* (1990) Intramuscular versus subcutaneous injection of unmodified insulin: Consequences for blood-glucose control in patients with type 1 diabetes mellitus. *Diabetic Medicine*, **7**, 335–342.
14. Edsberg, B., Herly, D., Hildebrandt, P., Kuhl, C. (1987) Insulin bolus given with a sprinkler needle: effect on absorption and glycaemic response to a meal. *British Medical Journal*, **294**, 1373–1376.
15. Malone, J.L., Lowitt, S., Grove, N.P., Shah, S.C. (1986) Comparison of insulin levels after injection by jet stream and disposable insulin syringe. *Diabetes Care*, **9**, 637–640.
16. Task Force in Jet Injectors, Council on Youth (1988) Position statement on jet injectors. *Diabetes Care*, **11**, 600–601.
17. Kuhl, C. (1988) Novo's research and development commitment to diabetes care. *Postgraduate Medical Journal*, **64** (suppl 3), 1–3.
18. Zimman, B., Perlman, K., Rodin, G. *et al.* (1984) Long-term open loop intravenous insulin infusion in Type 1 diabetes: feasibility, problems and promise. *Clinical and Investigative Medicine*, **7**, 199–204.
19. Selam, J.L., Giraud, P., Mirouze, J., Saeidi, S. (1985) Continuous peritoneal insulin infusion with portable pumps: factors affecting the operative life of the chronic catheter. *Diabetes Care*, **8**, 34–38.
20. Kritz, H., Hagmueller, G., Lovett, R., Irsigler, K. (1983) Implanted constant base rate insulin infusion devices for Type 1 diabetic patients. *Diabetologia*, **25**, 78–81.
21. Knatterud, G., Fisher, M. (1985) Report from the International Study Group on Implantable Insulin Delivery Devices. *Diabetes Care*, **8**, 308.
22. Selam, J.L., Charles, M.A. (1989) Devices for insulin use. *Diabetes Care*, **13**, 955–980.
23. Point Study Group (1988) One-year trial of remote-controlled implantable insulin infusion system in Type 1 diabetic patients. *Lancet*, **1**, 866–869.
24. Selam, J.L. (1988) Development of insulin pumps: long is the road. *Diabetic Medicine*, **5**, 724–733.
25. Vehlo, A., Froguel, P., Sternberg R. *et al.* (1989) *In vitro* and *in vivo* stability of electrode potentials in needle-type glucose sensors. *Diabetes*, **38**, 164–171.
26. Zeller, H., Novak, P., Landgrof, R. (1987) Blood-glucose measurements by means of infrared spectroscopy under physiological conditions. (Abstract) *Artificial Organs*, **2**, 315A.

27. Vehlo, G., Froguel, P., Thevenot, D.R., Reach, G. (1988) *In vivo* calibration of a subcutaneous glucose sensor for determination of subcutaneous glucose kinetics. *Diabetic Nutrition and Metabolism*, **3**, 227–233.
28. Marliss, E.B., Murray, F.T., Stokes, E.F. *et al.* (1977) Normalisation of glycaemia in diabetics during meals with insulin and glucagon delivery by the artificial pancreas. *Archives of Internal Medicine*, **137**, 639–649.
29. Hu, Y.F. (1987) The potential of islet transplants as a cure for human diabetes. *Journal of Diabetic Complications*, **4**, 115–119.
30. Mullen, Y., Clare-Salzer, M., Stein, E., Clark, W. (1989) Conference report: Islet transplantation for the cure of diabetes. *Pancreas*, **4**, 123–135.
31. Steel, C.M. (1987) Can molecular and cell biology offer a cure for diabetes? *Diabetic Medicine*, **4**, 9–12.
32. Squifflet, J.P., Sutherland, D.E.R., Florack, G. *et al.* (1988) Current status of pancreas transplantation. *Advances in Nephrology*, **17**, 343–362.
33. Sutherland, D.E.R., Moudry, K.C., Fryd, D.S. (1989) Results of Pancreas Transplantation Registry. *Diabetes*, **38** (suppl 1), 46–54.
34. Kinmonth, A.L., Mograth, G., Reckless, J.P.D. and the Nutrition Subcommittee of the Professional Advisory Committee of the British Diabetic Association (1989) Dietary recommendations for children and adolescents with diabetes. *Diabetic Medicine*, **6**, 537–547.
35. Brink, S. J. (1988) Pediatric, adolescent, and young-adult nutrition issues in IDDM. *Diabetes Care*, **11**, 192–280.
36. Kinmonth, A.L., Angus, R.M., Jenkins, P.A. *et al.* (1982) Whole foods and increased dietary fibre improve blood-glucose control in diabetic children. *Archives of Disease in Childhood*, **57**, 187–194.
37. Anderson, R.M., Donelly, M.B., Cressond, C.P., Debrick, R.F. (1989) Development of diabetes attitude scale for health-care professionals. *Diabetes Care*, **12**, 120–127.
38. Laron, Z., Galatzer, A., Amir, S. (1979) A multidisciplinary, comprehensive, ambulatory, treatment scheme for diabetes mellitus in children. *Diabetes Care*, **2**, 342–348.
39. Steffes, M.W., Chavers, B.M., Bilous, R.W., Maner, S.M. (1989) The predictive value of microalbuminuria. *American Journal of Kidney Diseases*, **XIII**, 25–28.
40. Karavanaki, K., Davies, A., Baum, J.D. (1990) The Avon Childhood Diabetes Study: Increased albumin excretion and relationship with blood pressure and glycaemic control. (Abstract) *British Paediatric Association*, 62nd annual meeting. P. 51
41. Morgensen, C.E. (1984) Microalbuminuria predicts clinical proteinuria and early mortality in maturity onset diabetes. *New England Journal of Medicine*, **310**, 356–360.
42. Viberti, G.C., Hill, R.D., Jarrett, R.J. *et al.* (1982) Microalbuminuria as a predictor of clinical nephropathy in insulin-dependent diabetes mellitus. *Lancet*, **1**, 1430–1432.
43. Rosenbloom, A.L., Silverstein, J.H., Lezotte, D. *et al.* (1981) Limited joint mobility in childhood diabetes mellitus indicates increased risk for microvascular disease. *New England Journal of Medicine*, **305**, 191–194.
44. Mitchell, E.A., Wealthall, S.R., Elliot, R.B. (1985) Tests for autonomic neuropathy in diabetic children. *Australian Paediatric Journal*, **21**, 105–109.
45. Gallai, V., Firenze, C., Mazzotta, G., Del Gatto, F. (1988) Neuropathy in children and adolescents with diabetes mellitus. *Acta Neurologica Scandinavica*, **78**, 136–140.
46. Viberti, G.C. (1989) Interventions based on microalbuminuria screening and low-protein diet in the treatment of kidney disease of diabetes mellitus. *American Journal of Kidney Diseases*, **XII**, 41–44.
47. Metcalfe, M.A., Baum, J.D. (1990) Incidence of childhood-onset diabetes under

the age of 15 years in the British Isles during 1988. *British Medical Journal.* (In press).
48. Riley, W.J., McLaren, N.K., Silverstein, J.H. (1988) The predictability of insulin-dependent mellitus. *Advances in Pediatrics*, **35**, 167–188.
49. Bonifazio, E., Bingley, P.J., Shattoch, M. *et al.* (1990) Quantification of islet-cell antibodies and prediction of insulin-dependent diabetes. *Lancet*, **335**, 147–149.
50. Eisenbath, G.S. (1986) Type 1 diabetes mellitus. A chronic auto-immune disease. *New England Journal of Medicine*, **314**, 1360–1368.
51. Karjalainen, J.K. (1990) Islet-cell antibodies as predictive markers for IDDM in children with background incidence of disease. *Diabetes*, **39**, 1144–1150.
52. Gotfredsen, C.F., Buschard, K., Frandsen, E.K. (1985). Reduction of diabetes incidence of BB Wistar rats by early prophylactic insulin treatment of diabetes prone animals. *Diabetologia*, **28**, 933–935.
53. Gottlieb, P.A., Rossini, A.A., Mordes, J.P. (1988) Approaches to prevention and treatment of IDDM in animal models. *Diabetes Care*, **11** (suppl 1), 29–36.
54. Position statement (1990) Prevention of type 1 diabetes mellitus. *Diabetes Care*, **13**, 1026–1027.
55. Bougneres, P.F., Carel, J.C., Castano L. *et al.* (1988) Factors associated with early remission of type 1 diabetes in children treated with cyclosporine. *New England Journal of Medicine*, **318**, 663–670.
56. Cook, J., Hudson, I., Harrison L.C. *et al.* (1989) Double-blind controlled trial of azathioprine in children with newly diagnosed type 1 diabetes. *Diabetes*, **38**, 779–783.
57. Herold, K., Rubenstein, A.H. (1988) Immunosuppression for insulin-dependent diabetes. *New England Journal of Medicine*, **318**, 701–703.
58. International Study Group of Diabetes in childhood and adolescents (ISGD) (1987) Warning against routine use of cyclosporine for newly diagnosed diabetics. *Lancet*, **ii**, 981.
59. Pozilli, P. (1988) Immunotherapy in type 1 diabetes. *Diabetic Medicine*, **5**, 734–738.

10 | Paediatric surgery

John Wagget
The Royal Victoria Infirmary, Newcastle upon Tyne

Surgery in childhood

Paediatric surgery is a very wide-ranging speciality, including all of the general abdominal surgery of childhood, urology, and surgery of the newborn infant. Within the umbrella of surgery in childhood, we have specialists in orthopaedic surgery, plastic surgery, ear-nose-and-throat surgery, and cardiac surgery. As it will not be possible to review all these areas, I will try and pick out some of the problems and areas where there are likely to be advances.

Pain control

One of the features common to all surgical procedures, and often forgotten, is the potential for causing pain.[1] Post-operative pain control should see important advances in the next decade. In the first instance, this may result from the better application of known methods and a change of attitude of the carers, nurses, paediatricians, anaesthetists, and surgeons. A recent report by the Royal College of Surgeons of England and the College of Anaesthetists highlights many of the problems and has a section especially on the needs of children.[2] Adoption of its recommendations would be a major advance for the 1990s.

Opioid infusions have been known to give better pain control than intermittent intramuscular injections, which are painful in themselves. In the older child, patient-controlled anaesthesia (PCA) can be used. Local anaesthesia and regional blocks have a major part to play in post-operative pain relief. In thoracotomies, the intercostal nerves can be infiltrated under direct vision before the chest is closed. Ilio-inguinal nerve blocks for herniotomy and undescended testis have proved useful, and other wounds can usefully be infiltrated locally.[3] For perineal operations, such as repairs for hypospadias or circumcision, epidural anaesthesia instituted immediately after the child is induced for general anaesthesia lessens the need for deep general anaesthesia, and also gives excellent pain relief for up to 12 hours post-operatively. At this time, oral analgesics can be introduced. The 'Green' report by the two Colleges[2] should be required reading for all doctors concerned with pain control.

Neonatal surgery

The speciality of paediatric surgery grew up around the surgery of the newborn, and the main advances in neonatal surgery we are likely to see are related to the use of antenatal ultrasound for diagnosis,[4] and to our understanding of the responses of the newborn to the stress of anaesthesia and surgery.[5,6] Antenatal ultrasound has already had a major impact on the management of babies ante-natally and post-natally. The urological abnormalities discovered by antenatal ultrasound, such as unilateral upper-tract distension and multi-cystic kidney, have already caused changes in our practice. Diagnostic pitfalls, however, have been described by Clarke *et al.*[7] who advise a full urological investigation before a diagnosis of multi-cystic kidney is made. These authors point out that a diagnosis based on ultrasound alone is especially susceptible to error. The management of multi-cystic kidneys has also caused discussion in surgical circles in the past few years. The previously accepted management was to excise the kidney in early life, but several centres have suggested a conservative approach. Some multi-cystic kidneys have been shown to get smaller over the first year of life, and it has been advocated that these be left alone.[8] However, the long-term worry concerns dysplastic renal tissue lying between the cysts having a potential for malignant change,[9] or the potential to cause hypertension, which leaves me still to advise early excision. A nephrectomy for multi-cystic kidney in the first month of life is a simple and straightforward procedure, especially if it can be carried out by the extra-peritoneal approach.

A pelvi-ureteric junction obstruction requires early surgery in order to preserve renal function. The problem arises in defining which children have a significant obstruction and not a dilated, stable, non-obstructed system. Ransley *et al.*[10] propose that if good function is demonstrated post-natally at three months, pyeloplasty should be deferred and only performed if function deteriorates, as judged by careful follow-up with ultrasound scan and the use of Diuretic ^{99m}Tc-DTPA scans. The problem of which kidneys benefit from surgery needs to be carefully considered by randomised long-term trials, if we are not to fall into the trap that we seem to have fallen into in the past with regard to surgery for ureteric reflux. Shanon and Feldman recently reviewed the literature on vesico-ureteric reflux and drew attention to the flawed trials carried out in this problematical area.[11] We should not repeat the mistakes in the newly defined problem areas in the 1990s.

The effects of surgery

The understanding of the effects of the intervention itself, anaesthesia and surgery, is still at an early stage and can be illustrated by the changes in the management of diaphragmatic hernia. This is a subject of great debate at the present time among paediatric surgeons and this debate is likely to continue into the 1990s. The accepted wisdom up to the early 1980s was that the operation for a baby's diaphragmatic hernia should be carried out immediately the diagnosis was made. The overall results of early surgery were bad, giving an overall survival rate of about 50% in most centres. A delayed approach was adopted in several centres in an uncontrolled way, the intention being to stabilise the baby's condition if possible over 24–48 hours, and then to carry out the operation as a planned procedure. Initial results show that this approach has at least no worse survival rates.[12] Two neonatal surgical units are presently carrying out a randomised trial to compare early versus delayed surgery.

Recent work by Bos *et al.*[13] might provide an explanation of why early surgery may be detrimental. Studies showing the impact of endogenous prostanoids in the peri-operative period indicate that surgery itself may provoke persistent pulmonary hypertension due to the release of thromboxane. It is suggested that this may be less likely to occur if surgery is delayed and the patient stabilised for 24–48 hours. Studies on the effects of anaesthesia and surgery in the term and pre-term infant show that their metabolic stress is different,[5] and also that changes in the management of anaesthesia affect these responses and, if properly managed, are associated with less stress and with improved clinical outcome.[6]

It is possible to salvage cases of diaphragmatic hernia that are dying on conventional ventilatory support by the use of extra corporeal membrane oxygenation (ECMO). However, the reported series so far lack satisfactory controls, and the criteria for ECMO seem to vary from one centre to another. A recent leading article in the *British Medical Journal* emphasised the need for such controlled trials. It is expensive and labour-intensive treatment. The suggestion of Sosnowski *et al.*[14] in the *BMJ* leader, that a small number of neonatal units are geared up to perform controlled trials, is a sensible one.

Ultrasound and prenatal diagnosis has also raised the possibility of fetal surgery for conditions such as diaphragmatic hernia, posturethral valves, and hydrocephalus. The reports so far do not show significant improvement in prognosis following *in-utero* procedures. In 200 fetuses with bilateral hydronephrosis, investigated by Harrison *et al.*, only five met criteria which they felt justified open fetal surgery. Three of these fetuses had the return of normal amniotic fluid dynamics, and all three survived the neonatal period and had adequate pulmonary function.[15] However, such surgery means that the mother has to undergo two major surgical procedures, and I think the justification for this is dubious.

The very low birth-weight infant has had its impact on neonatal surgery, mainly in the areas of management of necrotising enterocolitis, post-haemorrhagic hydrocephalus, and the management of inguinal hernias. Necrotising enterocolitis is still an enigma for the physicians and surgeons concerned. With established disease, a decision about timing of operative intervention is a difficult one, dependent on many factors, but particularly on the general condition of the baby, the local findings on clinical examination of the abdomen, and whether the baby is responding to antibiotics and supportive measures. In the 1990s we need better epidemiological studies to define the role of possible vascular mediators, and to predict more accurately the outcome of necrotising enterocolitis. Some form of non-invasive telemetric monitoring of gastro-intestinal motility, and multi-centre trials on the prevention of necrotising enterocolitis, should be priorities for the 1990s.[16]

Urology

In paediatric urology, one of the common problems is that of hypospadias, and here the emphasis has been towards one-stage surgery and to do the operation at about one to two years of age. One-stage surgery involves excising the chordee and using the prepucial flap, either as a free graft or based on the pedicle, bringing it round on to the ventral surface and suturing it into a tube. These advances have been possible by the use of magnification during the surgery, and the use of much finer suture materials. The use of soft silastic stents in the urethra rather than catheters into the bladder has also been an advance, since the stents need less management, and it is possible in certain circumstances to allow children to go home at an earlier stage following surgery. The thinking behind the moves towards early surgery and discharge is to lessen the physical and psychological impact on the child.

There is also an increasing trend to manage undescended testis earlier in the child's life, and certainly within the first two years after birth.[17] Here, we have to strike a balance between the preservation of spermatogenesis by early surgery and the possibility of damage to testicular vessels in the very small infant. There is almost certainly a trade-off between early surgery and damage to the testicular vessels, but there are no accurate figures available on this.

The other problem in relation to undescended testis that is causing concern in surgical circles is the question of the definite increase in the orchidopexy operations carried out, in relationship to the true incidence of undescended testes. The major problem regarding the diagnosis of undescended testes has been the difficulty in differentiating between true non-descent and the retractile testis. The other clinical problem is that of the ascending testis, and this has only been recognised as a distinct entity in the past few years.[18] Its incidence is unknown. It is also important to differentiate between palpable and non-palpable testes, since the non-palpable testis is often more difficult to bring into a satisfactory position in the scrotum and there is also a higher incidence of malformation of the vas and epididymis.[19] In the non-palpable testis which lies within the abdomen, re-plantation by microvascular surgery probably gives the best chance of a useful viable testis.[20]

Transplantation surgery

Transplantation is an area where our attitudes must change, and adoption of the presently available methods could make a major impact. Here, I make a plea for all paediatricians and paediatric surgeons to consider all dying patients as potential donors for kidney, liver, heart, and cornea, unless there are specific contra-indications.

In liver transplantation, the technique of reduction of liver size[21] means that more donors will be made available for the younger child, and the age limit in transplantation can be brought down. Cardiac transplantation in infancy has shown good short-term results and may become effective therapy for lethal cardiac disease.[22]

With the continuing development of fibre-optics, we are now able to look further into ever-smaller orifices, and ureteroscopy and nephroscopy, which are at present only available to adults, will become available to children. Arthroscopy is a rapidly developing field for both diagnosis and treatment with much less disturbance than open surgery to joints. This is especially true in investigation of knee-joint problems in children.

The laparoscope in abdominal surgery will be more widely used for diagnosis and treatment. For example, in experimental animals, liver trauma has been treated with success by laparoscopic treatment by sealing tears in the liver with tissue glue.

References

1. Lloyd-Thomas, A.R. (1990) Pain management in paediatric patients. *British Journal of Anaesthesia*, **64**, 85–104.
2. Working Party Report (1990) *Pain after surgery*. Commission on the Provision of Surgical Services: Royal College of Surgeons of England, College of Anaesthetists, London.
3. McNicol, L.R., Martin, C.S., Smart, N.G., Logan, R.W. (1990) Pre-operative bupivacaine for pyloromyotomy pain. *Lancet*, **i**, 54–55.
4. Scott, J.E.S., Renwick, M. (1990) Northern Region Fetal Abnormality Survey Results 1987. *Journal of Paediatric Surgery*, **4**, 394–397.
5. Anand, K.J.S., Brown, M.F., Causon, R.C. *et al.* (1985) Can the human neonate mount an endocrine and metabolic response to surgery? *Journal of Paediatric Surgery*, **20**, 41–48.
6. Anand, K.J.S., Sippell, W.G., Aynsley-Green, A.A. (1987). Randomised controlled trial of fentanyl anaesthesia in pre-term babies undergoing surgery: effects on the stress response. *Lancet*, **i**, 243–248.
7. Clarke, N.W., Gough, D.C.S., Cohen, S.J. (1989) Neonatal urological ultrasound: Diagnostic accuracies and pitfalls. *Archives of Disease in Childhood*, **64**, 578–580.
8. Bachman, H., Winkielman, J., Olding, H. (1988). Unilateral multi-cystic kidney dysplasia: Follow-up during the first two years of life. *Contributions of Nephrology*, **67**, 188–192.
9. Jung, W.H., Peters, C.A., Madell, J. *et al.* (1990) Flow cytometric evaluation of multi-cystic dysplastic kidneys. *Journal of Urology*, **144**, 413–415.
10. Ransley, P.G., Dhillon, H.K., Gordon, I. *et al.* (1990) The post-natal management of hydronephrosis diagnosed by pre-natal ultrasound. *Journal of Urology*, **144**, 584–587.
11. Shanon, A., Feldman, W. (1990) Methodologic limitations in the literature on vesico-ureteral reflux. A critical review. *Journal of Paediatrics*, **117**, 171–178.
12. Shanbhogue, L.K.R., Tam, R.K.H., Ninan, G., Lloyd, D.A. (1990) Pre-operative stabilisation in congenital diaphragmatic hernia. *Archives of Disease in Childhood*, **65**, 1043–1044.
13. Bos, A.P., Tibboel, D., Hazebrook, F.W.J. *et al.* (1990) Congenital diaphragmatic hernia: impact of prostanoids in the perioperative period. *Archives of Disease in Childhood*, **65**, 994–995.
14. Sosnowski, A.W., Bonser, S.J., Field, D.J. *et al.* Extra corporeal membrane oxygenation. Britain needs units equipped to perform the procedure and a controlled trial. *British Medical Journal*, **301**, 303–304.
15. Longaker, M.T., Adzick, N.S., Harrison, M.R. (1989) Foetal obstructive uropathy. *British Medical Journal*, **299**, 325–326.
16. McLead, R.E. (1990) Neonatal necrotising enterocolitis: current concepts and controversies. *Journal of Paediatrics*, **117**, S1–S74.
17. Gough, M.H. (1989) Cryptorchidism. *British Journal of Surgery*, **76**, 109–112.
18. Atwell, J.D. (1985) Ascent of the testis: fact or fiction. *British Journal of Urology*, **57**, 474.
19. De Palma, L., Carter, D., Weiss, R.M. (1988) Epididymal and vas deferens. Immaturity in cryptorchidism. *Journal of Urology*, **140**, 1194–1196.
20. Hanyson, C.B., Kaplan, G.W., Scherz, H.C. *et al.* (1990) Microvascular autotransplantation of intra-abdominal testis. *Journal of Urology*, **144**, 506–507.

21. Sokal, E.M., Veyckemans, F., de Ville de Goyet, J. *et al.* (1990) Liver transplantation in children less than 1 year of age. *Journal of Paediatrics*, **117**, 205–210.
22. Boucek, M.M., Kanakiyeh, M.S., Mathis, C.M. *et al.* and the Loma Linda University Pediatric Heart Transplant Group (1990). Cardiac transplantation in infancy: donors and recipients. *Journal of Pediatrics*, **116**, 171–176.

11 | Paediatric gastroenterology

P. J. Milla
Institute of Child Health, and Hospital for Sick Children, London

During the past few years paediatric gastroenterology has come of age. What was once an obscure subspecialty has emerged as a specialised field of medicine based upon an impressive expansion of knowledge related to the structure, function, and development of the gastrointestinal tract. This rapid increase of our understanding of the pathophysiology of many gastrointestinal disorders, often combined with spectacular technological developments enabling us to observe hitherto mysterious events in the gut, has laid the foundations for a higher level of professional expertise amongst paediatricians. In this short review I will highlight a number of general concepts which are of importance in paediatric gastroenterology, and those developments of the past five years which seem to me either to have altered, or probably will alter, the practice of the paediatrician dealing with gastrointestinal disorder.

Childhood and its effects on gastrointestinal disease

Childhood is a period of growth and of integrated and complex maturation of tissues, both of which are genetically determined. The susceptibility of children to disease processes and their response to them are often conditioned by the stage of maturation of a whole range of developmental processes. Such conditioning may result in symptoms which are in response not only to normal developmental events but also to the impact that gastrointestinal disease may have on the patient of a particular age, or to the profile of gastrointestinal disorder in the child. Examples of the effects of particular stages of development will be readily evident in many of the advances described below, but an obvious example of a normal developmental event is the jaundice seen for the first two or three days of life in many healthy full-term infants as the child's capacity to conjugate bilirubin matures. The profile of disease in the infant is different from that in the adolescent or adult. For example, obvious blood in the stool of an adult may indicate a colonic neoplasm but in an infant is more likely to suggest a Meckel's diverticulum.

Lastly, by virtue of its state of development, the child may be particularly vulnerable to disorders such as enteric infection. Since the immune system and mucosal function continue to mature after birth, the intestine of young infants is highly susceptible to infection. Such infection is particularly hazardous for young infants as it results in systemic dehydration and electrolyte imbalance due to the lack of reserve absorptive function, dependence on parents and nurses for an adequate fluid intake, and immaturity of compensating mechanisms. Disease which also limits food intake, or in which there is excessive faecal nutrient loss, will also cause failure to thrive (poor weight gain, delayed growth and development) relatively early in infants compared to older children. However, the impact of gastrointestinal disease on nutritional status is particularly noticeable in any period of rapid growth and maturity, and this occurs not only in infancy but also in adolescence.

The gastrointestinal tract is a complex organ with obvious topographical variations in function. The acquisition of energy for normal growth and development is largely carried out by digestion and absorption of nutrients in the small intestine with some conservation of malabsorbed nutrients in the colon. Disease or dysfunction of these parts of the gut occurs commonly in children who are not thriving, usually resulting in protracted diarrhoeal disease.

The small intestine and protracted diarrhoeal disease

The small intestine is the major site of digestion and absorption of nutrients, water, and electrolytes in the gut. Disease therefore frequently results in chronic diarrhoea and malnutrition. The disorders

Table 1. Protracted diarrhoea of infancy.

Aetiology	% of cases
Food sensitive enteropathy	56
Congenital and inherited defects	20
Autoimmune enteropathy	10
Colitis	2
Tumours	1
Structural anomalies	1
Idiopathic	10

causing diarrhoea are heterogeneous in nature,[1] but in over 80% an enteropathy is involved. In about 70% of the total number of patients a cause can be identified.[1] The remaining unexplained cases almost certainly represent a range of several different conditions and have a high mortality;[2] the average consultant paediatrician might see one such patient every year. Table 1 lists the causes at present known. In the past five years some progress has been made with previously unexplained cases and new methods of diagnosis explored in commoner conditions, especially coeliac disease.

Enteropathies

In over 80% of children with chronic diarrhoea and failure to thrive an enteropathy is involved. In about 60% this is as a result of sensitivity to foods due to a variety of causes, of which post-infectious and associated immunodeficiency appear to be the commonest. Nearly always the food sensitivity is transient and disappears after the age of two to three years.[3] The commonest food inducing such a transient food sensitive enteropathy is cow's milk, but we now know that other foods such as egg, fish, rice, chicken, and wheat may also induce an enteropathy.[4] In the 20% of cases of protracted diarrhoea in which no cause can be identified, at least two-thirds were previously due to an unidentified enteropathy which had a high morbidity and mortality. In recent years some progress has been made in elucidating the nature of such idiopathic enteropathic processes, and two new conditions have been described. For one of these, treatment has been devised.

Auto-immune enteropathy

Isolated cases of idiopathic protracted diarrhoea of infancy have been described in which circulating auto-antibodies to gut enterocytes have been shown by classic indirect immunofluorescent techniques.[5,6] These initial reports suggested that an auto-immune disorder with characteristics similar to those in other well-recognised organ-specific auto-immune diseases, such as hypothyroidism thyrotoxicosis or insulin-dependent diabetes mellitus, might account for some of the hitherto unexplained cases of protracted diarrhoea of infancy.

Mirakian[7] and her colleagues investigated and reported a large series of children with protracted diarrhoea of infancy for which a cause could not be found despite extensive investigation. Circulating auto-antibodies to enterocytes were detected by indirect immunofluorescence in 14 out of 25 patients with idiopathic protracted diarrhoea of infancy. Similar antibodies were not found in 50 children without gastrointestinal disease, 10 children with coeliac disease, and in only three out of 56 patients with chronic inflammatory bowel disease. In over 900 other non-gastrointestinal disease controls no enterocyte antibodies were found. The enterocyte antibodies were mainly IgG and were directed usually at a brush border antigen but sometimes to a cytoplasmic antigen. Other organ-specific and non-organ-specific autoantibodies were often found. High antibody titres, together with complement fixing ability and other organ-specific auto-antibodies, were associated with more severe disease and a worse prognosis. Diagnosis is dependent on the demonstration of at least an enteropathy, but often there is a pan-gut inflammatory disease, and circulating antibodies directed against enterocytes. The disorder should be suspected in those infants with protracted diarrhoea in whom more than one region of the gut is affected, who have not responded to simple dietary occlusion therapy, and/or have evidence of other organ-specific or non-organ-specific auto-immune disease.

A variety of treatments have been used, including oligo-antigenic diets, intravenous nutritional support where required, and immunomodulatory and immunosuppressive regimes. Of the latter, combinations of prednisolone and azathioprine or cyclosporin have proved most effective, but the numbers of patients seen are too small for controlled trials to be undertaken. At the present time it is recommended that when such a condition is suspected, the patient should be referred to a specialist centre.

Congenital microvillus atrophy

Between 1978 and 1985 a number of reports of infants with lethal protracted diarrhoea appeared. Some of these infants suffered from a condition that Schmitz[8] termed 'congenital microvillus atrophy'. Patients suffering from this condition usually present with diarrhoea from birth or within the first week of life. In some cases maternal polyhydramnios suggests diarrhoea *in utero*. The initial reports suggested that this condition might be inherited as an autosomal recessive trait, and certainly this appears to be true of some families.[9]

The diarrhoea is secretory in nature with a high electrolyte content, and continues despite withholding oral nutrition and providing adequate parenteral nutrition. The diagnosis is made on intestinal biopsy material. In the small intestine there is a uniform hypoplastic villus atrophy with a loss of villus height without crypt hyperplasia, resulting in thin mucosa but no increased inflammatory infiltrate in the lamina propria. Ultrastructural studies using the electron microscope reveal dramatic and unique changes. The surface epithelial cells have shortened infrequent microvilli, increased lysosomal bodies, and membrane-bound inclusions containing obvious microvillar components. These microvillous inclusions are the most obvious major diagnostic feature. Crypt enterocytes contain increased numbers of secretory granules but are otherwise normal. Colonic epithelium, where examined, has shown similar findings.

It has been suggested that this disorder is due to an abnormality of the cytoskeleton supporting the apical brush border membrane.[10] At the present time no effective treatment is known and the majority of patients have ultimately died either from the intractable diarrhoea or from the complications of parenteral nutrition.

Coeliac disease

This condition is the commonest cause for an enteropathy outside infancy. Its diagnosis is, however, somewhat clumsy and is based upon a set of rigorous criteria known as the 'ESPGAN' criteria, as shown in Table 2. These criteria arose from a meeting of the European Society for Paediatric Gastroenterology and Nutrition in 1969,[11] because of the difficulty sometimes encountered in arriving at a firm diagnosis. As discussed above, we now know many foods which in infancy may induce an enteropathy, and additionally these are usually transient conditions. Thus the ESPGAN criteria have proved a valuable guide to diagnosis and have stood the test of time. The heart of these criteria is the biopsy-controlled gluten challenge. In children over the age of three years, when an initial biopsy shows a crypt hyperplasia subtotal villus atrophy, who clinically respond to a gluten-free diet, it is highly likely that they suffer from coeliac disease, and many have questioned the need for children to undergo a biopsy-controlled gluten challenge. There are three circumstances where such a challenge is desirable:

1. if there is doubt about the original diagnosis, ie no initial diagnostic biopsy or biopsy inadequate or not characteristic;
2. if the child was under the age of three years at initial diagnosis;
3. if the patient or parent wishes to abandon the diet.

Table 2. Criteria for the diagnosis of coeliac disease (ESPGAN criteria).

1. Histologically abnormal small intestinal mucosa (usually subtotal villous atrophy).
2. Clinical and histological response to a gluten-free diet.
3. Histological with or without clinical relapse following gluten challenge.

New diagnostic tools

Gliadin antibodies

The presence of IgA antigliadin antibodies in the peripheral circulation may provide information which is diagnostically useful especially in association with a gluten challenge. This serological approach has been particularly used in countries where non-coeliac enteropathy is very uncommon, and in those communities has separated normal individuals from those with coeliac disease with a high degree of specificity.[12] However, in those parts of the world such as northern Europe where non-coeliac enteropathy, at least in infancy, is common, or in the developing world where small intestinal damage following acute gastroenteritis is common, positivity in such enteropathies occurs and specificity is considerably lower. It is only by the use of the ESPGAN criteria that a clear diagnosis is possible under those circumstances.[13]

Intra-epithelial lymphocytes

The change in density of intra-epithelial lymphocytes (IEL) in coeliac disease in response to gluten has been regarded as useful in the diagnosis in both children and adults, though it is not specific. Recent studies using monoclonal antibodies have shown the distinctive nature of intra-epithelial lymphocytes and that most of them are suppressor-cytotoxic phenotype, ie they are CD3 CD8 +ve. However, a small population is subset negative; that is, both CD8 and CD4 negative. In normal small intestine about 5% are CD3+CD8−CD4− but in coeliac disease nearly 30% fall into this category.[14] Further studies of IEL show that the T-cell receptor that they express may be of either the α/β dimer or the γ/δ dimer. Two groups have now shown that in normal mucosa about 10% of IELs express γ/δ receptors but in coeliac disease over 30% express γ/δ receptors when the mucosa is in relapse, and when in remission with morphologically normal mucosa the high proportion of IELs bearing γ/δ receptors remains.[15,16] Thus if those observations are confirmed it may become possible to diagnose coeliac disease on a single jejunal biopsy.

Transplantation

Transplantation of kidney, heart and lung, bone marrow, and liver are now established forms of treatment for chronic progressive organ failure which will inevitably result in death. In gastroenterology liver transplantation has been transformed in recent years from a highly experimental procedure to one which, although many problems remain, is now becoming a form of treatment to be considered in those with liver disease who might die without transplantation in under two years.[17]

Liver transplantation

Data from the European Liver Transplant Register indicate that of 3,614 transplants, 612 were done in children, and of 1,000 liver transplants performed since cyclosporin became available, 334 have been done in children.[18] Actuarial analysis in those over the age of one year showed a one-year survival rate of 74% and a five-year survival rate of 64%. The five-year survival rate for those transplanted under the age of one year was considerably lower at 37%.

Indications for liver transplantation are shown in Table 3. Major complications in those transplanted under the age of one year include primary non-function of the graft, sepsis, and vascular thrombosis.[18] Thirty percent require retransplantation. Results tend to be better in those electively transplanted rather than given emergency transplants. Post-transplant infection is a major problem. In the early stages endogenous recipient infection (eg tuberculosis), infection transmitted with the graft (eg hepatitis), cytomegalovirus, and wound infections are the main problems. Later cytomegalovirus, E-B virus and hepatitis together with opportunistic infections emerge as problems. Those patients with good graft function and minimal immunosuppression are at risk of community infections such as pneumococcus and meningococcus. The optimal immunosuppressive regimes with minimal side-effects and no rejection or infection remain to be defined.

Small intestinal transplantation

Children who have ultra-short bowel syndrome or untreatable small intestinal diseases sometimes are left in the position of depending

Table 3. Liver disorders of children undergoing liver transplantation.

Biliary atresia	52%
Metabolic disease	15%
Cholestatic disorders	8%
Cirrhosis	7%
Acute hepatic failure	7%
Other	11%

Figures derived from the European Transplant Register

upon parenteral nutrition for the rest of their lives. The availability of home parenteral nutrition has revolutionised the outlook for these patients and their families. Such treatment is not, however, without the continued threat of serious complications, and is expensive. A logical form of treatment for such patients is small bowel transplantation. Experience to date has only accrued from a few centres, notably Pittsburgh and Paris. The recent experience in Paris has for the most part been somewhat depressing, but there are a few areas where progress is being made.

Small intestinal transplantation was carried out in six children. The first graft was removed at eight hours for ischaemic reasons and the child reverted to the home parenteral nutrition. Early or delayed graft rejection occurred in all the remaining grafts, and despite treatment three were ultimately removed for chronic rejection. However, in four grafts, the patients tolerated up to 90% of their required enteral calorie intake.[19] This experience, together with the success of duodenal grafts as part of pancreatic transplantation, provides both experimental and ethical justification for seriously considering small intestinal transplantation where it is clear that the underlying cause of serious chronic gut failure is untreatable.[20]

Gastrointestinal motility

Until ten years ago there were virtually no studies of gastrointestinal motility in children. With advances in the physiology of gastrointestinal smooth muscle and enteric nerves, and the recognition of the importance of patterns of organisation of smooth muscle contraction, a new impetus to the understanding of gastrointestinal motility in man occurred. Systematic studies of motility were conducted in children, the results of which are now beginning to affect paediatric practice. The role of disordered motility in gastrointestinal disease in children, and how an understanding of the motor disorder has affected clinical management, is perhaps best illustrated by considering gastro-oesophageal reflux and related diseases.

Gastro-oesophageal reflux

Regurgitation of feeds because of gastro-oesophageal reflux (GOR) is common in young infants and in most is little more than an inconvenience. In some, however, regurgitation is symptomatic and results in the serious symptoms shown in Table 4. Carre[21] showed that 60% of infants who regurgitated stopped by 18 months of age with most symptoms settling by the age of 9 months. Thirty percent continued

Table 4. Presentation of gastro-oesophageal reflux and related disease.

Regurgitation symptoms	
Failure to thrive	– Impaired calorie intake due to excessive vomiting. Refusal to eat.
Anaemia Haematemesis Agitation and pain on feeding	– Oesophagitis, with or without stricture formation.
Recurrent respiratory disorder	– Apnoea and asthma, associated with reflux. Pneumonia—aspirated refluxed material.

to have symptoms until at least four years of age and 10% developed one or more of the complicating disorders shown in Table 4.

Gastro-oesophageal reflux may occur because of a variety of defects of function and structure of the oesophagus and diaphragm. It is clear, however, that a difference in pressure between the stomach and oesophagus is important, as is failure of the mechanisms to prevent flow down that pressure gradient. Thus the lower oesophageal sphincter (LOS) and motility of the oesophagus are important. Three groups of disorder occur:

1. low basal sphincter pressure;
2. transient LOS relaxation—either synchronous or asynchronous with swallowing;
3. transient increases in intra-abdominal or gastric pressure.

In most of us some GOR occurs after a meal due to rise of gastric pressure, with reflux occurring when there is complete relaxation of the LOS, as in swallowing. In the normal individual such refluxed material is rapidly cleared from the oesophagus by secondary peristalsis. In children with symptomatic GOR most reflux episodes are due to transient LOS relaxations which are asynchronous with swallowing.[22] However, in those infants who merely 'spit up' the mechanism is different. Here infants reflux synchronously with swallowing and the LOS seems to be relaxed for a longer period of time than normal. Thus their reflux is due to an exaggeration of physiological reflux that occurs after eating. Low basal sphincter pressures are unusual in GOR and are only found in severe oesophagitis or neurological disorders. Thus the idea of GOR being caused by a lax cardio-oesophageal sphincter is not borne out by scientific study. Whether oesophagitis occurs or not is dependent on the ability of the infant to clear the oesophagus of refluxed acid. In infants with symptomatic GOR acid-clearance times are prolonged, with evidence of disordered oesophageal motility which is most severe in those with oesophagitis.[22] There is some evidence to suggest underlying diseases of the motor control mechanism.[23] In term and preterm neonates there is evidence of gestationally dependent changes in the LOS.[24] Carre's studies clearly showed that infants with GOR followed a different developmental profile from those who did not regurgitate, and this would seem most commonly to be related to the development of control of the LOS during swallowing. In those with symptomatic GOR the developmental delay is not confined to the LOS but also involves the oesophageal body and seems to be very much more profound. Thus whether GOR is trivial or serious is dependent upon the nature of the underlying disorder of oesophageal motor activity rather than the presence or absence of a hiatus hernia, which is merely a radiological description of the behaviour of the intra-abdominal segment of the oesophagus and is seen with equal frequency in trivial or symptomatic GOR.

Investigation of the child suspected of having GOR is in three stages: demonstration of the presence and severity of GOR, the presence of complications, and the presence of underlying disorders which might give rise to GOR.

Demonstrations of presence and severity

The 'gold' standard at the present time is undoubtedly 24-hour ambulatory oesophageal pH monitoring with computerised data capture and analysis. Barium meal and scintiscanning both have serious drawbacks. In the former GOR is missed in up to 40% of studies, and in the latter the patient needs to lie still for at least one hour.

Presence of complications

A number of investigations are required: a full blood-count for iron deficiency anaemia, a chest X-ray, a search for fat-laden macrophages in the sputum where aspiration is suspected, and endoscopy with biopsy to detect oesophagitis. Where GOR is associated with fits or apnoea a pH study combined with apnoea monitoring, sleep studies, or an EEG may be very useful.

Presence of underlying disease

Gastro-oesophageal reflux that presents atypically may be the first indication of a cerebral tumour, and thus a CAT or MRI scan may be required. Disturbance of gastric emptying, as for instance in pyloric stenosis or a malrotation, may be associated with GOR and thus there is no place for a barium swallow in the investigation of GOR, but a barium meal with limited follow-through is helpful in defining the anatomy of the foregut. Suspected pseudo-obstructive disorders require specialist gastroenterological investigation.

Management

Gastro-oesophageal reflux may be controlled by a number of interventions: positioning, thickening of feeds, pharmacological agents, and surgery. The tendency for GOR in infants to resolve spontaneously has led to confusion regarding the indications for treatment and their merit. Some indications of the type of treatment that is likely to be successful can be gained from a knowledge of the severity of the reflux. Those in whom over 30% of a 24-hour period is spent with oesophageal pH below 4 will almost always ultimately require surgery, though a trial of intensive medical treatment should be carried out first.[24] Those with moderate (10–20%) or mild (5–10%) symptoms will usually be helped by medical means until such time as development of the oesophageal smooth muscle and myenteric plexus has proceeded to the point where reflux is no longer a problem.

Specific medical treatments have recently been reviewed and will not be considered here further.[25] Where medical treatment has failed surgery should be seriously considered and the arguments for and against this have also been the subject of recent debate.[25,26] In the past five years the nature of GOR in children and its association with the ontogeny of oesophageal motor function has been understood. More specific approaches to management are being developed related to objective assessment of GOR and related disease.

The future

Over the next five years it is clear that a number of developments will take place, some of which will have an impact on the practice of the physician who has occasion to deal with serious gastrointestinal disease.

Small intestinal diseases

The advent of monoclonal antibody techniques has revolutionised our ability to diagnose and treat some disorders. The therapeutic use of monoclonal antibodies is considered in Chapter 8. In gastrointestinal disorders they are likely to be of use in transplantation and in severe enteropathies associated with auto-immune disease and serious immunodeficiency disorders. In specialist centres diagnostic use of such antibodies as outlined for coeliac disease will become routine and should become available at regional and district level. It is likely that the nature of at present poorly understood or idiopathic enteropathies will become clearer as knowledge of factors related to growth and the structure of enterocytes increases.

Transplantation

Even though liver transplantation is now at a level of success comparable to other transplanted organs, a number of problems remain which are being energetically tackled by combined multi-centre studies. This is especially the case in terms of graft rejection and graft-versus-host disease. It is likely that improved conditioning and post-transplant regimes will be developed to deal with these problems.

In childhood liver transplantation, donor organ availability remains a major problem. However, the use of part-organ grafting and the development of extended *in vitro* preservation will do much to alleviate this problem. Small intestinal transplantation remains experimental but there are a number of observations which suggest that what a few years ago appeared to be a near impossible task may well in the 1990s become a clinical possibility in selected centres.

Gastrointestinal motility

The past ten years have seen the emergence of an understanding of the role of gastrointestinal motility in some disease processes in children. However, such knowledge has only been gathered by the use of difficult invasive techniques which hardly allow repeated use. Non-invasive methods are and will be developed to allow not only diagnosis but also objective monitoring of therapeutic interventions. One such method is that of surface electrogastrography, which is now at an advanced stage of development. In this method electrical activity of the stomach is recorded in a manner analogous to that of an electrocardiogram.

It is clear that much gastrointestinal disorder of infants is related to the state of development of the gut; this is particularly true of gastrointestinal motility, yet our state of knowledge regarding this is extremely fragmentary. It is likely that this area, together with studies to understand the nature of gastrointestinal neuromuscular disease, will develop during the 1990s.

References

1. Larcher, V.F., Shepherd, R., Francis, D.E.M., Harries, J.T. (1977) Protracted diarrhoea of infancy. Analysis of 82 cases with particular references to diagnosis and management. *Archives of Disease in Childhood*, **52**, 597–605.
2. Candy, D.C.A., Larcher, V.F., Cameron, D.J.S. *et al.* (1981) Lethal familial diarrhoea. *Archives of Disease in Childhood*, **56**, 15–23.
3. Walker-Smith, J. (1975) Cow's milk protein intolerance. Transient food intolerance of infancy. *Archives of Disease in Childhood*, **50**, 347–350.
4. Walker-Smith, J. (1986) Food sensitive enteropathies. *Clinical Gastroenterology*, **15**, 55–69.
5. McCarthy, D.M., Katz, S., Gazze, L. *et al.* (1978) Selective IgA deficiency associated with total villous atrophy of the small intestine and an organ-specific antiepithelial cell antibody. *Journal of Immunology*, **120**, 932–937.
6. Savage, M.O., Mirakian, R., Wozniak, E.R. *et al.* (1985) Specific auto-antibodies to gut epithelium in two infants with severe protracted diarrhoea. *Journal of Paediatric Gastroenterology and Nutrition*, **4**, 187–195.
7. Mirakian, R., Richardson, A., Milla, P.J. *et al.* (1986) Protracted diarrhoea of infancy: evidence in support of an auto-immune variant. *British Medical Journal*, **292**, 1132–1136.
8. Schmitz, J., Ginies, J.L., Arnaud-Batlandier, F. *et al.* (1982) Congenital microvillus atrophy: a rare cause of neonatal intractable diarrhoea. *Pediatric Research*, **16**, 1014.
9. Phillips, A.D., Jenkins, P., Raafat, F., Walker-Smith, J.A. (1985) Congenital microvillus atrophy: specific diagnostic features. *Archives of Disease in Childhood*, **60**, 135–140.
10. Carruthers, L., Dourmashkin, R., Phillips, A. (1986) Disorders of the cytoskeleton of the enterocytes. *Clinical Gastroenterology*, **15**, 105–121.
11. Meeuwisse, G. (1970) Diagnostic criteria in coeliac disease. *Acta Paediatrica Scandinavica*, **59**, 461.
12. Burgin-Wolff, A., Gaze, H., Lentze, M., Nussle, D. (1991) Gliadin and endonysium antibody determinators in childhood coeliac disease. In *Proceedings of International Coeliac Symposium*, ed Kumar, P., Walker-Smith, J.A. Oxford, Blackwell Scientific Publications (in press).
13. Suleman, G.I. (1978) Coeliac disease in Sudanese children. *Gut*, **19**, 121.
14. Spencer, J., MacDonald, T., Diss, T.C. *et al.* (1989) Changes in intra-epithelial lymphocyte sub populations in coeliac disease and enteropathy associated T cell lymphoma. *Gut*, **30**, 339–346.
15. Spencer, J., Diss, T.C., Walker-Smith, J.A. *et al.* (1991) T-cell receptor suppression by intra-epithelial lymphocytes in normal and coeliac jejuvum. *Gastroenterology* (in press).
16. Saidahm, E., Arato, A., Verkasolo, M. (1991) Constant increase of gamma/delta + T cells in coeliacs. *Pediatric Research* (in press).
17. Shaw, B.W., Wood, R.P., Kaufmann, S.S. *et al.* (1988) Liver transplant therapy for children (2 parts). *Journal of Paediatric Gastroenterology and Nutrition*, **7**, 157–166, 797–815.
18. Iwatsuki, S., Starzl, T.E., Todo, S. *et al.* (1988) Experience in 1000 liver transplants under cyclosporine-steroid therapy: a survival report. *Transplant Proceedings*, **20** (suppl 1), 498–504.
19. Goulet, O., Revillon, Y., Jan, D. *et al.* (1991) Small intestinal transplantation in children. *Pediatric Research* (in press).
20. Schraut, W.M. (1988) Current status of small bowel transplantation. *Gastroenterology*, **94**, 525–538.
21. Carre, I.J. (1959) The natural history of the partial thoracic stomach (hiatus hernia) in children. *Archives of Disease in Childhood*, **34**, 344–353.

22. Mahony, M.J., Migliavacca, M., Spitz, L., Milla, P.J. (1988) Motor disorders of the oesophagus in gastro-oesophageal reflux. *Archives of Disease in Childhood*, **63**, 1333–1338.
23. Eckardt, V.F. (1988) Does healing of oesophagitis improve oesophageal function? *Digestive Disease Sciences*, **33**, 161–165.
24. Da Dalt, L., Mazzoleni, B., Montini, G. *et al.* (1989) Diagnostic accuracy of pH monitoring in gastro-oesophageal reflux. *Archives of Disease in Childhood*, **64**, 1421–1426.
25. Milla, P.J. (1990) Reflux vomiting. *Archives of Disease in Childhood*, **65**, 996–999.
26. Spitz, L. (1982) Surgical treatment of gastro-oesophageal reflux in severely mentally retarded children. *Journal of the Royal Society of Medicine*, **75**, 525–529.

12 | Infectious diseases

Michael Levin
St Mary's Hospital Medical School, London

Introduction

Infectious diseases account for a large proportion of paediatric hospital admissions and out-patient consultations. To some extent all paediatricians are specialists in the infectious diseases of children, and are familiar with the management of common infections. However, over the past two decades there have been a large number of advances, which have increased the need for subspecialist expertise in infectious diseases.

Several new infectious diseases have been recognised, some of which have emerged as important paediatric problems (Table 1). These include human immunodeficiency virus (HIV) infection, the staphylococcal and streptococcal toxic shock syndromes, Lyme disease, Brazilian purpuric fever, Kawasaki disease, and Erhlichiosis. In addition to the recognition of new syndromes and diseases, the aetiological agents of several well-established paediatric diseases have been identified, human parvo-virus has been shown to be the cause of Fifth disease, human herpes virus 6 is probably the cause of roseola infantum, retroviruses have been established as causing not only the acquired immune deficiency syndrome, but also tropical spastic paraparesis. Among bacterial diseases, toxin-producing staphylococci have been identified as the cause of the toxic shock syndrome, verotoxin-producing *E. coli* as the cause of the haemolytic uraemic syndrome, and *Borrelia burgdorferi* is now established as the cause of Lyme disease.

While the discovery of new diseases and new infectious organisms are exciting advances, the changing epidemiological pattern of well-recognised children's infections are of great importance to all paediatricians. Epidemics of meningococcal disease continue to occur in several parts of the world. The incidence of streptococcal disease is again increasing, and a number of outbreaks of rheumatic fever in affluent societies have been reported. Increasing foreign travel and immigration have resulted in tropical and imported infections being

Table 1. New infectious agents and diseases

Disease	*Causative agent*
AIDS	HIV 1 HIV 2
Tropical spastic paraparesis	HTLV 1
Spongiform encephalopathy	Prions
Roseola infantum	(HH6) Human herpes virus 6
Fifth disease	Human parvo-virus B19
Lyme disease	Borrelia burgdorferi
Toxic shock syndrome	Staphylococcal toxic shock toxin
Non-A non-B hepatitis	Hepatitis C
Kawasaki disease	??
Streptococcal toxic shock syndrome	Group A streptococcus
Atypical pneumonia	Chlamydia pneumoniae
Legionnaires disease	Legionella pneumophila
Cat-scratch disease	Cat-scratch bacillus
Ehrlichiosis	Ehrlichia canis
Brazilian purpuric fever	Haemophilus aegyptius
Diarrhoea	Cryptosporidia
Haemolytic uraemic syndrome	Verotoxin-producing *E. coli*

seen with increasing frequency in all countries. The child returning from a package holiday in Spain may acquire a salmonella infection or an infection due to a penicillin-resistant pneumococcus. Travellers to Africa or the Far East may return with viral haemorrhagic fevers, malaria, dengue, Japanese B encephalitis, and a wide range of other tropical infections. Expertise and knowledge of the range of infections seen world-wide are therefore increasingly required in all countries, as is advice on vaccination and health precautions for travellers.

Advances in other paediatric subspecialties have introduced a new spectrum of infectious diseases. Increasing use of immunosuppressive treatments in haematology and oncology, renal transplantation, cardiac and liver transplantation, as well as advances in neonatology and paediatric surgery, have resulted in a wide variety of unusual opportunistic infections. A major component of the work of infectious disease specialists in the 1990s is the management of opportunistic infections in immunocompromised patients.

An increasing array of anti-microbial agents active against bacteria, viruses, fungi, and parasites have become available. New diagnostic tools have been developed, including monoclonal antibodies, nucleic-acid probes, and the polymerase chain reaction technology (PCR). The increasing understanding of cell and molecular biology has also opened up new avenues for research on the pathogenesis and pathophysiology of infectious diseases. Recognition of the role of host inflammatory responses in the causation of tissue and organ damage in infection has introduced the possibility of immunotherapy and pharmacological manipulation of the inflammatory response as treatments for infectious diseases. Infectious diseases specialists are involved in the production, evaluation, and introduction of new vaccines into clinical practice. It would clearly be impossible to discuss all of these advances, and this paper will therefore focus on only a few aspects which are of particular relevance to the general paediatrician.

New diseases and new infectious agents

The childhood exanthems are a group of diseases which illustrate some of the recent developments in paediatric infectious diseases. Fifteen years ago a child presenting with fever, an erythematous macular rash, and conjunctivitis would usually have been suffering from measles. With the introduction of measles vaccine, and more recently of the measles-mumps-rubella (MMR) vaccine, measles has now become an increasingly rare disease in the United Kingdom, and a new spectrum of infectious diseases need to be considered in the differential diagnosis of the febrile child with an erythematous rash.

The staphylococcal toxic shock syndrome

In 1978 Dr James Todd, working at the Children's Hospital in Denver, reported seven children who presented with fever, erythematous rash, strawberry tongue, conjunctival injection, ulceration of the lips and oropharynx, shock, and multi-organ involvement.[1] Desquamation was observed during the convalescent phase of the disease. The illness appeared to be distinct from previously recognised disorders, and was linked to colonisation or infection with *Staphylococcus aureus*.

In the early 1980s many thousands of cases were reported in the United States, mostly in young women. Careful epidemiological investigations established that menstruation and tampon use were risk factors for the disease, and publicity given to the Tampon Association has led to the disorder being considered largely a problem of adult women. However, cases have continued to occur which are not associated with menstruation, and many of these non-menstrual cases are children. The staphylococcal toxic shock syndrome has been recognised with increasing frequency in the United Kingdom and is an important disease to diagnose and to distinguish from other exanthems.[2]

The toxic shock syndrome usually presents with an acute onset of fever, diarrhoea, confusion, and the characteristic erythematous rash and mucous membrane lesions. In severe cases shock may develop rapidly together with multi-organ failure. Haematological and biochemical findings reveal impaired renal and liver function, anaemia, thrombocytopenia, abnormal coagulation, hypocalcaemia, and elevated muscle enzymes. In some cases there is no specific focus of infection, but *Staphylococcus aureus* may be found colonising the nasopharynx or mucous membranes. In other cases focal infection of surgical wound sites, abrasions, cuts, or the sinuses, are present.

Dr James Todd suggested in his original report that the toxic shock syndrome might be due to an unusual toxin produced by the staphylococcus.[1] This observation has subsequently been confirmed and it now appears that the disorder is caused by a number of related enterotoxins produced by the staphylococcus, the most common of which is called toxic shock toxin 1 (TSS1).[3] Under specific growth conditions, the toxin is produced and is absorbed into the circulation where it causes an intense inflammatory response. TSS1 has been shown to be a potent inducer of cytokine production by macrophages and many of the physiological derangements observed in this illness are probably the result of a widespread activation of host inflammatory mediators.

Although the toxic shock syndrome may be rapidly fatal, if the condition is recognised and appropriately treated, the majority of affected children are likely to survive. Severe cases necessitate admission to an intensive care unit, with aggressive management of shock, replacement of circulating volume, and treatment of organ failure. An important component of treatment is the detection and elimination of the focus of staphylococcal infection.[2,4]

Streptococcal toxic shock syndrome and invasive streptococcal disease

For a generation of paediatricians in the United Kingdom and other developed countries, rheumatic fever, post-streptococcal nephritis, and serious illness due to the group A streptococcus has become a rarity. The decline in importance of the streptococcus as a pathogen was generally attributed to improved living standards and the widespread use of antibiotics. However, it now appears that streptococcal infections undergo spontaneous changes in their epidemiology,[5] as there has been a recent resurgence in rheumatic fever and other serious streptococcal infections in developed countries.[6] Furthermore two new streptococcal-related syndromes have emerged over the past few years.

Streptococcal toxic shock syndrome has features similar to those of the staphylococcal toxic shock syndrome, and presents with shock, multiorgan failure, an erythematous rash which desquamates in the convalescent phase, and mucous membrane and conjunctival involvement.[7] Group A streptococci are isolated from blood or tissues, and probably induce disease by production of one or more toxins. The disease may be fulminant and fatalities have occurred despite aggressive management and intensive care.[8] Another recently reported streptococcal related disorder is that of invasive group A streptococcal infections which have been increasingly reported in young children. Septicaemia, empyema, soft tissue and lymph node infections due to this organism appear to have become more prevalent in many countries in recent years.[9]

Lyme disease

The disorder now known as Lyme disease first came to medical attention when parents in the town of Old Lyme in Connecticut, USA, became concerned that a large number of cases of 'juvenile rheumatoid arthritis' were being diagnosed in their community. Subsequent epidemiological investigations confirmed a greatly increased prevalence of an inflammatory joint disease in the area surrounding the town and implicated exposure to forested areas and tick bites in the causation of the disorder.[10] The suspicion that the disorder was caused by an infectious agent transmitted by tick bites was confirmed when the causative agent, a spirochaete now called *Borrelia burgdorferi*, was isolated from both affected patients and the insect vector, the tick *Ixodes dammini*.[11] A few days to weeks after the bite of an infected tick, the characteristic skin lesion, erythema chronicum migrans, develops. This is an erythematous skin lesion which begins as a red maculopapule and spreads circumferentially, with partial clearing centrally. The initial lesion usually surrounds the site of the bite but secondary lesions may appear in other areas. Skin lesions are often accompanied by fever, headache, generalised achiness, lymphadenopathy, and fatigue. These early symptoms subside and are followed weeks to months later by neurological, cardiac, musculo-skeletal, or arthritic symptoms.[12]

The spectrum of neurological abnormalities ranges from aseptic meningitis to severe encephalitis or peripheral nerve disease. Joint symptoms include arthralgias, intermittent attacks of arthritis, and chronic erosive sinovitis. The most common cardiac disorder is fluctuating atrio-ventricular block, but acute myopericarditis occurs in a significant proportion of patients.

Untreated, the disease may follow a chronic relapsing and remitting course with persistent symptoms over many years. Lyme disease in its early stages can be treated with oral penicillin, tetracycline, or erythromycin. Patients with established disease and central nervous system involvement are more refractory to treatment and may require parenteral treatment with high doses of penicillin or a third-generation cephalosporin.[13] Because of the varied symptoms and signs caused by *Borrelia burgdorferi*, the possibility of Lyme disease must be entertained in the differential diagnosis of children presenting with a wide range of symptoms. Although the disorder is more prevalent in the wooded areas of the east coast of the United States, it has been reported throughout Europe and is being recognised with increasing frequency in children who have not travelled outside the United Kingdom.

Kawasaki disease

Since the first descriptions of Kawasaki disease in Japan 20 years ago, the disorder has emerged as an important childhood entity with a world-wide distribution.[14] The illness typically affects infants and young children and presents with fever, lymph-node enlargement, polymorphous rash, reddening of the palms and soles, peripheral oedema, conjunctival injection, and changes in the oral cavity and mucous membranes. Desquamation usually occurs in the second and third weeks of the illness. The clinical features overlap those of staphylococcal and streptococcal toxin diseases, and also have features in common with measles, leptospirosis, and Rocky Mountain spotted fever.

Although the aetiology of Kawasaki disease remains unknown the epidemiological features are consistent with an infective aetiology.[15] The disorder comes in epidemics which occur in most countries on a three-yearly basis. In Japan, where over 80,000 cases have been reported, careful epidemiological studies have documented a wave-like spread of the epidemic from one part of the island to another. These features, together with the defined age group of children affected, indicate that the disease is due to an infectious agent. One of the exciting challenges for paediatricians and infectious diseases physicians in the 1990s is to identify the causative agent of this disease.

The major complication of Kawasaki disease is a widespread arteritis with a particular predilection for the coronary arteries and other extra-parenchymal muscular arteries. Coronary-artery aneurysms occur in 40% of cases and fatal myocardial infarction occurs in approximately 1% to 2% of cases.[16]

Carefully conducted therapeutic trials in Japan and in the United States have convincingly demonstrated that intravenous immunoglobulin given in the early phases of the disease can significantly reduce the likelihood of coronary-artery aneurysms developing.[17] For this form of treatment to be applied, the diagnosis needs to be established in the first 10 days of the illness, and this requires a greatly increased awareness of the disorder.[18]

Fifth disease

Fifth disease is a mild febrile illness with a reticular rash and a characteristic slapped-cheek appearance. An infectious aetiology for the illness has been suspected for many years. However, it is only over the past few years that the causative agent has been identified as being human parvo-virus (B19).[19] A great deal has been learnt about the spectrum of disease caused by this organism, which has also been shown to cause aplastic crises in children with haemolytic disorders, chronic and relapsing arthropathy, and fetal infection.[20,21] Parvo-virus infection during pregnancy may result in the condition of fetal hydrops or spontaneous abortion. New information on the biology of this virus is emerging rapidly and the full spectrum of disease it causes will probably only become apparent in subsequent years

Roseola infantum

Another febrile exanthem of young children for which a causative agent has now been identified is roseola infantum.[22] This disorder occurs in young infants with short febrile illness, followed by an erythematous macular exanthem. A newly discovered herpes virus, human herpes virus 6, has emerged as the cause of roseola infantum, and like other herpes viruses may cause a persistent latent infection. Although little is so far known about this virus it is likely that it will be found to be responsible for other clinical syndromes.[23]

Haemolytic uraemia syndrome

The haemolytic uraemia syndrome (HUS) is now the most common cause of acute renal failure in children in many countries, and has long been suspected of having an infectious aetiology. Epidemiological studies conducted during the 1970s and early 1980s clearly established that the most common form of HUS affects infants and young children, invariably follows a diarrhoeal prodrome, and occurs in epidemics.[24] A major advance in the understanding of this disorder came in 1983 when Karmali *et al.* reported an association between the haemolytic uraemic syndrome and the presence in the stool of a strain of *E. coli* which produced an unusual cytotoxin now termed verotoxin.[25]

Studies from several different countries have now confirmed the association of HUS with verotoxin producing *E. coli*.[26] In the past few years much has been learnt about the biology of verotoxin producing *E. coli*, and their role in the haemolytic uraemic syndrome.[27] There are two distinct verotoxins, VT1 and VT2, which are produced not only by *E. coli* but also by a variety of other enteric pathogens. VT1 is identical to shigatoxin produced by *Shigella dysenteriae* type 1, whereas VT2 is structurally and antigenically distinct. VT1 consists of an A subunit with a molecular weight of 32,000 and 5 copies of a B subunit of molecular weight 7,700. After binding to specific receptors, the A subunit is separated from the B subunit, enters the cell, and inhibits protein synthesis, leading ultimately to cell death. Verotoxin appears to be toxic for endothelial cells and may produce a disease similar to the haemolytic uraemic syndrome after injection into experimental animals.[24,27]

The isolation of the causative agent of the haemolytic uraemic syndrome and the increased understanding of the pathophysiology of this disorder which has followed, raise the exciting possibility that treatments to prevent or reverse this serious disorder will be developed over the next decade.[24]

HIV infection and AIDS

In the relatively short period since the first clinical descriptions of the acquired immune deficiency syndrome, a spectacular increase in knowledge of this disorder and the causative HIV virus has been achieved. Within two years of the clinical recognition of the syndrome, the aetiological agent was established as being the retrovirus now called HIV 1. Research teams throughout the world have now elucidated its structure, mode of replication, and many aspects of the pathophysiology of HIV infection.[28]

Although the incidence of HIV infection in children is much lower than in adults, there is likely to be a progressive increase in the number of children with HIV infection, as the virus spreads more widely in the heterosexual population.[29] In many countries in Africa, such as Uganda, Zaire, Zambia, and Zimbabwe, HIV infection accounts for a large proportion of all paediatric inpatient admissions. In the UK, the number of infected children remains small, but their impact on all aspects of paediatric practice is likely to be far greater than the numbers would suggest.

Two major groups of children are affected by the HIV virus: haemophiliacs and recipients of blood transfusions, and infants born to HIV-positive mothers. While the numbers of those acquiring the disease through infected blood products are unlikely to increase further now that screening of blood and heat treatment of factor VIII are available, the number of children acquiring the disease through vertical transmission is expected to increase progressively.[29]

Many people have the image of HIV-infected children as presenting with a fulminant and rapidly fatal disorder. While this is true of a proportion of infants who become ill and may die in the first months of life, it has been increasingly recognised that the disorder may be compatible with prolonged survival. Approximately 20% of infants born to HIV-positive mothers are infected by the virus and remain HIV-positive after 18 months of age when maternally acquired antibodies would normally have disappeared.[30] Many infected children remain free of symptoms for several years, and survival into the teens is being increasingly reported.

The presenting symptoms of HIV-infected children are non-specific, and may be easily confused with those of any other childhood disorders: repeated upper respiratory tract infections; lymphadenopathy; recurrent fever; diarrhoea; and failure to thrive.[31] As these symptoms are also seen in many children who are not infected by HIV, who present to casualty departments and paediatric units, the possibility of HIV infection will need to be considered increasingly in paediatric practice. Bacterial infections are a major problem in HIV-infected children. Septicaemia, meningitis, pneumonia, and soft-tissue infections may be the presenting feature of the illness. The causative organisms are usually *S. pneumoniae* or *H. influenzae* as they are in children without HIV, but in addition infection due to a wide range of the gram-positive and gram-negative pathogens may also occur.[32]

Opportunistic infections present a major challenge in the management of HIV-infected children. Children presenting with tachypnoea and pulmonary infiltrates may be suffering from pneumonia or pneumonitis caused by a very wide range of bacteria, viruses, fungi, or parasites[33] (Table 2). Empiric treatment regimes are unlikely to cover all the possible pathogens, and it is essential for successful therapy to establish the aetiological agent. This requires not only familiarity with the spectrum and clinical features of opportunistic infections, but also access to microbiology and virology laboratories familiar with the diagnostic techniques required to identify the unusual pathogens.

Table 2. Opportunistic infections in HIV-infected children

Bacteria	*Protozoa*
S. pneumoniae	Pneumocystis carinii
H. influenzae	Toxoplasma gondii
Salmonella	Cryptosporidium
Pseudomonas	Giardia lamblia
Staphylococcus	Entamoeba histolytica
Klebsiella	Blastomyces hominis
Mycobacterium tuberculosis	
Atypical mycobacteria	*Fungi*
Mycoplasma	
Chlamydia	Candida species
Nocardia	Cryptococcus neoformans
Listeria	Histoplasmosis
	Aspergillus species
Viruses	
CMV	
Herpes simplex	
Varicella zoster	
Adenovirus	
RSV	
Influenza	
Measles	
Epstein Barr virus	

A major advance in the diagnosis of opportunistic lung infections in children has been the development of fibre-optic bronchoscopy, and the procedure of broncho-alveolar lavage, which enables the diagnosis of the causative agent to be established without recourse to open-lung biopsy in many cases. Using bronchoscopy or, if necessary, open-lung biopsy, an aetiological agent can be established in a high proportion of cases, and appropriate treatment started.[34] Of major importance is the distinction between opportunistic infections and the entity of lymphocytic interstitial pneumonitis (LIP) which occurs in a high proportion of HIV-infected children. LIP presents insidiously, with tachypnoea and cough, and may progress slowly to respiratory failure. Chest X-ray characteristically shows a reticular-nodular pattern which is often associated with hilar lymphadenopathy. Epstein Barr virus has been implicated in the aetiology of LIP, and the disorder may respond to steroids as well as to AZT.[35]

Central nervous system involvement occurs in many HIV-infected children. Developmental delay, loss of developmental milestones, or spastic paraparesis may be the presenting features.[36] The neurological disorder is often a direct result of HIV infection of the central nervous system, but it is essential to distinguish this from opportunistic infections such as cerebral toxoplasmosis, cryptococcal meningitis, and other bacterial and fungal infections.

Persistent diarrhoea and failure to thrive are important features of HIV infection and may be caused by a range of different infectious agents. A number of new pathogens, including cryptosporidium and *Blastomyces hominis*, have emerged as problems in HIV-infected children. Persistent diarrhoea may also be due to CMV colitis, other chronic viral infections, or persistent bacterial infection.[37]

The treatment of HIV-infected children necessitates aggressive diagnosis and treatment of opportunistic infections. Paediatricians who see only an occasional HIV-infected child and are unfamiliar with the management of opportunistic infections in immunocompromised children are unlikely to diagnose and treat the range of unusual pathogens appropriately. In addition to the management of opportunistic infection, specific treatments for HIV infection are becoming available.[38] AZT (zidovudine) has been shown to be beneficial in adults and is already being used in trials on children. Other drugs such as dideoxyinosine (DDI) are also under trial. Intravenous immunoglobulin infusions and the use of steroids for LIP have also been advocated, but there is, as yet, no evidence from controlled trials of their efficacy. Decisions as to when to institute anti-viral drugs, or treatment with immunoglobulin, at which stage of the disease they should be started, and how to assess and evaluate their effect are difficult, and require experience in the manifestations and progression of the disorder as well as familiarity with the rapidly changing literature.[38]

Although the medical problems presented by HIV-infected children are considerable, the social and emotional problems faced by these children are of even greater magnitude. HIV-infected children may come from families in which the parents are ill or dying. Parents may be drug users, and may be unable to comply with treatment. Problems of fostering and adoption arise frequently, and affected children may face isolation and victimisation in their schools and communities.

In planning services for HIV-infected children two opposing priorities need to be considered. In view of the complexity of the medical problems, centralisation of care in regional centres which are familiar with the spectrum of the disease and the diagnosis and management of opportunistic infections would be desirable. Infectious diseases specialists would play a major role in the care of HIV-infected children in regional centres. However, in view of the social and psychological problems faced by these children it is essential that as much of the care as possible be based close to home, in local district hospitals and the community. In order to reconcile these conflicting needs, a model of shared care should be developed. Regional paediatric infectious diseases units would be available to assess children and plan their treatment as well as admitting children with severe opportunistic infections for diagnosis and treatment. However, the regional units would refer children back to their local hospital where most of the day-to-day care would be undertaken. Close liaison between the regional units and the district and community services would be essential for comprehensive care. As long as the numbers of children infected by the HIV virus in the UK remain relatively small, it is unlikely that each district hospital would have sufficient expertise in the management of the disorder to undertake optimal care, and the sharing of care with a regional specialist unit would help to improve the overall management of the disorder.

For each of the new diseases and new infectious agents discussed above, a similar pattern has been followed: clinical recognition of a new syndrome has been followed by epidemiological studies which have suggested an infectious aetiology. Detailed studies undertaken by infectious diseases and microbiology units have identified the causative agent, and the molecular and cellular biology of the organism and its interaction with the host have then been elucidated. Finally treatments have been developed and the possibility of a vaccine to prevent the disorder then explored. Infectious diseases specialists have been involved in all phases of the process and have provided the link between the clinical problem and the basic science required for its solution.

Antimicrobial treatment

An ever-expanding armamentarium of new antimicrobial agents has been developed in recent years. A list of only some of these compounds is shown in Table 3. Clinicians are overwhelmed with information and advertisements for new antibiotics, including the third-generation cephalosporins, quinolones, macrolides, and extended spectrum penicillins. Antiviral therapy, having for many years been an area where few compounds were available, has now come of age with the development of a number of new drugs which have potent antiviral activity. Acyclovir is highly effective against herpes simplex virus,[39] and the new agent gancyclovir shows promise in the treatment of cytomegalovirus infection.[40] Ribavirin is active against a number of viruses and has already entered clinical use in the treatment of respiratory syncytial virus (RSV) infections[41] and Lassa fever.[42] AZT, DDI, and other anti-retroviral agents have now entered clinical use.[38] In the field of anti-fungal agents fluconazole and intraconazole have shown promise in the treatment of systemic fungal infections. There has also been progress in the field of anti-parasitic drugs with the introduction of paziquantel for the treatment of schistosomiasis and quinghaosu for the treatment of malaria.

New chemotherapeutic agents are emerging so rapidly that it is difficult to be fully up-to-date on the range of drugs available. Infectious diseases specialists are playing a major role in the evaluation of new antimicrobial agents, assessment of their advantages in relationship to existing treatments, and monitoring their toxicity. With increasing numbers of imported infections and opportunistic infections in immunocompromised patients a major component of the work of infectious diseases specialists will be to guide paediatricians and other paediatric subspecialists in the treatment of infection and the choice of antimicrobial agent.

Host pathogen interactions

One of the most exciting areas in the field of infectious diseases is that of research on the pathophysiology and pathogenesis of infectious diseases. The tools of molecular and cell biology have enabled the process by which micro-organisms damage the host to be studied and understood. There has been increasing recognition that the damage to tissues and organs observed in infectious diseases may be caused not only by the pathogen, but also by triggering of host inflammatory responses by toxins or products released by the infectious agent.

In the case of meningococcal sepsis or endotoxic shock, endotoxin triggers the release from macrophages of the cytokines, tumour necrosis factor (TNF), and interleukin I (IL I). These cytokines amplify the inflammatory response and recruit neutrophils, platelets, and other leukocytes to the inflammatory reaction. Inflammatory mediators are released from these effector cells which are responsible for disruption of the normal homeostatic function of the vascular endothelium and other tissues.[43]

Recognition of the role played by host inflammatory pathways in the pathophysiology of sepsis has led to immunotherapy and pharmacological manipulation of these responses. Therapeutic trials with anti-inflammatory agents such as steroids have documented a beneficial effect in a number of infections, including bacterial meningitis.[44,45] Furthermore, the use of monoclonal antibodies directed either at

Table 3. New antimicrobial agents

AGENTS	USE
Antibiotics	
2nd generation cephalosporins	
Cefoxitin Cefotetan	Gram −ve/gram +ve infections
3rd generation cephalosporins	
Ceftriaxone Cefotaxime Ceftazidime Ceftizoxime	Broad cover for gram −ve and gram +ve infections very active against H. influenzae N. meningitidis and S. pneumoniae
Oral cephalosporins	
Cefixime Axetil-cefuroxime	Oral therapy of gram +ve and gram −ve infections
Mecillinam Aztreonam	Gram −ve sepsis Similar spectrum to aminoglycosides
Imipenem/cilastatin	Very broad spectrum antibiotic
Sulbactam/ampicillin Clavulanic acid/amoxicillin	Treatment of infections with Beta lactamase producing organisms
Ciprofloxacin	Active against gram +ve and gram −ve organisms including pseudomonas
Roxithromicin	Active against gram +ve organisms and toxoplasmosis
Antiviral agents	
Amantadine	Prophylaxis and treatment of influenza
Trifluorothymidine	Herpes simplex eye infections
Acyclovir	Herpes simplex, and varicella zoster infections
Adenine arabinoside	Herpes simplex and varicella zoster infections
Ribavirin	RSV bronchiolitis, Lassa fever
Zidovudine (AZT)	HIV infection

2′3 Dideoxyinosine (DDI)	Potential use for HIV infection
2′3 Dideoxycytidine (DDC)	Potential use for HIV infection
Gancyclovir (DHPG)	Cytomegalovirus infection
Phosphonoformate (Foscarnet)	Cytomegalovirus infection
Antifungals	
Fluconazole	Candida, and cryptococcal infection
Intraconazole	Aspergillus and candida infections paracoccidiomycosis
Terbinafine	Dermatophyte infections
Antihelminthic	
Ivermectin	Onchocerca volvulis
Praziquantel	Broad spectrum including *Schistosomiasis*, cysticercosis, fluke infections
Albendazole	Broad spectrum antihelminthic
Antiprotozoal agents	
Qinghaosu	Plasmodium falciparum
Trimetrexate	Pneumocystis carinii
Difluoromethylornithine	Trypanosomiasis Pneumocystis carinii
Allopurinol	Leishmaniasis
Nifurtimox	Chagas disease

endotoxin or at inflammatory mediators such as TNF have been beneficial in improving the prognosis in experimental septicaemia and endotoxic shock.[46,47] It is likely that during the next decade anti-inflammatory and immunomodulating therapy will become an important part of the treatment of infectious diseases.

Vaccination

The ultimate goal in the practice of infectious diseases must be to prevent the serious infectious diseases of childhood. A large number of new vaccines have been developed using the tools of molecular biology

Table 4. Some new vaccines under trial or available

Acellular pertussis
Haemophilus B capsular polysaccharide
Haemophilus B polysaccharide/protein conjugate vaccines: i Capsular polysaccharide/tetanus toxoid conjugate ii Capsular polysaccharide diphtheria toxoid conjugate iii Capsular polysaccharide/N. meningitidis outer membrane conjugate iv Haemophilus B oligosaccharide/mutant diphtheria toxin conjugate
Pneumococcal polysaccharide
Varicella zoster
Rotavirus
Oral typhoid
Hepatitis B
Cytomegalovirus
Japanese B encephalitis
Human diploid cell rabies vaccine
E. coli J5 Anti endotoxin vaccine

and the increased understanding of the pathobiology of infection (Table 4). Infectious diseases specialists have been involved in all phases of the development of new vaccines and in their assessment in clinical trials. As the number of vaccines available increases there will be a growing need for experts who can advise on their use as well as conduct trials and monitor their beneficial and potentially toxic effects.

Conclusions

Only a small proportion of the advances in the field of infectious diseases has been discussed in this chapter. However, it should be apparent that infectious diseases is an exciting and dynamic specialty which closely links clinical practice with the basic sciences. In order to deal with the range of new diseases, new treatments, and new insights into infectious processes, all major paediatric centres in the country will require a paediatric infectious diseases specialist to advise on the management of infection, undertake research in the field of infectious diseases, and participate in the evaluation of new treatments and vaccines. Infectious diseases specialists will not only need to have thorough training in paediatrics but will also require a detailed knowledge of microbiology, immunology, pharmacology, and epidemiology. At present there is not a single established training post in paediatric infectious diseases in the United Kingdom. In order to ensure that highly trained clinicians and scientists are available to meet the infectious challenges of the 21st century there is an urgent need to establish and fund training posts which will provide comprehensive training in the clinical and scientific aspects of paediatric infectious diseases.

References

1. Todd, J., Fishaut, M., Kapral, F., Welch, T. (1978) Toxic shock syndrome associated with phage-group 1 staphylococci. *Lancet*, **2**, 1116–1118.
2. Buchdahl, R., Levin, M., Wilkins, B. *et al.* (1985) Toxic shock syndrome. *Archives of Disease in Childhood*, **60**, 563–567.
3. Schlievert, P.M. (1989) Role of toxic shock syndrome Toxin 1 in toxic shock syndrome. *Reviews of Infectious Diseases*, **ii** (suppl), 107–109.
4. Chesney, P.J. (1989) Clinical aspects and spectrum of illness of toxic shock syndrome: overview. *Reviews of Infectious Diseases*, **ii** (suppl 1), 1–7.
5. Bisno, A.L., Shulman, S.T., Dajani, A.S. (1988) Rise and fall (and rise) of rheumatic fever. *Journal of the American Medical Association*, **259**, 728–729.
6. Westlake, R.M., Graham, T., Edwards, K.M. (1990) An outbreak of acute rheumatic fever in Tennessee. *The Pediatric Infectious Diseases Journal*, **9**, 97–100.
7. Stevens, D.L., Tanner, M.H., Winship, J. *et al.* (1989) Severe group A streptococcal infections associated with a toxic shock-like syndrome and scarlet fever toxin A. *New England Journal of Medicine*, **321**, 1–7.
8. Cone, L.A., Woodard, D.R., Schlievert, P.M., Tomory, G.S. (1987) Clinical and bacteriologic observation of a toxic shock-like syndrome due to streptococcus pyogenes. *New England Journal of Medicine*, **317**, 146–149.
9. Harnden, A., Lennon, D. (1988) Serious suppurative Group A streptococcal infections in previously well children. *The Pediatric Infectious Disease Journal*, **7**, 714–718.
10. Steere, A.C., Malawista, S.E., Syndman, D.R. (1977) Lyme arthritis: an epidemic of oligo-articular arthritis in children and adults in three Connecticut communities. *Arthritis and Rheumatology*, **20**, 7–17.
11. Burgdorfer, W., Barbour, A.G., Hayes, S.F. *et al.* (1982) Lyme disease – A tick-born spirochetosis. *Science*, **216**, 1317–1319.
12. Stechenberg, B.W. (1988) Lyme disease: the latest great imitator. *The Pediatric Infectious Disease Journal*, **7**, 402–409.
13. Dattwyler, R.J., Halperin, J.J., Volkman, D.J., Luft, B. J. (1988) Treatment of late Lyme borreliosis—randomised comparison of ceftriaxone and penicillin. *Lancet*, **i**, 1191–1194.
14. Kawasaki, T. (1967) Acute febrile mucocutaneous syndrome with lymphoid involvement with specific desquamation of the fingers and toes. *Japanese Journal of Allergy*, **16**, 178–222.
15. Yanagawa, H., Nakamura, Y., Kawasaki, T., Schigematsu, I. (1986) Nationwide epidemic of Kawasaki disease in Japan during winter of 1985–86. *Lancet*, **ii**, 1138–1139.
16. Rowley, A.H., Gonzales-Crussi, F., Shulman, S.T. (1988) Kawasaki syndrome. *Review of Infectious Diseases*, **10**, 1–15.

17. Newburger, J.W., Takahashi, M., Burns, J.C. *et al.* (1986) The treatment of Kawasaki disease with intravenous gamma globulin. *New England Journal of Medicine*, **315**, 341–347.
18. Shulman, S.T., Bass, J.L., Bierman, F. *et al.* (1989) Management of Kawasaki syndrome: a consensus statement prepared by North American participants of The Third International Kawasaki Disease Symposium, Tokyo, Japan, December 1988. *The Pediatric Infectious Disease Journal*, **8**, 663–667.
19. Anderson, M.J., Jones, S.E., Fisher Hock, S.P. (1983) Human parvovirus, the cause of erythema infectiosum (Fifth Disease). *Lancet*, **i**, 1378.
20. Anand, A., Gray, E.S., Brown, T. *et al.* (1987) Human parvo-virus infection in pregnancy and hydrops fetalis. *New England Journal of Medicine*, **316**, 183–186.
21. Torok, T.S. (1990) Human parvo-virus B19 infections in pregnancy. *The Pediatric Infectious Disease Journal*, **10**, 772–776.
22. Yamanishi, K., Okuno, T., Shiraki, K. (1988) Identification of human herpes virus 6 as a causal agent for exanthem subitum. *Lancet*, **i**, 1065–1067.
23. Yoshiyama, H., Suzuki, E., Yoshida, T. *et al.* (1990) Role of human herpes virus 6 infection in infants with exanthema subitum. *The Pediatric Infectious Disease Journal*, **9**, 71–74.
24. Levin, M., Walters, M.D.S., Barratt, T.M. (1989) Haemolytic uraemic syndrome. *Advances in Paediatric Infectious Diseases*, **4**, 51–82.
25. Karmali, M.A., Petric, M., Steele, B.T., (1983) Sporadic cases of haemolytic uraemic syndrome associated with faecal cytotoxin and cytotoxin producing *E. coli* in stools. *Lancet*, **i**, 619–620.
26. Milford, D.V., Taylor, C.M., Guttridge, B. *et al.* (1990) Haemolytic uraemic syndromes in the British Isles 1985–8: association with verocytotoxin producing *Escherichia coli*. Part 1: clinical and epidemiological aspects. *Archives of Disease in Childhood*, **65**, 716–721.
27. Milford, D.V., Taylor, C.M. (Annotation) (1990) New insights into the haemolytic uraemic syndromes. *Archives of Disease in Childhood*, **65**, 713–715.
28. Gallo, R.C. (1987) The AIDS virus. *Scientific American*, **256**, 46–56.
29. Oxtoby, M.J. (1990) Perinatally acquired human immunodeficiency virus infection. *The Pediatric Infectious Disease Journal*, **9**, 609–619.
30. European Collaborative Study (1988) Mother to Child transmission of HIV Infection. *Lancet*, **ii**, 1039–1042.
31. Pahwa, S. (1988) Human immunodeficiency virus infection in children: nature of immunodeficiency, clinical spectrum and management. *The Pediatric Infectious Disease Journal*, **7**, 561–571.
32. Kranski, R., Borkowsky, W., Bonk, S. *et al.* (1988) Bacterial infections in human-immunodeficiency-virus – infected children. *The Pediatric Disease Journal*, **7**, 323–328.
33. Scott, G.B., Hutto, C., Makuch, R.W. *et al.* (1989) Survival in children with perinatally acquired human immunodeficiency virus type 1 infection. *New England Journal of Medicine*, **321**, 1791–1796.
34. de Blic, J., Blanche, S., Danel, C. *et al.* (1989) Bronchoalveolar lavage in HIV-infected patients with interstitial pneumonitis. *Archives of Disease in Childhood*, **64**, 1246–1250.
35. Rubinstein, A., Bernstein, L.J., Charytan, M. *et al.* (1988) Corticosteroid treatment for pulmonary lymphoid hyperplasia in children with the acquired immune deficiency syndrome. *Pediatric Pulmonology*, **4**, 13–17.
36. Epstein, L.G., Sharer, L.R., Oleske, J.M. *et al.* (1986) Neurological manifestations of human immunodeficiency virus infection in children. *Paediatrics*, **78**, 678–687.
37. Smith, P.D., Lane, H.C., Gill, V.J. (1988) Intestinal infections in patients with AIDS. Etiology and response to therapy. *Annals of Internal Medicine*, **108**, 328–333.
38. Pizzo, P.A., Wilfert, C.M. (1990) Treatment considerations for children with human immunodeficiency virus infection. *The Pediatric Infectious Disease Journal*, **9**, 690–699.

39. Whitley, R., Alford, D., Hirsch, M.S. *et al.* (1986) Vidarabine versus acyclovir in herpes simplex encephalitis. *New England Journal of Medicine*, **314**, 144–149.
40. Keay, S., Bissett, J., Merigan, T.C. (1987) Gancyclovir treatment of cytomegalovirus infections in in-iatrogenically immunocompromised patients. *Journal of Infectious Diseases*, **156**, 1016–1021.
41. — (1986) Ribavirin therapy for respiratory syncytial virus infections: Report of a scientific workshop. *The Pediatric Infectious Diseases Journal*, **9** (suppl), 67–124.
42. McCormick, J.B., King, I.J., Webb, P.A. *et al.* (1986) Lassa fever: effective therapy with ribavirin. *New England Journal of Medicine*, **314**, 20–26.
43. Levin, M. (1990) The Inflammatory response to infection. in *Infection in the Newborn*. Ed J de Louvois, D. Harvey, John Wiley and Sons, 1–12.
44. Lebel, M.H., Bishara, F.J., Syrogiannopoulos, G. A. (1988) Dexamethasone therapy for bacterial meningitis. *New England Journal of Medicine*, **319**, 964–971.
45. Girgis, N.I., Farid, A., Mikhail, I.A. *et al.* (1989) Dexamethasone treatment of bacterial meningitis in children and adults. *The Pediatric Infectious Disease Journal*, **8**, 848–851.
46. Tracy, K.J., Fong, Y., Hesse, D.G. *et al.* (1987) Anti-cachectin/TNF monoclonal antibodies prevent septic shock during lethal bacteraemia. *Nature*, **330**, 662–664.
47. Nys, M., Cloes, J.M., Demonty, J., Joassin, L. (1990) Protective effects of polyclonal sera and of monoclonal antibodies active against *Salmonella minnesota* Re 595 lipopolysaccharide during experimental endotoxemia. *Journal of Infectious Diseases*, **162**, 1087–1095.

13 | Respiratory disease: wheezing disorders

Michael Silverman
Department of Paediatrics and Neonatal Medicine, Royal Postgraduate Medical School, Hammersmith Hospital, London

Introduction

Many advances in the diagnosis and management of childhood respiratory illness in the 1980s have been on a small scale, but because of the clinical importance of this group of diseases, added together they represent an important advance in the field of child health. Improved understanding of mechanisms and pathogenesis of wheezing diseases has stemmed from advances in a number of techniques. Both in the realms of clinical epidemiology and of cell biology, there have been contributions to improved management. In this review I hope to illustrate the way in which clinical research has contributed to better understanding, and has been translated into more effective management. Where possible, I shall indicate trends which may have important implications for the management of wheezing disorders in childhood, for the 1990s.

Prevalence and aetiology

It has been consistently demonstrated throughout the 1980s that in the industrialised world, the prevalence of childhood asthma has steadily increased.[1,2] Admissions to hospital with the diagnosis of asthma have increased several-fold,[3] far more than could be explained by diagnostic transfer,[4] with the decline in use of the term 'bronchitis' to describe wheezing in young children.[5] In addition, in older children and young adults there has been an increase in the absolute mortality in England and Wales.[6] In relation to the total number of cases, however, the mortality rate may in fact have declined slightly. Surprisingly, in the youngest age group for which figures are available (one to four years) mortality has declined both relatively and in absolute terms, in spite of the fact that in this age group our management skills are at their weakest.[6]

Along with an increase in symptom prevalence, repeated population surveys at 15-year intervals have demonstrated an increase in the level of bronchial responsiveness in populations of schoolchildren.[2] There is thus consistent evidence that both asthma and its most important physiological marker, bronchial responsiveness, have become more prevalent.

A number of lines of evidence suggest that fetal and early neonatal environment may be critical in the expression of asthma in susceptible individuals. Carefully conducted population studies in Tucson, USA, starting in early pregnancy and continuing with physiological and clinical observations throughout early childhood, have demonstrated that those infants who are destined to develop wheeze in association with respiratory infections start life with smaller airways than those children who do not wheeze in infancy.[7] Recent unpublished data (R. Castile, Boston, USA, personal observations) have shown that one important factor in determining lung size at birth is fetal exposure to maternal cigarette-smoking. In this study, lung function in the newborn period in otherwise healthy infants was diminished in proportion to the random, maternal, urinary cotinine level during pregnancy, suggesting, perhaps, a causal relationship. Urinary cotinine is a good indicator of the quantity of cigarettes smoked. These measurements confirm previous epidemiological evidence that maternal smoking during pregnancy is associated with early childhood respiratory illness.[8] Most studies have shown boys to be more affected by postnatal smoke exposure than girls;[9] the effect is proportional to dose.[10]

The development of atopic sensitisation is clearly important in established asthma in children at school age, most of whom are atopic. In 1990 the first evidence was presented that both sensitisation and subsequent asthma were determined by the level of house-dust mite exposure in the first year of life.[11] It has been proposed that the current domestic environment may be an important factor leading to the increase in the development of sensitisation, since carpeted, centrally heated houses form the ideal environment for house-dust mite to flourish. Visible mould on the walls is associated with a 3.5-fold increase in the likelihood of wheeze.[12] Overcrowding may be another factor.[13]

The propensity to mount an IgE response to inhaled antigen is clearly important in asthma. In fact, the relationship between the age-related IgE level and severity of asthma for schoolchildren is very close.[14] Recent research has come close to identifying a gene determining the IgE response in asthma.[15] There may be additional hereditary factors. Bronchial responsiveness in asthmatic families can be segregated into hypo- and hyper-responsive categories, suggesting a single-gene mode of inheritance.[16,17]

These observations have major implications for preventive health care programmes in the 1990s. The prevalence of wheezing in young children is so common that even a small reduction in maternal smoking is likely to have a major effect on the prevalence of lower respiratory tract illnesses in young children. Moreover it is likely that methods of reducing exposure to house-dust mite in the first year, by modifying the domestic environment, could be increasingly important in attempts to prevent or delay the onset of atopic sensitisation and subsequent asthma in susceptible individuals. It may soon be possible to identify susceptible individuals, to judge from progress in the recognition of the gene which determines atopic status.

Classification of wheeze

In the 1970s the tendency to label all recurrently wheezy children as asthmatic seemed important, in order to ensure that appropriate treatment was provided. It was felt that by labelling children with the term 'wheezy bronchitis', encouragement might be given to prescribe antibiotics rather than topical bronchodilators and anti-inflammatory agents (such as sodium cromoglycate and topical corticosteroids). These observations were reinforced by careful studies of older children, such as that of Williams and McNichol, which suggested that children with a history of wheezy bronchitis were epidemiologically very similar to those with a history of standard childhood asthma.[18] Recently, however, a number of follow-up studies have shown that, for instance, recurrent wheezing which follows acute bronchiolitis is unrelated to atopic hypersensitivity, and follows a different pattern from that of atopic childhood asthma (see review reference 19). Moreover there is increasing evidence that there is a condition which can only be termed 'wheezy bronchitis' in which episodic symptoms occur in association with viral respiratory tract infections, and in the absence of intercurrent wheeze or cough.[19] Is the distinction between 'wheezy bronchitis' and 'regular atopic asthma' important?

The prognosis for children with recurrent wheeze associated with upper respiratory tract infections is clearly entirely different from that of regular, atopic, childhood asthmatics. Moreover, it may well be that the pathophysiology and hence the treatment should be different. Clearly both groups respond to bronchodilators, and in fact it is now quite clear that even in the youngest age group, the physiology of the airways is such that the bronchodilators might be expected to be effective.[20] However, the indications for long-term topical anti-inflammatory agents in children up to three years old are unknown and it is possible that by lumping together the two groups within clinical trials, as has generally been done up to now, clinical research workers have failed to come up with clear guidelines to the management of either group.

Over the next few years it could become increasingly apparent that there are different sub-groups of wheezy pre-school children. Perhaps children with recurrent wheezy bronchitis or post-bronchiolitic wheeze and regular atopic asthmatics will become distinguishable from each other and from children who wheeze following preterm birth[21] or in association with recurrent gastro-oesophageal reflux.

Treatment

The *classes of drugs* used to treat wheezy children have changed little over the past 20 years.[22] Recently, theophylline preparations have become less fashionable, as the high prevalence of side-effects has become appreciated. The group of long-acting β_2 adrenergic agents is likely to become available for paediatric use over the next few years. Since we have been urged not to rely excessively on *regular* β-adrenergic agents in treating the day-to-day symptoms of childhood asthma, it is difficult to see what role these agents might have. Their most likely application will be for nocturnal symptoms.

The controversy about the role of inhaled β agonists in infancy may be close to resolution. Conflicting evidence from different studies must be due to study design. Future work must take into account the following variables: the age of subjects, the severity of disease, the acuteness of the illness, the means of administration (oral, parenteral, nebulised aerosol or metered-dose aerosol), the dose administered, and the likely dose received.[23] It is clear that nebulised[24] and parenteral[25] bronchodilators are sometimes effective in acute, severe infantile asthma, and in laboratory studies.[20] On balance, the evidence favours ipratropium bromide for treating wheezy infants.

The emphasis on airway inflammation in the pathogenesis of asthma has led to the widespread use of *topical inhaled corticosteroids* for even mild asthma in adults. Although we are encouraged by adult physicians to rely more heavily on topical steroids in treating children, there is clearly a simple, dose-related suppression of the adrenal function which has to be considered in every case.[26,27,28] No guidance has been proposed to evaluate the risk-benefit ratio in the use of topical steroids in children.

While topical steroid therapy has clearly benefited 'middle-aged' childhood asthmatics, their place in the management of wheezy infants and preschool children is controversial. For instance, of recent clinical trials of budesonide in preschool children, nebuliser therapy (500mcg twice daily) was ineffective,[29] low-dose metered-dose inhaler (MDI) with spacer (200mcg twice daily) had a marginal effect,[30] while high-dose MDI and spacer therapy (400mcg twice daily) was clearly beneficial.[31] Leaving aside differences between studies in the age distribution of subjects and the problems of classification of asthma (see above), it seems likely that both the dose administered and the mode of administration (ie the proportion of the dose deposited in the respiratory tract) may be important considerations in treatment.

Another area of controversy concerns the efficacy of corticosteroid therapy for acute severe airway obstruction, including acute bronchiolitis, in young infants. A recent, large, double-blind study again suggests that systemic corticosteroids are ineffective[32] while, paradoxically, another study suggested that inhaled topical steroids given for a few weeks after recovery from acute bronchiolitis may have beneficial effects several months later.[33] In the present situation, I do not feel that corticosteroid therapy, topical or systemic, is appropriate for a first episode of acute bronchiolitis.

New forms of therapy for persistent, severe, steroid-dependent asthma, a particular problem in teenage girls, may be expected over the next few years. Low-dose weekly *methotrexate* has been shown to be extremely effective for this type of problem in adults, with relapse on withdrawal of therapy.[34] This is merely a pointer to possible future developments.

While the pharmacopoeia has not altered significantly, our therapeutic skills have improved considerably. A number of papers have described techniques which are available for the *administration of topical agents by inhalation* to young children.[35–39] The evidence that drug deposition from metered aerosol/spacer devices may be almost as effective as the dose delivered by nebuliser, and more efficient at delivering small (<5 micron) droplets, gives a rationale for replacing home nebulisers with spacers.[40,41] Although as yet there are no satisfactory commercially available spacer/face-mask devices for aerosol administration, a number of prototype devices are available.[36–40] It is to be expected that during the 1990s, sophisticated devices which take account of the tidal volume and breathing frequency of infants and young children will become available. Whether metered-dose inhalers in their present form will continue to be available once chlorofluorocarbon propellants are withdrawn, remains to be seen.

A number of *consensus statements* dealing with the management of common clinical problems have been published recently. Among them, the consensus statement on the management of childhood asthma[22] points to other trends in therapeutics. In particular the reliance on increased doses of bronchodilators administered by aerosol in acute severe asthma, in combination with anticholinergic agents, has been justified by therapeutic studies.[42] This has meant a reduction in the need for parenteral bronchodilators and for intensive care. Continuous bronchodilator administration for the most severe cases has even been advocated,[43] although experience shows that side-effects are troublesome under these circumstances. Hyperactivity and tremor are particular problems.

Another trend in therapeutics which is to be welcomed is the introduction of *self-management plans*. The National Asthma Campaign in the UK has been in the forefront of the advocacy of written, simple management plans for parents and children. Thus either on the basis of symptoms or with additional measurements of peak flow rate, short-term variations in therapy can be made by families themselves, or even by school teachers. The limits have to be set by contract between child, parents, and doctor, depending on the likelihood of compliance by the family. There is as yet no evidence that some of the suggested manoeuvres in self-management plans (for instance the doubling of inhaled steroids at the first sign of an upper respiratory infection) are of any benefit. The results of trials to clarify these points can be expected over the next year or two.

Conclusion

The major changes which can be expected in the management of wheezing disorders over the next two years will probably continue to be brought about by small changes in the types and efficacy of existing classes of anti-asthma drugs. In particular, in the youngest age groups, appropriate therapeutic devices which deliver adequate doses to the respiratory tract are probably the key to effective treatment.

The long-term prognosis of childhood asthma is worse than formerly suspected.[44–46] Many would consider it a lifelong disorder. It is therefore clear that the greatest long-term advances are likely to come in the field of prevention, particularly from efforts to reduce maternal smoking during pregnancy, and from techniques to eliminate the house-dust mite from the home environment in the first few years of life, for those infants who, by the techniques of molecular genetics, can be shown to be predisposed to atopy. Prospects for gene therapy, already a possibility for single gene defects such as α-1 anti-trypsin deficiency, and a probability for cystic fibrosis, seem to be a long way ahead for wheezing disorders in children.

References

1. Burney, P. (1988) Why study the epidemiology of asthma. *Thorax*, **43**, 425–428.
2. Burr, M.L., Butland, B.K., King, S., Vaughan-Williams, E. (1989) Changes in asthma prevalence: two surveys 15 years apart. *Archives of Disease in Childhood*, **64**, 1452–1456.
3. Anderson, H.R. (1989) Increase in hospital admissions for childhood asthma: trends in referral, severity and readmissions from 1970 to 1985 in a health region of the United Kingdom. *Thorax*, **44**, 614–619.
4. Burney, P.G.J., Chinn, S., Rona, R.J. (1990) Has the prevalence of asthma increased in children? Evidence from the national study of health and growth 1973–86. *British Medical Journal*, **300**, 1306–10.
5. Hill, R., Williams, J., Tattersfield, A., Britton, J. (1989) Change in the use of asthma as a diagnostic label for wheezing illness in school children. *British Medical Journal*, **299**, 898.
6. Anderson, H.R. (1989) Is the prevalence of asthma changing? *Archives of Disease in Childhood*, **64**, 172–175.
7. Martinez, F.D., Morgan, W.J., Wright, A.L. *et al.* (1989) Diminished lung function as a predisposing factor for wheezing respiratory illness in infants. *New England Journal of Medicine*, **319**, 1112–1117.
8. Taylor, B., Wadsworth, J. (1987) Maternal smoking during pregnancy and lower respiratory tract illness in early life. *Archives of Disease in Childhood*, **62**, 786–791.
9. Murray, A.B., Morrison, B.J. (1989) Passive smoking by asthmatics: its greater effect on boys than on girls and on older than on younger children. *Pediatrics*, **84**, 451–459.
10. Neuspiel, D.R., Rush, D., Butler, N.R. *et al.* (1989) Parental smoking and post-infancy wheezing in children: a prospective cohort study. *American Journal of Public Health*, **79**, 168–171.
11. Sporik, R., Holgate, S.T., Platts-Mills, T.A.E., Cogswell, J.J. (1990) Exposure to house-dust mite allergen (Der p1) and the development of asthma in childhood. *New England Journal of Medicine*, **323**, 502–507.
12. Strachan, D.P. (1988) Damp housing and childhood asthma: validation of reporting of symptoms. *British Medical Journal*, **297**, 1223–1226.
13. Wright, A.L., Holberg, C.J., Martinez, F.D. *et al.* Group Health Medical Associates (1989) Breast feeding and lower respiratory tract illnesses in the first year of life. *British Medical Journal*, **299**, 946–949.
14. Burrows, B., Martinez, F.D., Halonen, M. *et al.* (1989) Association of asthma with serum IgE levels and skin-test reactivity to allergens. *New England Journal of Medicine*, **320**, 271–277.
15. Cookson, W.O.C.M., Sharp, P.A., Faux, J.A., Hopkin, J.M. (1989) Linkage between immunoglobulin E responses underlying asthma and rhinitis and chromosome 11q. *Lancet*, **1**, 1292–1295.
16. Longo, G., Strinati, R., Poci, F., Fumi, F. (1987) Genetic factors in nonspecific bronchial hyperreactivity. *American Journal of Diseases of Children*, **141**, 331–334.
17. Hopp, R.J., Bewtra, A.K., Biven, R. *et al.* (1988) Bronchial reactivity pattern in nonasthmatic parents of asthmatics. *Annals of Allergy*, **61**, 184–186.
18. Williams, H., McNichol, K.N. (1969) Prevalence, natural history and relationship of wheezy bronchitis and asthma in children. An epidemiological study. *British Medical Journal*, **4**, 321–325.
19. Wilson, N.M. (1989) Wheezy bronchitis revisited. *Archives of Disease in Childhood*, **64**, 1194–1199.
20. Silverman, M. (1989) Airway responsiveness in infancy. *Clinics in Experimental Allergy*, **19**, 345–348.
21. Lucas, A., Broke, O.G., Cole, T.J. *et al.* (1990) Food and drug reactions, wheezing and eczema in preterm infants. *Archives of Disease in Childhood*, **65**, 410–415.

22. Warner, J.O., Gotz, M., Landau, L.I. *et al.* (1989) Management of asthma: a consensus statement. *Archives of Disease in Childhood*, **64**, 1065–1079.
23. Collis, G.G., Cole, C.H., LeSouef, P.N. (1990) Dilution of nebulised aerosols by air entrainment in children. *Lancet*, **336**, 341–343.
24. Mallol, J., Barrueto, L., Girardi, G. *et al.* (1987) Use of nebulised bronchodilators in infants under 1 year of age. *Pediatric Pulmonology*, **3**, 298–303.
25. Lowell, D.I., Lister, G., Koss, H.V., McCarthy, P. (1987) Wheezing in infants: the response to epinephrine. *Pediatrics*, **79**, 939–945.
26. Prahl, P., Jensen, T., Bjerregaard-Andersen, H. (1987) Adrenocortical function in children on high-dose steroid aerosol therapy. *Allergy*, **42**, 541–544.
27. Bisgaard, H. (1988) Adrenal function in children with bronchial asthma treated with beclomethasone dipropionate and budesonide. *Journal of Allergy and Clinical Immunology*, **81**, 1088–1095.
28. Priftis, R., Milner, A.D., Conway, E., Honour, J.W. (1990) Adrenal function in asthma. *Archives of Disease in Childhood*, **65**, 838–840.
29. Van Bever, H.P., Schuddinck, L., Wojciechowski, M., Stevens, W.J. (1990) Aerosolised budesonide in asthmatic infants: a double blind study. *Pediatric Pulmonology*, **9**, 177–180.
30. Bleeson, J.G.A., Price, J.F. (1988) Controlled trial of budesonide given by the nebuhaler in preschool children with asthma. *British Medical Journal*, **297**, 163–166.
31. Bisgaard, H., Munck, B.L., Neilsen, J.P., Petersen, W., Ohlsson, S.V. (1990) Inhaled budesonide for treatment of recurrent wheezing in early childhood. *Lancet*, **336**, 649–651.
32. Springer, C., Bar-Yishay, E., Uwayyed, K. *et al.* (1990) Corticosteroids do not affect the clinical or physiological status of infants with bronchiolitis. *Pediatric Pulmonology*, **9**, 181–185.
33. Carlsen, K.H., Leegaard, J., Larsen, S., Orstavik, I. (1988) Nebulised beclomethasone diproprionate in recurrent obstructive episodes after acute bronchiolitis. *Archives of Disease in Childhood*, **63**, 1428–1433.
34. Shiner, R.J., Nunn, A.J., Chung, K.F., Geddes, C.M. (1990) Randomised, double-blind, placebo-controlled trial of methotrexate in steroid-dependent asthma. *Lancet*, **336**, 137–140.
35. Pedersen, S. (1986) How to use a rotahaler. *Archives of Disease in Childhood*, **61**, 11–14.
36. Mallol, J., Barrueto, L., Girardi, G., Toro, O. (1987) Bronchodilator effect of fenoterol and ipratropium bromide in infants with acute wheezing: use of MDI with a spacer device. *Pediatric Pulmonology*, **3**, 352–356.
37. O'Callaghan, C., Milner, A.D., Swarbrick, A. (1989) Spacer device with face-mask attachment for giving bronchodilators to infants with asthma. *British Medical Journal*, **298**, 160–161.
38. Conner, W.T., Dolovich, M.B., Frame, R.A., Newhouse, M.T. (1989) Reliable salbutamol administration in 6–36 month old children by means of a metered-dose inhaler and aerochamber with mask. *Pediatric Pulmonology*, **6**, 263–267.
39. Bisgaard, H., Ohlson, S. (1989) PEP-spacer: an adaptation for administration of MDI in infants. *Allergy*, **44**, 363–364.
40. Salmon, B., Wilson, N.M., Silverman, M. (1990) How much aerosol reaches the lungs of infants and toddlers? *Archives of Disease in Childhood*, **65**, 401–403.
41. O'Callaghan, C. (1990) Particle size of beclomethasone dipropionate produced by two nebulisers and two spacing devices. *Thorax*, **45**, 109–111.
42. Reisman, J., Galdes-Sebalt, M., Kazim, F. *et al.* (1988) Frequent administration by inhalation of salbutamol and ipratropium bromide in the initial management of severe acute asthma in children. *Journal of Allergy and Clinical Immunology*, **81**, 10–20.

43. Portnoy, J., Aggarwal, J. (1988) Continuous terbutaline nebulisation for the treatment of severe exacerbations of asthma in children. *Annals of Allergy*, **60**, 368–371.
44. Kelly, W.J.W., Hudson, I., Phelan, P.D. *et al.* (1987) Childhood asthma in adult life: a further study at 28 years of age. *British Medical Journal*, **294**, 1059–1061.
45. Strachan, D.P., Anderson, H.R., Bland, S.M., Peckham, C. (1988) Asthma as a link between chest illness in childhood and chronic cough and phlegm in young adults. *British Medical Journal*, **296**, 890–893.
46. Gerritsen, J., Roeter, G.H., Postma, D.S. *et al.* (1989) Prognosis of asthma from childhood to adulthood. *American Review of Respiratory Disease*, **140**, 1325–1330.

14 | Method and myth in the treatment of cystic fibrosis

Richard E. Olver
Department of Child Health, University of Dundee, Ninewells Hospital and Medical School, Dundee

Introduction

It was my original intention to write a comprehensive review evaluating treatment policy for all the major system disorders of cystic fibrosis (CF). However, it soon became clear that such an approach was over-ambitious, and it proved to be more difficult than I had anticipated to sort out CF treatment based on scientific method from that based on myth. I have therefore limited the scope of this paper to the question of drug treatment in CF lung disease (those wanting an overview of current CF management are referred to the Personal Practice section of *Archives*[1]). The decision to focus on lung disease in CF is not difficult to justify. Lung disease is a fundamental determinant of morbidity and mortality in CF, yet uncertainty and confusion characterise our approach to the use of the therapeutic tools we have at our disposal. Furthermore, the discovery of the abnormal transport regulatory protein and the associated defect of epithelial ion transport in CF makes this a particularly appropriate time to look at possible future developments in therapy – such as the introduction of drugs which modify ion transport and somatic gene therapy.

Antibiotic use – general considerations[2–5]

Penicillin, the first effective anti-staphylococcal antibiotic, became available in the early 1940s, and gentamicin, the first effective anti-pseudomonal drug, became available in 1963. There have been large numbers of clinical trials of antibiotic treatment in CF (Michel[2] lists 79 trials of anti-pseudomonal therapy between 1980 and 1987), and it is perhaps surprising to find that the use of antibiotics in CF remains an area of controversy, not consensus. No two paediatricians use the same protocol. Part of the problem is that the indications for antibiotic treatment and the timing, duration, and route of administration are all variables. Antibiotics may be used for continuous prophylaxis, or given as soon as a pathogen is found in the sputum and then repeated at regular intervals (irrespective of clinical condition), or they can be administered only for clinical exacerbations. Add to this the alternatives of monotherapy or combination therapy given orally, intravenously, or by inhalation, and you have 16 feasible permutations. Given the bewildering choice, it is clear that the development of optimum treatment protocols requires the careful co-ordination of clinical trials. This approach, which characterises research into childhood malignancy, has been sadly lacking in CF. Furthermore, it has to be said that the design of the majority of published clinical antibiotic trials has been poor. It is obvious that open studies can be of only limited value, but even those trials that claim to be randomised, controlled, and blind often suffer from one or more defects – small numbers, lack of stratification for disease severity, confounding variables not controlled for and use of multiple outcome measures – all of which leads to difficulty in reaching statistically and clinically valid conclusions. In general, controlled studies have followed, not preceded, established practice.

Despite disagreements about the most appropriate regimes for antibiotic use in CF, there is near unanimity in the view that CF patients require higher total doses of antibiotics as a result of altered pharmacokinetics[3] (compared to non-CF controls, patients with CF have higher antibiotic distribution volumes per unit bodyweight and more rapid antibiotic elimination). This requirement applies irrespective of the type of drug being prescribed, β-lactam or aminoglycoside. Each of these groups of drugs has its own strengths and weaknesses. For β-lactams[4] there is a wide margin between therapeutic and toxic blood levels (wide therapeutic index), but allergic reactions are not uncommon. β-lactams do not, in general, exhibit a post-antibiotic effect on gram-negative bacteria (ie bacterial killing ceases when the drug is no longer present in significant concentration) and hence dosing regimes need to be such that blood levels are kept at or above the mean inhibitory concentration (MIC) throughout much of the period of treatment. Usually administration of large doses given four times a day can achieve this and continuous infusion is not necessary. For aminoglycosides,[3,4] there is a narrow margin between therapeutic and toxic levels (narrow therapeutic index), and monitoring of blood levels is essential. Aminoglycosides exhibit a strong post-antibiotic effect on gram-negative and gram-positive bacteria, and intermittent dosing (8- or 12-hourly) is therefore the ideal. Both the post-antibiotic effect and the rate of bacterial killing are strongly dose-related. In general, for aminoglycosides, peak levels of 8–12mg/l and trough levels of 1–2mg/l are desirable. For the reasons given earlier, this will usually entail the use of high daily doses.

β-lactams and aminoglycosides have complementary antibacterial actions – the former group disrupting the bacterial cell wall and allowing access of the latter to the ribosomes where protein synthesis is inhibited. Presumably these mechanisms form the basis of the synergy between the two groups, which can be clearly demonstrated *in vitro* but does not seem to confer clear clinical benefit.[5]

The introduction of quinolones such as ciprofloxacin represents a major extension of the antibiotic armamentarium. They provide an effective means of oral therapy with 70% bioavailability[6] and good penetration into airway secretions. Ciprofloxacin is effective in the treatment of *P. aeruginosa, S. aureus,* and *H. influenzae*, but prolonged monotherapy may lead to the development of resistance.

Antibiotic use for specific infections

S. aureus infection predominated as the major cause of lung infection when CF was first described, but ceded this position to *P. aeruginosa* in the early 1960s.[7] Prevalence of chronic staphylococcal infection is variable (10–30%) and declines with age. Use of anti-staphylococcal antibiotics as routine prophylaxis is widespread, but there are very few data to show that this practice is clinically useful and there is some concern that it may induce *P. aeruginosa* colonisation. However, benefit from prophylaxis can be inferred from a blind crossover study[8] in which cephalexin, a drug with little activity against *H. influenzae* and none against *P. aeruginosa*, was used for four-monthly periods. During treatment periods there was an increased rate of weight gain and a decreased frequency of respiratory infections and hospitalisation of those initially colonised with *H. influenzae* or *S. aureus*.

Most United Kingdom CF centres give continuous anti-staphylococcal prophylaxis, but an alternative policy of aggressive treatment of positive sputum culture is pursued by the Danish CF centre, with seemingly good results.[9] Their standard treatment of *S. aureus* infection – dicloxacillin (or rifampicin in cases of penicillin allergy) given with sodium fusidate and probenecid for 14 days – is reported to eradicate *S. aureus* in about 70% of cases. Treatment failures receive repeat courses and persistent failure is managed with prolonged administration of the same antibiotics or a course of intravenous (IV) clindamycin plus sodium fusidate. On average each patient receives two anti-staphylococcal treatments per year, and as a result less than 10% of patients attending the Danish CF centre are reported as being infected with *S. aureus* for more than six months.

The prevalence of *P. aeruginosa* has increased since the introduction of effective anti-staphylococcal treatment and is reported in between 50–80% of patients attending CF centres.[7] Chronic infection is more frequent in specialised centres than elsewhere (eg 57% at the Danish CF centre versus 27% elsewhere in Denmark[7]), and infection occurs at a younger age. Eventually most patients become infected with *P. aeruginosa* which is then impossible to eradicate. Persistence of infection *in vivo* during treatment with antibiotics to which the organism is sensitive *in vitro* may be related to the poor penetration of antibiotics into the airway, growth of pseudomonas in microcolonies surrounded by a protective mucoid exopolysaccharide, and defective mucociliary clearance.

The traditional and still widespread indication for the use of anti-pseudomonal antibiotic therapy is an acute exacerbation of pulmonary infection. In such exacerbations, *P. aeruginosa* has been reported[7] as being implicated in about 50% of cases, *S. aureus* in about 19%, and *H. influenzae* in 14%. However, non-bacterial triggers such as viral infections[10] are also important and, since treatment of acute exacerbations may include intensification of chest physiotherapy, it has taken an exceptionally well-designed placebo-controlled study to show that antibiotics improve lung function during an acute exacerbation more than bronchodilators and chest physiotherapy alone. In a study from Minnesota[11], patients received bronchodilators and chest physiotherapy, and at four days were stratified on the basis of their initial forced vital capacity (FVC) and randomised to receive intravenous tobramycin and ticarcillin or placebo for a further 14 days (in addition to continued bronchodilators and chest physiotherapy). During this period, the antibiotic group showed significantly greater reductions in the density of pseudomonas and other bacteria in sputum and greater increases in FVC, forced expiratory volume $(FEV)_1$ and forced expiratory flow-rate ($FEF_{25-75\%}$) than the placebo group. Reduction in the density of pseudomonas in sputum correlated significantly with each of the measures of lung function. Interestingly, two weeks after cessation of antibiotics the density of sputum bacteria had returned to admission levels but the effect on lung function was prolonged and FVC, FEV_1, and $FEF_{25-75\%}$ did not return to initial values for 8, 9, and 4.6 months respectively.

An alternative to what might be called the 'reactive' policy of treating acute exacerbations with antibiotics is the 'pro-active' policy of the Danish CF centre which was introduced in 1976[12] in an attempt to prevent pulmonary damage by *P. aeruginosa* which might otherwise have occurred by the time an acute exacerbation became clinically apparent. The group's preferred treatment consists of 14-day courses of intravenous tobramycin plus a β-lactam at three- to four-monthly intervals irrespective of the patient's clinical condition. However, because of resistance or hypersensitivity reactions to β-lactams,

Table 1. Doses of some useful antibiotics in cystic fibrosis

	Route	mg/kg per 24 h	Doses per day	Maximum daily dose (g)
β-lactams				
Amoxycillin	O	50	3–4	
Ampicillin	IV	150	3–4	
Augmentin	O	50	3–4	
Azlocillin	IV	300–400[d]	3–4	20
Aztreonam	IV	150	3–4	8
Ceftazidime	IV	150–200[d]	3–4	12
Flucloxacillin	O	50–100[c]	3–4	
	IV	150	3–4	
Imipenem-Cilastin	IV[a]	50–60[d]	3–4	4
Piperacillin	IV	300–400[d]	3–4	20
Ticarcillin	IV	500–600[d]	3–4	30
Others				
Ciprofloxacin	O	40	2–3	2
	IV[a]	10	2	0.8
Clindamycin	IV[a]	25–30[d]	3–4	3
Erythromycin	O	50	3–4	2
Rifampicin	O	15–20[d]	1	
Sodium Fusidate	O	50	3–4	2
Tobramycin[b]	IV	10	2–3	
By Nebuliser		Total dose/24 hr		
Colistin	Inhal	2 million units[e]	2	
Methicillin	Inhal	1000 mg[e]	2	
Tobramycin	Inhal	160 mg[e]	2	

[a] Infuse over 20–30 minutes.
[b] Aminoglycoside of first choice. Adjust dose after 3 days to achieve peak of 8–12 mg/l and trough of 1–2 mg/l. Gentamicin and netilmicin dosage as for tobramycin.
[c] Use lower dose if given with sodium fusidate; consider adding probenecid (15 mg/kg per 24 h) to maintain high blood levels.
[d] Use the lower dose *above* 5 years.
[e] Halve dose *under* 5 years.

approximately 25% of treatment courses have consisted of monotherapy with tobramycin. In recent years, nebulised colistin and/or oral ciprofloxacin between IV courses has been added to the regime. As is so often the case in CF, the change in policy in 1976 did not follow any kind of controlled study, yet it has to be said that the effect of survival looks impressive. In the period 1971–5, during which patients received anti-pseudomonal antibiotics for acute exacerbations, survival of those chronically infected with *P. aeruginosa* was 54%, while in the five-year period following 1976, survival rose to 82%. However, these data need to be interpreted with caution. A recent paper[13] from the CF centre in Toronto, based on observations made in 502 patients over the period 1975–88, reported five-year survival rates of between 89–98% and ten-year survival rates of 78–87% in patients first infected with *P. aeruginosa* between birth and seven years – all of whom received anti-pseudomonal antibiotics during acute exacerbations but not on a regular pro-active basis. It may well be that the differences in treatment policies between these two centres are more apparent than real, and that in practice a low threshold for treating acute exacerbations may be similar to a regular pro-active policy.

Aminoglycosides and β-lactams show synergy *in vitro* and this combination of antibiotics was used by the Minnesota and Danish groups. However, there is no convincing evidence that combination therapy is superior to monotherapy in terms of clinical response,[14] nor evidence that development of resistance is any less frequent.[5] This is an important point because monotherapy, being simpler to administer, is the policy of choice for home intravenous treatment (see below).

P. cepacia is an uncommon isolate from the sputum of patients with CF,[7] but it has on occasion posed a significant problem in at least one large CF centre where it was noted to be associated with a poor prognosis in a proportion of patients. Segregation of infected patients in hospital and the maintenance of good hygienic practices are important measures in preventing cross-infection. *P. cepacia* exhibits multiple drug resistance (including resistance to colistin), but cefuroxime may sometimes be effective.[2]

H. influenzae is probably the least harmful of the pathogens commonly isolated from patients with CF.[4] Oral amoxycillin is the drug of choice but, where β-lactamase resistance develops, the addition of clavulanic acid or a switch to erythromycin is usually effective in achieving eradication.

Home intravenous antibiotic therapy

Home IV antibiotic therapy, whether it be for acute exacerbations or regular pro-active treatment, is an attractive proposition for a number of reasons.[15] Firstly (and most obviously) it causes less disruption to the child's life and reduces the time spent away from home and school. Secondly, it is cheaper. Thirdly, at least theoretically, it reduces the risk of cross-infection.

In a controlled, but non-randomised, open study[16] comparing combination antibiotic therapy administered in hospital with the same regime administered at home, both forms of treatment for acute exacerbations were equally effective as judged by the improvement in pulmonary function tests. However, the narrow therapeutic index of aminoglycosides and the consequent need to monitor blood levels makes these drugs unsuitable for home therapy. The low MICs for *P. aeruginosa* demonstrated by newer cephalosporins such as ceftazidime and cefsulodin, coupled with the wide therapeutic index shared by β-lactams in general and their proven efficacy when given as IV monotherapy,[2] doubtless explains why these drugs are fast becoming the first choice for home IV treatment.

The role of inhaled antibiotics[17]

Nebuliser therapy provides a means of achieving high concentrations of antibiotic at the surface of the lung epithelium and in sputum which are not possible by oral or IV administration. As long ago as the 1940s, aerosol penicillin was used to treat staphylococcal infection in CF, but it was not until the 1980s that placebo-controlled studies of nebulised anti-pseudomonal antibiotics were carried out. In general these have shown that regular inhaled antibiotic combinations (eg carbenicillin and gentamicin[17]) and monotherapy (eg colistin,[18] ceftazidime, or tobramycin) are effective in terms of improved pulmonary function and reduced number of hospital admissions. Colistin, a drug which is rarely given IV because of toxicity, offers the advantage of a low-frequency of *P. aeruginosa* resistance. Used as monotherapy, this drug is prescribed as an adjunct to regular IV antibiotic therapy by the Danish CF centre in order to retard deterioration between IV courses,[18] and interest in its use is increasing in the UK. Inhalation antibiotic therapy may also have a role in infants and young children in whom pseudomonas infection is mild/moderate and home IV therapy impracticable – the only alternative being hospitalisation. Whatever antibiotics are used for inhalation therapy, the choice of nebuliser system is absolutely crucial – a point often overlooked by those prescribing this form of treatment. The system must be capable of delivering the bulk of the drug in droplets $< 5\mu m$ diameter if it is to reach and deposit in the small airways.[19] Ultrasonic nebulisers are generally incapable of meeting this requirement but the majority of jet nebulisers, coupled to a pressurised air supply capable of flows of at least 10 litres per minute, *when working under load*, can. High flow rates are also necessary in order to keep the duration of nebuliser therapy short, and hence improve compliance, and to maximise the amount of drug nebulised. In the context of home treatment, these requirements dictate[20] the use of a powerful compressor such as the Maxi Mark III (Medix) or possibly the CR60 (Medic-Aid). One other important variable is the size of antibiotic 'fill'. Because of the dead space inherent in the design of the jet nebuliser, 3–4ml fills result in a greater proportion of the drug being nebulised compared to a 2ml fill.[21]

Antibiotic resistance[22,23]

Emergence of resistant strains may be the result of selection of resistant variants or mutation or, in the case of β-lactams, induction of β-lactamase. Because of the availability of effective alternatives, resistance by *S. aureus* or *H. influenzae* to first-line antibiotics is rarely a clinical problem. Resistance exhibited by *P. aeruginosa* may be short-lived and resistant strains usually disappear within a few months of discontinuing the relevant antibiotic. Antibiotic sensitivity patterns may fluctuate during therapy[5] and the emergence of resistant strains shows no correlation with clinical response. These observations may be related in part to the poor reproducibility of MIC measurements for pseudomonas (plus or minus one dilution is regarded as good), and the fact that *in vitro* culture conditions bear little relation to the *in vivo* environment. Nevertheless, resistance is rarely absolute and, when confronted with a mixed resistance pattern, it would seem sensible to pick one or more antibiotics to which the organism is said to be sensitive. Not surprisingly, resistance tends to be less in respect of the newer antibiotics, and this is presumably one explanation for their popularity.[5] Emergence of a multiply resistant organism in an ill patient requiring antibiotic therapy is an indication for use of high-dose combination therapy with a β-lactam and aminoglycoside in hospital.

Bronchodilators and steroids

In relation to CF, George Bernard Shaw's character (allegedly modelled on Sir Almroth Wright) was clearly wrong when he suggested that the 'one genuinely scientific treatment for all diseases . . . is to stimulate the phagocytes . . . drugs are a delusion' (*The Doctor's Dilemma*, 1906). In fact, the phagocytes are working overtime in CF and it is the lysosomal enzymes and oxygen radicals liberated by polymorphonuclear leucocytes which cause the chronic inflammation and progressive lung damage characteristic of CF.[24] Airway damage assists the penetration of foreign antigens through the epithelial barrier and so contributes to the high frequency of atopy and airway lability in CF. All patients with CF should be regularly assessed for reversible airways obstruction (including exercise-induced wheezing) and treated in the usual way with bronchodilators and sodium cromoglycate/inhaled steroids. Sudden onset or worsening of wheeze, associated with fever, an increased eosinophil count, and pulmonary infiltrates suggests the development of bronchopulmonary aspergillosis. Some patients respond to bronchodilators but others require treatment with oral steroids. Systemic steroid therapy has also been used in an attempt to control the chronic inflammatory response and consequent tissue damage associated with chronic lung infection. In a small double-blind randomised trial over four years,[25] CF patients treated with alternate day prednisone (2mg/kg, to a maximum of 60mg total) were significantly better as judged by a variety of clinical measures (including height, weight, and hospital admissions), pulmonary function tests, and serological indices (ESR and IgG).

Drugs designed to modify ion transport

Discovery of the defect in chloride channel regulation in CF[26] has focussed attention on the exciting possibility of developing drugs specifically designed to restore the normal balance of ion transport across the airway epithelium. The hydration of airway secretions is physiologically regulated by changes in the balance between the driving force provided by active transport of chloride towards the lumen of the lung and that provided by active sodium transport in the reverse direction. Thickened bronchial mucus and defective mucociliary clearance, which leads in turn to obstructive airways disease and chronic infection in CF, are associated with diminished chloride permeability of the apical (lumenal) surface of airway epithelial cells and excess sodium absorption. These observations have prompted a trial of nebulised amiloride (a sodium channel-blocker used clinically as a diuretic) to restore the normal hydration of airway secretions by reducing the absorption of sodium and the water osmotically linked to it. In a small double-blind randomised crossover study[27] in CF adults, the CF research group in North Carolina has demonstrated a reduction in sputum viscosity and a slowing in the rate of decline of FVC during amiloride treatment periods ($FEF_{25-75\%}$ was not measured). Amiloride does have antibacterial effects, and the finding of similar quantitative pseudomonas counts in sputum during active and placebo treatment periods does not exclude this as a possible contributory factor. The use of amiloride in this way is currently the subject of a multi-centre study in North America.

Possibilities of increasing chloride permeability arise from another study[28] by the North Carolina group which has demonstrated that, of the three intracellular regulatory mechanisms for chloride secretion – Ca^{2+}, cAMP dependent protein kinase A and protein kinase C – the calcium regulatory mechanism is retained. The finding that increasing intracellular Ca^{2+} concentration is effective in initiating chloride secretion by CF airway epithelium opens up therapeutic possibilities.

Somatic gene therapy has come a step nearer with the recent publication of a paper[29] showing that infection of a CF airway epithelial cell line with a virus/plasmid system which expresses recombinant DNA coding for the normal CF transmembrane regulatory protein (CFTR) results in restoration of the normal CF secretory response to isoprenaline and cAMP (mediated by protein kinase A). Major problems have to be surmounted before this technique can be used *in vivo* but it is no longer fanciful to predict that in the foreseeable future it may be possible to deliver a CFTR expression system to the lung epithelium of CF patients, perhaps by means of aerosol inhalation, and so restore normal function.

Summary and conclusions

In spite of the poor quality of much of the data, there can be no doubt that antibiotics have an important role to play in the treatment of CF. The main difficulty lies in knowing which permutations of drugs and delivery systems to use. My own practice, which is based on no more than an educated guess as to what represents optimum treatment in CF, is as follows.

S. aureus. For all pre-school age children: continuous flucloxacillin prophylaxis with addition of sodium fusidate for breakthrough infection. School age: flucloxacillin plus sodium fusidate for positive cultures with repeated or prolonged therapy (± probenecid) if infection persists (rifampicin plus sodium fusidate if penicillin allergic). Intravenous clindamycin plus sodium fusidate for symptomatic infection with *S. aureus* if standard oral therapy fails.

P. aeruginosa. Pre-school age: daily nebulised tobramycin or colistin with addition of IV antibiotics (eg azlocillin plus tobramycin or ceftazidime alone) given in hospital for acute exacerbations. Regular, pro-active, 14-day courses of antibiotics (as above) at three- to four-monthly intervals in hospital if acute exacerbations are frequent or clinical deterioration rapid. School age: regular, pro-active monotherapy (eg ceftazidime) at three-monthly intervals at home with daily inhalation therapy (tobramycin or colistin) or oral ciprofloxacillin between IV courses. Aztreonam shows no cross hypersensitivity with other penicillins and can be used as an alternative in an allergic patient.

Definition of the role of systemic steroid therapy in CF to inhibit the hyperimmune response, and consequent lung damage, will have to await the outcome of a large multi-centre study currently under way in North America. Until then, the only clear indication for such therapy is bronchopulmonary aspergillosis.

In conclusion, I can do no better than quote from the final paragraph of Tim David's review[1] which runs as follows: 'Much of the current treatment of cystic fibrosis is based on dogma masquerading as science. Single-centre studies cannot answer important therapeutic questions, such as the value of antipseudomonal or antistaphylococcal regimens. The energy devoted to endless arguments about whether patients ought to attend special centres would be better used to initiate a nationally co-ordinated multi-centre study of specific therapeutic regimens. Highly successful precedents for this approach exist in the Medical Research Council trials of leukaemia treatment, and the United Kingdom Children's Cancer Study Group trials of solid tumour treatment.'

In short, much of what we do in CF is based on myth – in the sense that there is precious little evidence to support our choice of treatment regimens. If we are to do better for our patients in the 1990s, a more rigorous application of scientific method will be required – both in the evaluation of current therapies and of those to come.

References

1. David, T. J. (1990) Cystic fibrosis. *Archives of Disease in Childhood*; **65**, 152–157.
2. Michel, B. C. (1988) Antibacterial therapy in cystic fibrosis: A review of the literature published between 1980 and February 1987. *Chest*; **94**, 129S–140S.
3. Horrevorts, A. M., Driessen, O. M. J., Michel, M. F., Kerrebijn, K. F. (1988) Pharmacokinetics of antimicrobial drugs in cystic fibrosis; aminoglycoside antibiotics. *Chest*; **94**, 120S–125S.
4. Mouton, J. W., Kerrebijn, K. F. (1990) Antibacterial therapy in cystic fibrosis. *Medical Clinics of North America*; **74**, 837–850.
5. Geddes, D. M. (1988) Antimicrobial therapy against Staphylococcus aureus, Pseudomonas aeruginosa, and Pseudomonas cepacia. *Chest*; **94**, 140S–144S.
6. Davis, R. L., Koup, J. R., Williams-Waren, J. *et al.* (1987) Pharmacokinetics of ciprofloxacin in cystic fibrosis. *Antimicrobial Agents and Chemotherapy*; **31**, 915–919.
7. Hoiby, N. (1988) Hemophilus influenzae, Staphylococcus aureus, Pseudomonas cepacia, and Pseudomonas aeruginosa in patients with cystic fibrosis. *Chest*; **94**, 97S–102S.
8. Loening-Baucke, V. A., Mischler, E., Myers, M. G. (1979) A placebo-controlled trial of cephalexin therapy in the ambulatory management of patients with cystic fibrosis. *Journal of Pediatrics*; **95**, 630.
9. Szaff, M., Hoiby, N. (1982) Antibiotic treatment of Staphylococcus aureus infection in cystic fibrosis. *Acta Paediatrica Scandinavica;* **71**, 821–826.
10. Wang, E. E. L., Prober, C. G., Manson, B. *et al.* (1984) Association of respiratory

viral infections with pulmonary deterioration in patients with cystic fibrosis. *New England Journal of Medicine*; **311**, 1653–1658.
11. Regelmann, W. E., Elliott, G. R., Warwick, W. J., Clawson, C. C. (1990) Reduction of sputum Pseudomonas aeruginosa density by antibiotics improves lung function in cystic fibrosis more than do bronchodilators and chest physiotherapy alone. *American Review of Respiratory Disease*; **141**, 914–921.
12. Pedersen, S. S., Jensen, T., Hoiby, N. *et al.* (1987) Management of Pseudomonas aeruginosa lung infection in Danish cystic fibrosis patients. *Acta Paediatrica Scandinavica*, **76**, 955–961.
13. Kerem, E., Corey, M., Gold, R., Levison, H. (1990) Pulmonary function and clinical course in patients with cystic fibrosis after pulmonary colonization with Pseudomonas aeruginosa. *Journal of Pediatrics*, **116**, 714–719.
14. Jackson, M. A., Kusmiesz, H., Shelton, S. *et al.* (1986) Comparison of piperacillin vs. ticarcillin plus tobramycin in the treatment of acute pulmonary exacerbations of cystic fibrosis. *Pediatric Infectious Diseases*, **5**, 440–443.
15. Gilbert, J., Robinson, T., Littlewood, J. M. (1988) Home intravenous antibiotic treatment in cystic fibrosis. *Archives of Disease in Childhood*; **63**, 512–517.
16. Donati, M. A., Guenette, G., Auerbach, H. (1987) Prospective controlled study of home and hospital therapy of cystic fibrosis pulmonary disease. *Journal of Pediatrics*; **111**, 28–33.
17. Hodson, M. E. (1988) Antibiotic treatment; aerosol therapy. *Chest*; **94**, 156S–160S.
18. Jensen, T., Pedersen, S. S., Garne, S. *et al.* (1987) Colistin inhalation therapy in cystic fibrosis patients with chronic Pseudomonas aeruginosa lung infection. *Journal of Antimicrobial Chemotherapy*; **19**, 831–838.
19. Newan, S. P., Woodman, G., Clarke, S. W. (1988) Deposition of carbenicillin aerosols in cystic fibrosis: effects of nebuliser system and breathing pattern. *Thorax*; **43**, 318–322.
20. Newman, S. P., Pellow, P. G. D., Clarke, S. W. (1986) Choice of nebulisers and compressors for delivery of carbenicillin aerosol. *European Journal of Respiratory Disease*; **69**, 160–168.
21. Newman, S. P., Pellow, P. G. D., Clay, M. M., Clarke, S. W. (1985) Evaluation of jet nebulisers for use with gentamicin solution. *Thorax*; **40**, 671–676.
22. van Klingeren, B. (1988) Antibiotic resistance in Pseudomonas aeuroginosa, Hemophilus influenzae, and Staphylococcus aureus. *Chest*; **94**, 103S–108S.
23. Hoogkamp-Korstanje, J. A. A., Spyker, J. (1988) Antibiotic resistance in Pseudomonas aeruginosa, Hemophilus influenzae, and Staphylococcus aureus – Discussion. *Chest*; **94**, 108S–109S.
24. Doring, G., Albus, A., Hoiby, N. (1988) Immunologic aspects of cystic fibrosis. *Chest*; **94**, 109S–114S.
25. Auerbach, H. S., Williams, M., Kirkpatrick, J. A., Colten, H. R. (1985) Alternate-day prednisone reduces morbidity and improves pulmonary function in cystic fibrosis. *Lancet*; **ii**, 686–688.
26. Welsh, M. J. (1990) Abnormal regulation of ion channels in cystic fibrosis epithelia. *FASEB Journal*; **4**, 2718–2725.
27. Knowles, M. R., Church, N. L., Waltner, W. E. *et al.* (1990) A pilot study of aerosolised amiloride for the treatment of lung disease in cystic fibrosis. *New England Journal of Medicine*; **322**, 1189–1194.
28. Boucher, R. C., Cheng, E. H. C., Paradiso, A. M. *et al.* (1989) Chloride secretory response of cystic fibrosis human airway epithelia: preservation of calcium but not protein kinase C- and A-dependent mechanisms. *Journal of Clinical Investigation*; **84**, 1424–1431.
29. Riche, D. P., Anderson, M. P., Gregory, R. J. *et al.* (1990) Expression of cystic fibrosis transmembrane conductance regulator corrects defective chloride channel regulation in cystic fibrosis airway epithelial cells. *Nature*; **347**, 358–363.

15 | Paediatric oncology: towards cure 'at least cost'

Alan W. Craft
Royal Victoria Infirmary, Newcastle upon Tyne

Introduction

The past 30 years have seen a steady improvement in the prognosis for children who have malignant disease. This has occurred primarily because of the use of cytotoxic chemotherapy which has been added to the other two modalities of surgery and radiotherapy. This vastly improved survival has enabled the paediatric oncologist to study the late effects of the treatment which was necessary for cure and thereby to modify treatment for subsequent generations of children. At a time when long-term survival was unlikely it was justified to adopt a policy of cure at almost 'any cost', but this has slowly changed to one where, for many tumour types, we are pursuing a philosophy of cure at 'least cost'. Much attention has been devoted to identifying different prognostic groups within tumour types, so that treatment can be intensified for those who still have a poor outlook, but reduced for those where the prospects for long-term survival are high. The mere fact that we are now able to talk about cure is also a considerable advance. In addition to changes in the philosophy of management there have been a number of practical advances in supportive care which have facilitated the administration of treatment.

Current survival rates

The improvements in survival which have occurred over the past 20 years along with the most recent five-year survival rates for different categories of malignant disease in children are shown in Table 1. These are data taken from the national registry of childhood malignancy held by the Children's Cancer Research Group in Oxford.[1] The figures given are for children diagnosed in 1980–82 and clearly do not represent the survival which we would expect for those diagnosed in 1990–92. However, they do show a clear pattern of improvement which has been sustained in subsequent years. In particular, many of those categories which have a relatively poor prognosis in Table 1 have shown considerable improvement in recent years. Although the use of chemotherapy has been the most important single factor in improving prognosis for children with cancer, two other points are particularly relevant. There has been an increasing trend over the past 20 years to centralise the care for children with cancer into major regional paediatric oncology centres. This has not been universal, so that it has been possible to study survival rates for those who are and those who are not referred to such specialist centres. The Childhood Cancer Research Group (CCRG) have shown quite clearly that there is a significant improvement for many categories of disease when their care is centralised.[2] Even for those diseases where better survival cannot be shown, eg Wilms' tumour, it has recently been demonstrated that patients not referred to specialist centres receive inappropriate treatment. In the case of Wilms' tumour, non-referred patients are usually treated according to outdated protocols of therapy which 'over-treat' most patients and therefore cause unnecessary and unwanted late effects.[3]

Because childhood cancer is such a rare disease advances can only come about by large co-operative studies. No one centre in the UK is large enough to conduct randomised studies on its own patients. For this reason there is collaboration between different centres, and

Table 1. Five-year percentage survival rates for principal types of childhood cancer diagnosed 1971–73 and 1980–82. (Data from National Registry of Childhood Tumours) (From Draper and Stiller, 1989).

	Years of diagnosis	
	1971–73	1980–82
Acute lymphoblastic leukaemia	37	64
Acute non-lymphoblastic leukaemia	4	19
Hodgkin's disease	76	91
Non-Hodgkin lymphoma	21	55
Brain and spinal tumours	42	50
Neuroblastoma	16	35
Retinoblastoma	87	86
Wilms' tumour	58	75
Osteosarcoma	18	35
Ewing's tumour	37	33
Rhabdomyosarcoma	26	48
Malignant gonadal germ cell tumours	50	84

the majority of children in the UK are entered into therapeutic studies run by either the Medical Research Council (MRC) or the United Kingdom Children's Cancer Study Group (UKCCSG). Once again there is clear evidence from the CCRG that children entered into such studies have a better chance of survival and of receiving the most up-to-date and appropriate therapy.[4]

Thirty years ago there were many children who presented with malignant disease in whom there was no prospect of long-term survival, and palliative care only was given. There is now virtually no child in whom a diagnosis of cancer is an automatic death sentence, and for most there is real hope of long-term survival and possible cure.

What is a cure?

Cure is the restoration of complete health and the prospect of living for a normal life-span. Figure 1 shows the prospects of living a further five years for children surviving five years from the diagnosis of cancer. It can be seen that for the vast majority of children, five-year survival is synonymous with long-term survival. A few late relapses will occur and a very small proportion of children will die as a late consequence of the treatment received, eg from second primary tumours which it is estimated will affect 3% of children by the time they have survived 15 years from the first.[5] Of course, many of these second

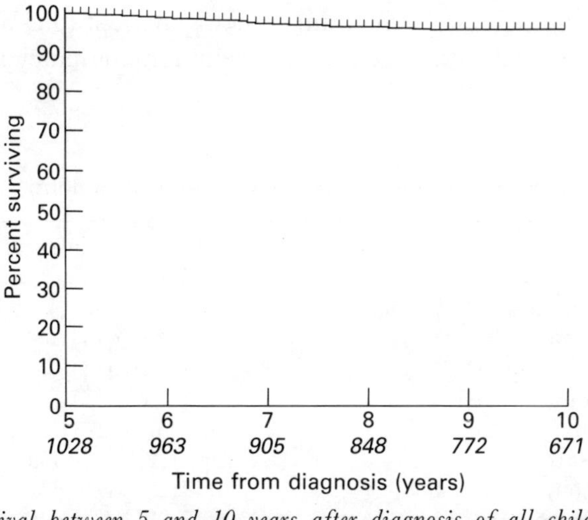

Fig. 1. *Survival between 5 and 10 years after diagnosis of all childhood cancer. Data from Northern Regional Children's Malignant Disease Registry. Figures at bottom (in italics) indicate population at risk.*

tumours can also be successfully treated. We are also beginning to identify those factors in treatment which predispose to second primary tumours. The combination of alkylating agents, eg cyclophosphamide and irradiation, has been recognised as an important aetiological factor[6] and this is now taken into account in the design of current protocols.

Diagnostic advances

1. Biological studies

The availability of fresh tumour tissue for biological studies is leading to a greater understanding of the nature of cancer in children, and also providing information which may well be of prognostic value. The cytogenetic profile of a tumour may be of diagnostic importance. An increasing number of specific chromosomal abnormalities are being associated with particular tumours and some of the more common are shown in Table 2.[7] Where the histological appearance of a tumour is equivocal, the presence of a recognised chromosomal translocation may aid the diagnosis eg 11:22 translocation in Ewing's tumour.[8]

Other biological studies which are possible and important include the study of oncogenes: eg, the presence of the oncogene N-myc in neuroblastoma is of great prognostic significance.[9] A single copy of the N-myc oncogene in a tumour usually indicates a good prognosis, whereas most of the tumours which have an unfavourable prognosis have multiple copies of this oncogene. It is therefore of great importance *not* to put all biopsy material into formalin but to place some in appropriate tissue-culture medium for cytogenetic studies and to freeze some for biological studies. For this reason, if malignancy is suspected

Table 2. Cytogenetic rearrangements in paediatric tumours.[7]

Solid Tumours	Cytogenetic rearrangements
Germ cell tumours	i(12p)
Retinoblastoma	del(13) (q14)
Osteogenetic sarcoma	del(13) (q14)
Wilm's tumour	del(11) (p13) ;t(3;17)
Neuroblastoma	del(1) (p32) (p36), DMs, HSRs
Rhabdomyosarcoma	3p, t(2;13) (q37;q14), t(2,11)
Ewing's sarcoma	t(11;22) (q24;q12)
Peripheral neuro-epithelioma	t(11;22) (q24;q12)
Synovial sarcoma	t(x;18) (q22.1;q11.2)

it is preferable to refer to the specialist centre before biopsy has been carried out. Many new diagnostic advances are likely to come from the study of such material.[10]

2. Imaging

The advent of computerised tomographic (CT) scanning has led to a vastly improved ability to delineate the extent of a tumour at diagnosis. While the appearance of a tumour on CT scanning can never give a pathological diagnosis, it defines very clearly where the tumour is, making surgery easier and the delivery of radiotherapy more accurate and efficient.[11] More recently, magnetic resonance imaging (MRI) has been developed and for certain areas of the body, eg the nervous system and bones, it appears to have superior imaging capability.[12]

3. Urinary catecholamine estimation

The diagnosis of neuroblastoma is often aided, and sometimes made, on the basis of raised levels of catecholamines in the urine. Traditionally a 24-hour urine has been necessary to determine the daily output of these substances. It has now been shown by several different groups that a 'spot' sample of urine is all that is required provided that the levels of catecholamines are related to creatinine,[13] as there is an excellent correlation between a 24-hour sample and a spot sample. If the two metabolites, homovanillic acid (HVA) and vanyl mandelic acid (VMA), are estimated then over 90% of cases of neuroblastoma will be identified[14] using a spot urine.

Advances in supportive care

1. Central venous catheters

Access to the circulation for the administration of cytotoxic drugs, antibiotics, and parenteral nutrition has always been one of the most difficult aspects of the care of children with cancer. Over the past five years the use of semi-permanent central venous catheters (CVC) has revolutionised this aspect of care.[15] These devices are inserted into a major vein, in either the neck or the groin, and then tunnelled under the skin to a suitable exit site, usually on the anterior chest or abdominal wall. For certain situations a subcutaneous 'port' of access is used with a reservoir attached to the CVC implanted under the skin.

The care of the catheter is important to prevent infections, and includes regular flushing with a heparin-containing solution. This can be achieved by most parents at home and allows the child the freedom to participate in any activity which he chooses, including swimming. Most children being treated for cancer become neutropaenic and immunosuppressed during the course of their treatment, and the presence of a central venous catheter increases the number of infections which a child will have. Many of these are due to colonisation of the catheter with *Staphylococcus albus*, and a recent study suggests that these can be abolished by the simultaneous administration of heparin and vancomycin.[16]

2. Local anaesthetic cream

For those children who still require repeated venepuncture, or for those who have a central venous catheter with an implanted port, the use of a local anaesthetic cream, EMLA, can considerably improve the quality of life and reduce needle phobia.[17]

3. Anti-emesis

One of the most distressing side-effects of cytotoxic chemotherapy is the emesis which occurs with the majority of these drugs. Cisplatin, which is being increasingly used, is particularly emetogenic, and considerable attention has been given to the development of effective regimes to combat this. These have included combinations of metoclopramide, prochlorperazine, and dexamethasone, none of which has proven universally effective and most having significant side-effects themselves, eg the distressing dystonic reactions associated with metoclopramide. However, an entirely new class of anti-emetics has now been developed, the 5HT-3 antagonists. The first of these to be released, odansetron, appears to be a highly effective anti-emetic,[18] and its relative value is now being assessed in comparative controlled trials.

Advances in therapy

There have been very few new chemotherapeutic agents developed in the past few years, and most of those currently in use have been with us for a long time. However, the timing and method of administration of each drug is now being optimised to obtain maximum therapeutic benefit with a minimum of side-effects. The recognition of prognostic factors has also enabled a better targeting of intensive therapy for those where there will be the major therapeutic gain. The following are examples of current therapeutic strategies: firstly for acute lymphoblastic leukaemia (ALL), where in general the prognosis has improved dramatically over the past 20 years; and secondly disseminated neuroblastoma, which remains one of the most difficult tumours to treat.

Acute lymphoblastic leukaemia

Figure 2 shows survival for children with ALL from the Northern Region who were diagnosed in four successive quinquennia. The improvement in survival can be largely attributed to increasingly intensive chemotherapy programmes and central nervous system irradiation used according to MRC therapeutic protocols. Over the past decade it has been recognised that survival has been achieved at a price, with many long-term survivors exhibiting considerable educational difficulties which can be attributed to the late effects of the central nervous system (CNS) irradiation. This is illustrated by Table 3, which shows the significant deficit in IQ for children treated for ALL when compared with those receiving chemotherapy for solid tumours.[19] In addition to the intellectual damage there is also clear

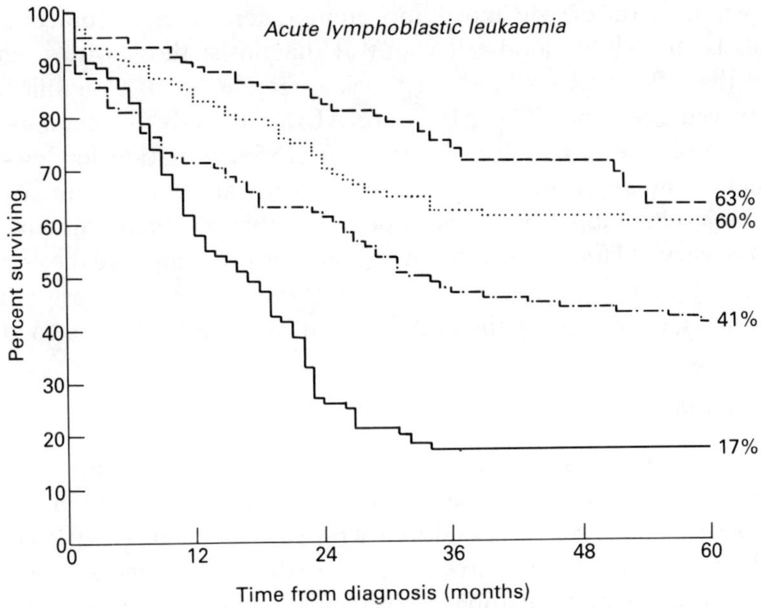

Fig. 2. *Survival for children with acute lymphoblastic leukaemia diagnosed in the Northern Region 1968–87 in four successive quinquennia. 104 children diagnosed between 1968 and 1972 inclusive* ———: *105 diagnosed between 1973 and 1977 inclusive* · — · — ·: *87 diagnosed between 1978 and 1982 inclusive* ········: *102 diagnosed between 1983 and 1987 inclusive* — — — .

Table 3. Mean IQ of patients and siblings with leukaemia or solid tumours (Twaddle *et al.*, 1986).[19]

	Before treatment estimate	4–6 years after treatment	7–8 years after treatment
Leukaemia			
Patients	104.3	99.2	98.3
Siblings	108.4	107.9	109.1
Solid tumour			
Patients	103.7	108.5	107.6
Siblings	107.2	108.6	110.6

evidence of late endocrine effects, with poor growth and subnormal growth hormone production in some children.[20] Because of this CNS damage the dose of cranial irradiation employed in most therapeutic protocols was reduced from 24Gy to 18Gy in the hope of mitigating these late effects. However, preliminary results suggest that intellectual and endocrine effects still occur,[21] so that for the new series of studies a different strategy of CNS prophylaxis is being employed.

Analysis of previous studies, both in the UK and elsewhere, has shown that the single most important determinant of outcome in ALL is the white-blood-cell count at diagnosis; those with a count less than $20 \times 10^9/l$ and also being female have a significantly improved outcome. The MRC UKALL XI study is therefore investigating the possibility of removing CNS irradiation for low-risk patients and replacing it with prolonged intrathecal and intensified systemic chemotherapy. It is hoped that this will maintain the excellent survival for these children and significantly improve the quality of life. Meanwhile, treatment is being intensified for those whose prognosis, as judged by the initial presenting features, is less good.

Neuroblastoma

While the overall survival for children with neuroblastoma has improved over the past 20 years (Fig. 3), this has largely been due to the better management of children with early-stage disease, ie stages I, II and IVs. Those who have widespread disease at diagnosis, ie stage IV, continue to have an appalling prognosis. The stage at presentation is therefore a very important prognostic determinant, as is age. More recently, biological factors associated with outcome have been identified, the most important being DNA ploidy, and N-myc gene amplification. A recent study from the United States has shown a clear correlation which appears to be independent of age and, to some extent, stage.[22] Those tumours which are diploid appear to have a worse prognosis than those which are hyperdiploid, and a single copy of the N-myc gene usually indicates a good prognosis. It seems likely, therefore, that there are actually two different types of neuroblastoma, one of which has an inherently good prognosis and the other a poor prognosis. Most of the improvements in survival have come from the good prognosis group. It now seems likely that only very minimal treatment is required for this group of patients, and certainly for stage I and II many centres are now using surgery alone to remove the primary tumour, and giving no further therapy.

Because of the appalling prognosis for stage IV disease, and for those with bad prognostic factors, treatment is being intensified for this group. The European Neuroblastoma Study Group (ENSG) has carried out a series of studies over the past few years, each of which has intensified the chemotherapy. These have culminated in a regime which employs both high-dose and rapid-schedule chemotherapy

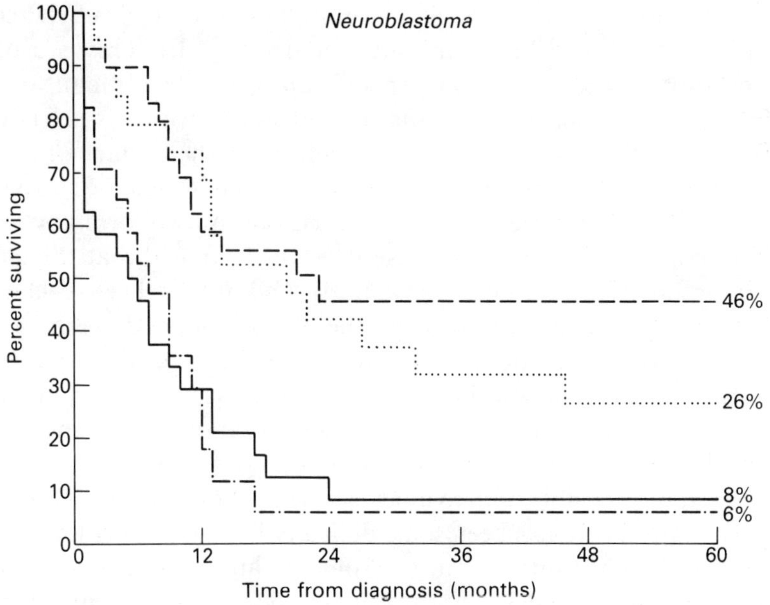

Fig. 3. *Survival for children with neuroblastoma diagnosed in the Northern Region 1968–87 in four successive quinquennia. 24 children diagnosed between 1968 and 1972 inclusive ———: 17 diagnosed between 1973 and 1977 inclusive ·—·—·: 19 diagnosed between 1978 and 1982 inclusive ·········: 29 diagnosed between 1983 and 1987 inclusive — — —.*

followed by further high-dose chemotherapy and autologous bone-marrow rescue.[23] The preliminary results of this approach are encouraging, with many more patients appearing to go into complete remission than have been seen in previous treatment protocols. The current approach in the ENSG is therefore to compare this new, extremely intensive regime with a more conventional high-dose chemotherapy regime in a randomised study. The outcome is awaited with interest.

Targeted therapy

Anti-cancer therapy acts by killing cells which are actively dividing. It follows, therefore, that not only are the malignant cells killed but a substantial number of normal dividing cells will also be damaged. The principle of anti-cancer treatment is to strike a balance between these two effects, allowing the normal cells to recover yet killing more of the cancer cells with each cycle of therapy. It has long been an ambition of scientists to produce a 'magic bullet' where the anti-cancer therapy was given only to the malignant cells. A great deal of effort has gone into investigating this possibility over the past few years, and clinical trials of promising agents are currently being carried out. The principle of most of these studies is that a substance is identified which will 'home in' onto the cancer cells. This is usually a monoclonal antibody to some specific antigenic determinant on the surface of the cancer cell, or another substance which is selectively taken up by the cancer cell. A radio-isotope is then attached to this substance and when it reaches its target the cell to which the substance is attached is irradiated. This principle has been used for many years in the treatment of thyroid disease where it is known that the gland takes up iodine-containing substances, and it has been relatively easy to adopt this approach using the radio-isotopes I^{131} and I^{132}.

Meta-iodobenzylguanidine (MIBG) is a substance which has been shown to be taken up specifically by neural crest tissue, and in particular neural crest tumours.[24] Most phaechromocytomas and many neuroblastomas take up this substance, and by attaching an I^{131} label to it, it is possible both to image a tumour and to provide targeted radiotherapy. There has been some difficulty in determining the correct dose of radiation to deliver to the tumour, and there are additional problems in that MIBG is not taken up exclusively by neural tissue. It can also affect normal bone marrow. More recently still, monoclonal antibodies have been produced which bind to certain brain tumours, and pilot studies of I^{131} labelling of these antibodies have been carried out in the therapy of leptomeningeal tumours.[25] This is one area of therapy which is likely to receive much greater attention in the future.

The future

Cytokines

The next few years will undoubtedly see refinements of therapy, and these are likely to be associated with a better understanding of the biology of cancer in children. Less and more-specific therapy will probably be given to those tumours which have an inherently good prognosis, and more-intensive and innovative techniques will be applied to those malignancies where we are currently not doing well. Although there have been some new chemotherapy agents over the past 20 years, there have been no new modalities of therapy. The next few years are likely to see the advent of a totally new class of therapeutic agent, the cytokines. It is now 10 years since interferon first received wide publicity as a possible anti-cancer agent. However, it never seemed to reach its projected therapeutic potential and this is almost certainly due to the fact that the interferon being used was of very poor quality.[26]

The revolution in genetic engineering which has occurred over the past few years has enabled large quantities of pure interferon and many other cytokines to be produced. Cytokines are polypeptides which either have a regulatory action on growing cells or support the proliferation and differentiation of precursor cells. The cytokines include interferon and interleukin which are both subdivided into various sub-groups. In addition there are haematopoietic colony-stimulating factors, tumour necrosis factors, and others. Table 4

Table 4. Cytokines in clinical use.

Supportive	
Erythropoietin	– anaemia of chronic renal failure and prematurity
GM-CSF/G-CSF	– congenital and chemotherapy-induced neutropaenia, – aplastic anaemia and AIDS
Cytotoxic	
TNF α	– refractory cancer
IFN α	– chronic leukaemias and hepatitis B
Modulatory	
IL 2	– refractory cancer
IFN γ	– leprosy

indicates some of the 30 substances which are currently recognised as cytokines, but this is a rapidly moving field of research and it is likely that there will be many changes in both the numbers, and recognised function, of cytokines over the next few years.

The availability of cytokines produced by industrially manufactured recombinant proteins has enabled many clinical studies to be carried out. These fall into three categories: supportive, cytotoxic, and immunoregulatory. Those used for support are the colony-stimulating factors which can reduce the period of neutropenia following the administration of cytotoxic chemotherapy. It is quite likely that the use of substances such as GM-CSF and G-CSF will allow considerable intensification of chemotherapy to be undertaken.[27] The interferons and tumour necrosis factor appear to have significant cytotoxic action without the concurrent administration of chemotherapy. Response rates of over 90% have been seen in hairy-cell leukaemia, and even in malignant melanoma, a cancer notoriously difficult to treat, response rates of 11% have been seen.[28]

Finally, there is the immunomodulatory function which is mediated by interleukin II and interferon. Both of these substances can augment the host's normal immune responses. A sub-group of normal lymphocytes, lymphokine activated killing cells (LAK cells), will kill cancer cells *in vivo*. There is growing evidence that these need the presence of various cytokines, and it is hoped that the natural killing ability may be augmented by the exogenous administration of cytokines. It seems very likely that 'the cytokines are coming'.[29]

Screening for neuroblastoma

The ability to detect cancer at the earliest possible stage has always been an aim of doctors trying to control cancer at any time of life. However, most paediatric malignancies do not lend themselves to screening, apart from neuroblastoma. There is considerable evidence that those children diagnosed with neuroblastoma within the first year of life have a significantly better prognosis than those diagnosed later, and that they require less therapy. The majority of neuroblastomas also secrete catecholamines and the metabolites of these can be detected in the urine. It therefore seems, at least from the theoretical point of view, that screening for neuroblastoma might be possible and potentially worth while.

A great deal of pioneering work has been carried out in Japan, initially by Sawada in Kyoto City, who in the early 1970s started screening projects.[30] The preliminary results were promising, and other centres in Japan further developed the methodology.[31] In 1984 the Japanese Government were convinced of the efficacy of screening for neuroblastoma, and since that date all six-month-old babies in Japan have been offered screening. Preliminary results suggest that screening can detect neuroblastoma at an early stage and that those so detected seem to have a much better prognosis than previously. However, there are considerable difficulties in the epidemiological interpretation of the Japanese studies, one of the major problems being that screening detects some tumours which would otherwise have spontaneously regressed.

Both the American Cancer Society and the International Paediatric Oncology Society have recently produced statements indicating that they do not believe that there is yet sufficient evidence for the universal implementation of screening for neuroblastoma, but that the evidence from Japan is suggestive that there may be some benefit and that the present requirements are for a small number of very large, well-designed, controlled studies which have as their end-point the death rate from neuroblastoma in screened and unscreened populations. One such study has recently started in Quebec,[32] and another is planned for five health authority regions of England and the whole of Scotland, following pilot studies in the north of England.[33] It will be at least seven to eight years before the results of these studies are available. Evaluation of the efficacy of neuroblastoma screening will not only include the possible saving of lives, but will also look at the cost of this, in both financial and human terms.

Conspectus

There have been tremendous advances in the management of children with cancer over the past 20 years, and many more children are now surviving. The present cohort of long-term survivors does include some children and young adults who have significant late effects of therapy. Current therapy is designed to minimise these side-effects, and the aim of future therapy must be to eliminate them altogether. We have moved from an era of 'cure at any cost' through one of 'cure at least cost', and hopefully the next few years will bring 'cure at no cost'. The ultimate goal, however, must be prevention, and hopefully over the next few years we will develop a better understanding of the nature of childhood cancer from which may develop preventive strategies.

References

1. Draper, G., Stiller, C.A. (1989) Cautious optimism. *Paediatric Nursing*, **May**, 22–23.
2. Stiller, C.A. (1988) Centralisation of treatment and survival rates for cancer. *Archives of Disease in Childhood*, **63**, 23–60.
3. Pritchard, J., Stiller, C.A., Lennox, E.L. (1989) Over-treatment of children with Wilms' tumour outside paediatric oncology centres. *British Medical Journal*, **299**, 835–6.
4. Stiller, C.A., Draper, G.J. (1989) Treatment, centre size, trial entry and survival in acute lymphoblastic leukaemia. *Archives of Disease in Childhood*, **64**, 798–807.
5. Hawkins, M.M., Draper, G.J., Kingston, J.E. (1987) Incidence of second primary tumours among childhood cancer survivors. *British Journal of Cancer*, **56**, 339–47.
6. Meadows, A.T., Baum, E., Fossati-Bellani, F. *et al.* (1985) Second malignant neoplasms in children: an update from the Late Effects Study Group. *Journal of Clinical Oncology*, **3**, 532–8.
7. Israel, M.A. (1989) Molecular and cellular biology of pediatric malignancies. In: Pizzo, P.A., Poplack, D.G., *Principles and Practice of Pediatric Oncology*; Philadelphia: Lippincott, 39–64.
8. Turc-Carel, C., Philip, I., Berger, M.P. *et al.* (1984) Chromosome study of Ewing's sarcoma cell lines. *Cancer Genetics, and Cytogenetics*, **12**, 1–19.
9. Seeger, R.C., Brodeur, G.M., Sather, H. *et al.* (1985) Association of multiple copies of N myc oncogene with rapid progression of neuroblastoma. *New England Journal of Medicine*, **313**, 1111–1116.
10. Pearson, A.D.J., Reid, M.M., Davison, E.V. *et al.* (1988) Cytogenetic investigations of solid tumours of children. *Archives of Disease in Childhood*, **63**, 1012–1015.
11. Parker, B.R. (1989) Imaging studies in the diagnosis of pediatric malignancies; in Pizzo, P.A., Poplack, D.G., *Principles and Practice of Pediatric Oncology*; Philadelphia: Lippincott, 127–148.
12. Kucharczyk, W., Brant-Zawadzki, M., Sobel, D. *et al.* (1985) Central nervous system tumours in children: Detection by magnetic resonance imaging. *Radiology*, **155**, 131–136.
13. Tuchman, M., Ramnaraine, M.R., Woods, W.G., Krivit, W. (1987) Three years of experience with random urinary homovanillic and vanillylmandelic acid levels in the diagnosis of neuroblastoma. *Pediatrics*, **79**, 203–205.
14. Laug, W., Siegel, S., Shaw, K. *et al.* (1978) Initial urinary catecholamine metabolite concentrations and prognosis in neuroblastoma. *Pediatrics*, **62**, 77–83.
15. Webber, T.R., West, K.W., Grosfeld, J.L. (1983) Broviac central venous catheterisation in infants and children. *American Journal of Surgery*, **145**, 202–204.
16. Schwartz, C., Henrickson, K.J., Roghmann, K., Powell, K. (1990) Prevention of bacteremia attributed to luminal colonisation of tunneled central venous catheters with vancomycin-susceptible organisms. *Journal of Clinical Oncology*, **8**, 1591–1597.
17. Clarke, S., Radford, M. (1986) Topical anaesthesia for venepuncture. *Archives of Disease in Childhood*, **61**, 1132–1134.
18. Pinkerton, C.R., Williams, D., Wootton, C. *et al.* (1990) 5-HT_3 antagonist odansetron—an effective outpatient anti-emetic in cancer treatment. *Archives of Disease in Childhood*, **65**, 822–825.
19. Twaddle, V., Britton, P.G., Kernahan, J., Craft, A.W. (1986) Intellect after malignancy. *Archives of Disease in Childhood*, **61**, 700–702.
20. Shalet, S.M., Clayton, P.E., Price, D.A. (1988) Growth and pituitary function in children treated for brain tumours or acute lymphoblastic leukaemia. *Hormonal Research*, **30**, 53–61.
21. Starceski, P.J., Lee, P.A., Blatt, J. *et al.* (1987) Comparable effects of 1800 and

2400 rad (18 and 24Gy) cranial irradiation on height and weight in children treated for acute lymphoblastic leukemia. *American Journal of Diseases of Children*, **141**, 550–52.
22. Look, A.T., Hayes, F.A., Shuster, J.J. *et al.* (1991) Clinical relevance of tumour cell ploidy and N-myc gene amplification in childhood neuroblastoma. *Journal of Clinical Pharmacology* (in press).
23. Pearson, A.D.J., Pinkerton, C.R., Craft, A.W. (1989) Ultra high dose induction regimen for disseminated neuroblastoma—'NAPOLEON'. *Proceedings of European Conference of Clinical Oncology*, **5**, 01134.
24. Hoefnagel, C.A., Voute, P.A., de Kraker, J., Marcuse, M.R. (1987) Radionucleotide detection and therapy of neural crest tumours using ^{131}I metaiodobenzylguanidine. *Journal of Nuclear Medicine*, **28**, 308–314.
25. Lashford, L.S., Davies, A.G., Richardson, R.B. *et al.* (1988) A pilot study of ^{131}I monoclonal antibodies in the therapy of leptomeningeal tumours. *Cancer*, **61**, 857–868.
26. Cantell, K., Gresser, I., De Maeyer, E. (1979) Why is interferon not in clinical use today? *Interferon*—I. London: Academic Press, 2–28.
27. Moore, M.A. (1990) Haematopoietic growth factors in cancer. *Cancer*, **65**, 836–844.
28. Foon, K.A. (1989) Biological response modifiers: the new immunotherapy. *Cancer Research*, **49**, 1621–1639.
29. Windebank, K.P. (1990) The cytokines are coming. *Archives of Disease in Childhood*, **65**, 1283–1285.
30. Sawada, T., Kidowaki, T., Sakamoto, I. *et al.* (1984) Neuroblastoma: Mass screening for early detection and its prognosis. *Cancer*, **53**, 2731–2735.
31. Nishi, M., Miyake, H., Takeda, T. *et al.* (1987) Effects of mass screening of neuroblastoma in Sapporo City. *Cancer*, **60**, 433–436.
32. Woods, W.G., Tuchman, M., Robinson, L.L. *et al.* (1990) Screening for neuroblastoma in North America. Preliminary results from the Quebec Project. *Medical and Pediatric Oncology*, **18**, 368.
33. Craft, A.W., Dale, G., McGill, A. *et al.* (1989) Biochemical screening for neuroblastoma in infants: A feasibility study. *Medical and Pediatric Oncology*, **17**(4), 373–378.

16 | Haematology

Ian M. Hann
Hospital for Sick Children, Great Ormond Street, London

Introduction

The past five years have seen an explosion in knowledge and its practical clinical application within the field of haematology. Predicting the future five years is an almost impossible task when one takes account of the current speed of change. I hope to present the most important areas of change and to deal with 'non-malignant' haematology.

Haematology has for many years been at the forefront of medical scientific advance, since the pioneering days when the structure of haemoglobin was described. All paediatricians are learning to cope with the modern era of molecular biology wherein almost every paper in haematological and other journals seems to need the cachet of a polymerase chain reaction (PCR). Most of us are having to go through a painful process of re-education, and nowhere is this more obvious than in haematology. Within a very short period of time this new science has leapt from the esoteric to the practical and essential. For this reason, I will concentrate on the area of prenatal diagnosis of haematological disorders which exemplifies the process. I have little doubt that gene therapy will come into being within the foreseeable future, and this has recently been discussed in excellent reviews[1] as well as in chapter 8 of this volume.

Neonatal coagulation

What else has happened of note? I believe that we have had to relearn a rather bitter lesson with regard to haemorrhagic disease of the newborn, ie that it is a very nasty process with severe morbidity and mortality.[2] Looking back, I find it hard to understand why some of us decided to give up prophylactic therapy. Oral administration appears an attractive alternative to parenteral therapy but the optimal dosage has still not been determined. I also believe that we should follow the American guidelines and give intramuscular Vitamin K_1

1 mg to breast-fed infants who develop diarrhoea lasting more than a few days. Infants who have a continuing risk of vitamin K deficiency, with malabsorption or biliary atresia, require regular supplements. Infants who receive antibiotics are also at risk.[2]

The level of knowledge of normal and disordered coagulation in the neonate has dramatically increased over the past five years.[2] The normal ranges of a wide variety of coagulants and anticoagulants are now well known and the processes leading to bleeding and thrombosis are becoming clearer. Although deficiencies of anticoagulants such as antithrombin III, protein C, and protein S are rare, the consequences can be disastrous, and management of these problems will improve in the near future.[2]

Blood transfusion

In the field of blood transfusion, serious problems have occurred which have, at long last, alerted doctors to the inherent dangers of blood products. We are now well aware of the problems of cytomegalovirus (CMV) infection in neonates and immunocompromised patients, particularly those undergoing various forms of transplantation. The availability of screened CMV antibody-negative blood products from the blood transfusion service (BTS) has made major inroads into this problem. We now have therapies such as gancyclovir and high-dose specific immunoglobulin which, along with rapid DNA probe diagnosis, have greatly improved the outcome in established disease.[3] Hepatitis C has been recently described, and hopefully it is only a matter of time before the other causes of non-A, non-B, non-C hepatitis are described. Hepatitis B vaccine has been a real therapeutic success in preventing disease in highly susceptible groups such as haemophiliacs. Heat treatment of factor VIII has reduced, but probably not abolished, the risk of all virus infections in these patients and we await the introduction of recombinant factor VIII within the next five years. The financial costs of this therapy will provide a major challenge to the production of new resources.

Human immunodeficiency virus infection should not recur as a problem in the new haemophilia population because of donor screening and product heat inactivation, but the future of existing infected children remains uncertain. It is of some comfort that the current progression rate to AIDS in the younger patients is currently running at the low rate of 2.5% per year.[4] Azidothymidine (AZT) therapy has produced further hope, but we do not know when to start this treatment and whether combinations with newer drugs such as dideoxyinosine (DDI) may reduce toxicity and increase efficacy. At present we institute therapy when the CD4-positive lymphocyte count falls below $0.2 \times 10^9/l$ or specific infections occur. These patients are given co-trimoxazole prophylaxis against *Pneumocystis* pneumonia and regular pentamidine inhalations if toxicity precludes the use of the former drug. The lives of families with these children are often desperate and a great deal of time and resources are spent in giving them the psychological support they need.

All paediatricians must now be aware of the hazards of blood-product therapy and of the legal requirements to monitor carefully their use as clearly set out under product liability legislation, which was long overdue. The search for alternative therapies is in its infancy but the impetus to perform proper studies is now in existence. We know that some children with bleeding disorders will respond to measures such as DDAVP therapy and the use of antifibrinolytics such as tranexamic acid. Important clinical research is under way to determine whether reduced blood loss and usage in cardiac and other surgery can be achieved by the use of 'cell savers' and aprotinin therapy. Similarly, we do not know whether the cheap plasma colloid substitutes are safe for use in children, and consequently trials are in progress. There is also a possibility that red-cell substitutes may become available.

The Blood Transfusion Service (BTS) in Great Britain has an excellent record of safety. Its improved donor screening programmes, along with a wide range of screening for infection of donated units, will help to plug the gap while the search goes on for better methods to inactivate viruses. Meanwhile, we should all use blood products with great caution and not, for instance, when haematinic therapy would suffice. The use of autologous stored blood in older children needs to be considered, and where applicable, appropriate funding for extra hospital blood-bank resources needs to be identified. I do not think that directed-donor transfusion (ie, from relatives or friends) could or should take on in this country. However, conservation of blood supplies by the use of small-volume packs should now be established in all units which are giving small transfusions, for example to neonates.

Prenatal diagnosis of blood disorders

The development of fetal blood sampling and analysis of fetal DNA obtained from amniotic fluid cells or chorion biopsy have revolutionised this area of medicine. There have been several recent reviews of this large and complex subject.[6,7,8,9] Various methods are available for diagnosis although DNA techniques performed on amniotic fluid cells or chorionic villi will gradually take over. Fetal blood sampling can be used for the diagnosis of genetic disorders of red cells, white cells, and platelets, as well as enzyme clotting factor deficiencies and globin chain synthesis disorders.

Fetal blood sampling

The method of Daffos,[10] using a 20-gauge needle under ultrasound guidance to obtain fetal blood, has been adopted by most centres. Procedure-related fetal loss using this technique has been reduced to 1% compared with 6–7% using fetoscopy. Blood thus obtained has been used to diagnose many haematological diseases but the largest experience is with structural haemoglobin variants and thalassaemias, using the globin synthesis rate measurement. Table 1 shows some of the disorders which can be identified using fetal blood. This table shows that various coagulation disorders can be diagnosed *in utero*, including rare ones such as autosomal recessive thrombocytopenia and Wiskott-Aldrich syndrome. Many red-cell disorders are amenable to a similar approach, and this has already been applied to the severe red-cell enzymopathies such as triose phosphate isomerase deficiency. White cells can also be obtained for the diagnosis of chronic granulomatous disease using the nitro blue tetrazolium (NBT) test.

Amniocentesis

Nowadays obtaining amniotic fluid is mainly of value because amniotic cells can then be used to produce fetal DNA. These cells can also be used for biochemical analysis of a wide variety of disorders so long as the enzyme is expressed, some of which are listed in Table 2.

A good example of the value of studies on amniotic cells is in Fanconi's anaemia. Culture of these cells with a DNA cross-linker, diepoxybutane, produces increased chromosome fragility. Attempts are now under way to treat affected siblings by taking the cord blood of proven unaffected HL-A matched fetuses and using it for transplantation.[11] It seems very likely that cells obtained by chorion biopsy will be equally useful in diagnosis.

Fetal DNA analysis

As stated previously, DNA can be obtained from chorionic villus sampling (CVS) or from amniotic fluid cells, although the latter method has only recently been applicable because the small amount of DNA produced can now be amplified using the polymerase chain

Table 1. Some disorders that can be identified by fetal blood sampling.

Haemoglobinopathies
Structural haemoglobin variants S, C, E Lepore
β thalassaemia
α thalassaemia, Hb Bart's hydrops
Other red cell disorders
Rhesus haemolytic disease
Specific enzyme defects
Hereditary erythroblastic multinuclearity with a positive acidified serum lysis test (HEMPAS)
Coagulation and related disorders
Haemophilia
Christmas disease
von Willebrand's disease
Other factor deficiencies
Thrombocytopenia
Wiskott-Aldrich syndrome
α_1-antitrypsin deficiency
White cell and related disorders
Chronic granulomatous disease
Genetic neutropenia
Immunodeficiency states
Cytogenetic analysis
Fanconi's anaemia
Bloom's syndrome
Xeroderma pigmentosa

reaction (PCR). These methods have revolutionised prenatal diagnosis of genetic disease and although this has mainly been applied to disorders of haemoglobin and coagulation, this will soon change.

The optimal way of obtaining CVS-derived DNA is controversial but it seems likely that the trans-abdominal approach may be increasingly used because it is available up to 13–14 weeks' gestation. With regard to the morbidity of CVS, the length of follow-up is insufficient to be certain but it appears to be a safe and acceptable procedure.

Methods for DNA analysis

A detailed discussion of this complex subject is not within the scope of this chapter and the reader is referred to several excellent reviews.[8,9]

Table 2. Some metabolic disorders identified by biochemistry of amniotic fluid cells.

Condition	*Enzyme*
Acatalasaemia	Catalase
Combined immunodeficiency disease	Adenosine deaminase
Glutathione synthetase deficiency	Glutathione synthetase
α-glutamylcysteine deficiency	α-glutamylcysteine synthetase
Methyltetrahydrofolate reductase deficiency	Methyltetrahydrofolate reductase
Tetrahydrofolate reductase deficiency	Tetrahydrofolate methyl transferase
Orotic aciduria	Orotate phosphoribosyl transferase Orotine 5-phosphate decarboxylase
Erythropoietic porphyria	Uroporphyrinogen synthetase
Coproporphyria	Coproporphyrinogen oxidase
Intermittent porphyria	Uroporphyrinogen 1-synthetase
Protoporphyria	Haem synthetase
Methaemoglobinaemia	NADH-linked diaphorase
Gaucher's disease	Ceramidase
Lesch-Nyhan syndrome	Hypoxanthine-guanine phosphoribosyl transferase (HGPRT)

Suffice it to say that the 'traditional' method of Southern blotting takes up to a week to produce a diagnostic result. However, the polymerase chain reaction has now been introduced and allows the amplification of a short DNA sequence over a few hours and the identification on gels or nylon filters, using non-radioactive oligonucleotide probes. This method may be applicable in the future following *in vitro* fertilisation, when the diagnosis could be established after testing a number of fertilised ova.

Overall results of prenatal diagnosis for blood disorders

Up to the end of 1982 the impact of prenatal diagnosis using fetal blood sampling in north Italy, Cyprus, Greece, and Sardinia, and among British Cypriots, had been a decline in the β thalassaemia birth rate to between 10 and 50% of that expected.[9] Among 3959 reported prenatal diagnoses the fetal loss rate was 6.2%, with 1.6% maternal complications, 6.5% premature deliveries, and an error rate of 0.8%. The results in other blood disorders are encouraging but are as yet only based on small numbers of procedures, mainly screening for bleeding disorders. At that time there were 208 procedures for haemophilia A, 19 for Christmas disease, and 4 for von Willebrand's disease. Another study in Greece between 1977 and 1988 reported the result of 3712 fetal blood-sample diagnoses. There were 17 definite and 3 probable errors, and 33 failures to get a sample. The fetal loss rate was 2.5%, which is a good result but still substantial.[9] Of course the other major problem with fetal blood sampling is the long period of uncertainty and the need for midtrimester termination of pregnancy, if indicated.

Fetal DNA analysis has now been in use for about a decade. In Sardinia, for example, where most cases of β thalassaemia major result from one mutation, over 1000 prenatal diagnoses have been carried out, more recently using dot-blot analysis. There were no misdiagnoses and fetal loss was in the region of 2%. In the UK up to the end of 1985 there had been over 600 prenatal diagnoses, mainly by analysis of restriction fragment length polymorphisms, in this population with many different β thalassaemia mutations. There were 14 fetal losses, 5 misdiagnoses, and 6 failures. First-trimester prenatal diagnosis is thus feasible and has an error rate of less than 1%. Errors can be minimised by excluding non-paternity using concurrent DNA fingerprinting technology. It seems likely that DNA analysis will be applied more widely to the prenatal diagnosis of other blood diseases, eg haemophilia A and Christmas disease. In fact, it could be used for any blood disorder for which a gene probe is now available (see Table 3).

Screening programmes

The antenatal clinic is where screening for blood diseases takes place. Most of these diseases are rare and thus screening will not become a routine part of antenatal programmes. It is likely that a family history for inherited blood disorders and a routine blood count will be the general practice, but where the gene frequency of haemoglobin disorders is high, screening for them will obviously be applicable. Within the UK at the present time this usually consists of screening for sickle cell disease in areas with susceptible populations (including people from the Mediterranean and Middle East), and in this situation it is also applied through neonatal blood screening.

When assessing the blood count results for the possibility of thalassaemia trait, the mean corpuscular volume (MCV) and mean

Table 3. Some of the haematological disorders for which gene probes are available.

Haemoglobin disorders	*Immunodeficiency*
α-globin	Adenosine deaminase
β-globin	
γ-globin	*Coagulation and thrombosis*
	Factor VIII
Red-cell enzyme deficiencies	Factor IX
Glucose-6-phosphate dehydrogenase	All other factors
Phosphoglycerate kinase	Antithrombin III
Pyruvate kinase	α_1-Antitrypsin (and variants)
	Protein C
Red-cell enzyme proteins	von Willebrand factor
Spectrins, actin, band 4.1.	
Miscellaneous	
Erythropoietin	
Transferrin and receptor	
Various cellular oncogenes	
Complement (various components)	
Haptoglobin	
Immunoglobins and T cell receptors	
Human T lymphocyte viruses (HTLV)	
Platelet derived growth factor; G-CSF; GM-CSF; various interleukins	

From D.J. Weatherall. In *Fetal and Neonatal Haematology* (eds Hann, I., Gibson, B., Letsky, E.). Baillière Tindall, London, 1990.

corpuscular haemoglobin (MCH) are crucial. Ideally, the cut-off values for further investigation are MCV 80fl, and MCH 27pg. Like all screening procedures this will entail a number of unnecessary investigations, but the cut-off is designed to avoid missing women with thalassaemia and only slightly reduced red-cell indices. The further tests consist of a haemoglobin A_2 level (HbA_2) which, if elevated, confirms β thalassaemia trait and indicates the need to test the husband. If both are carriers, appropriate genetic counselling should be instituted. If the woman has thalassaemic indices and normal HbA2, the father must be tested. If he also has thalassaemic indices the couple must be urgently investigated in a specialist laboratory. If he does not, the urgent investigation is not required. Tests to see whether they are heterozygous for both α and β thalassaemia, or if they have α thalassaemia or β thalassaemia with normal HbA2, should however be carried out.

With regard to other inherited blood diseases, their rarity dictates the need for further studies only when there is a positive family history. Coagulation disorders have already been mentioned and gene probes are available for the diagnosis of haemophilia A and Christmas disease. In addition, red-cell enzymes can be assayed by fetal blood sampling, but gene probes for first trimester diagnosis of severe enzymopathies are increasingly becoming available.

Most developed countries have concentrated their resources for prenatal diagnosis of the common haemoglobinopathies in central laboratories. This works well so long as communications are clear and rapid and so long as expertise in counselling patients about the potential outcome of at-risk pregnancies is also developed. If the latter does not occur the patients are left confused and improperly educated, and the whole purpose of prenatal testing is compromised. Laboratories are rapidly developing the sequencing methods for identifying unusual β thalassaemia mutations and those which lead to less severe disease forms. However, the RFLP linkage techniques will still have to be applied to those families in which mutations cannot be identified. Thus it seems likely that they will have to retain the ability to carry out fetal blood sampling and globin-chain synthesis for the rare cases where DNA analysis is not possible.

Haematopoietic growth factors

Within a bewilderingly short space of time the growth factors for blood cells, which hitherto were apparently mythical compounds used by tissue culture researchers to make their colonies grow, have been defined, multiplied, cloned, and produced as potential therapeutic compounds. There is little doubt that they will soon become an important part of our therapeutic armamentarium. In order to understand their rôle one has to have a grasp of normal blood development.

To put it simply, the pluripotent stem cell is capable of self-renewal as well as replication. Thereafter, there is differentiation down the lymphoid and myeloid lines. Lymphocytes of mainly T and B type are produced from the former and the other blood elements from the latter (Fig. 1). Indicated on this figure are the various precursor colony forming units which can be grown in tissue culture bottles. Although the stem cells are most difficult to grow because various accessory cells and 'feeder layers' are required to mimic real life, the Dexter long-term colony assay gives us insight into the inner domains of the bone marrow and, along with the other simpler assays for more mature precursors, has facilitated the fundamental understanding of bone-marrow growth differentiation and control. A simplified diagram of the action of colony stimulating factors is shown in Fig. 2. In fact, the process is a complex one with many checks and controls with which all crucial human processes are endowed. The next step is therefore to apply these compounds to the management of disorders in which the bone marrow has failed to follow this orderly process. This seems superficially easy but there are potentially large drawbacks

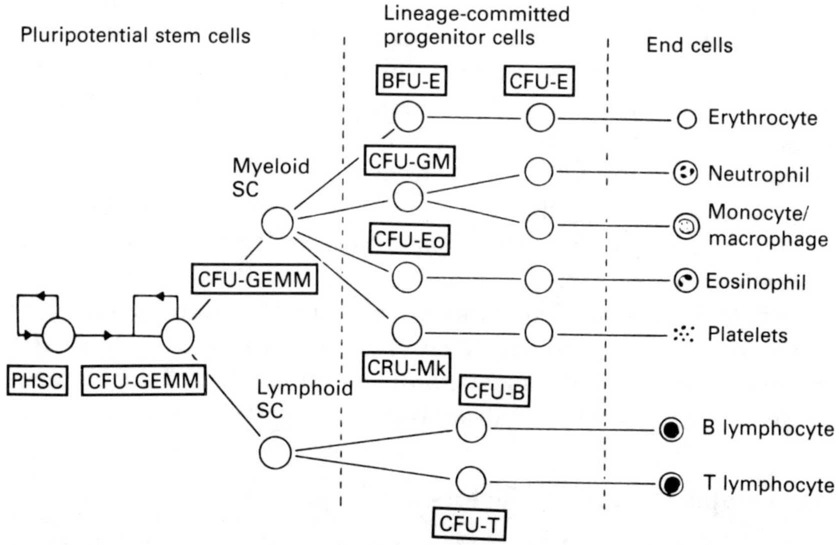

Fig. 1. *Development of haemopoiesis. CFU = colony forming unit; BFU = burst forming unit; PHSC = pluripotential haemopoietic stem cell; GEMM = granulocyte, erythroid, monocyte, megakaryocyte; E = erythroid; GM = granulocyte, macrophage; Eo = Eosinophil; Mk = megakaryocyte; B = B cell; T = T cell.*

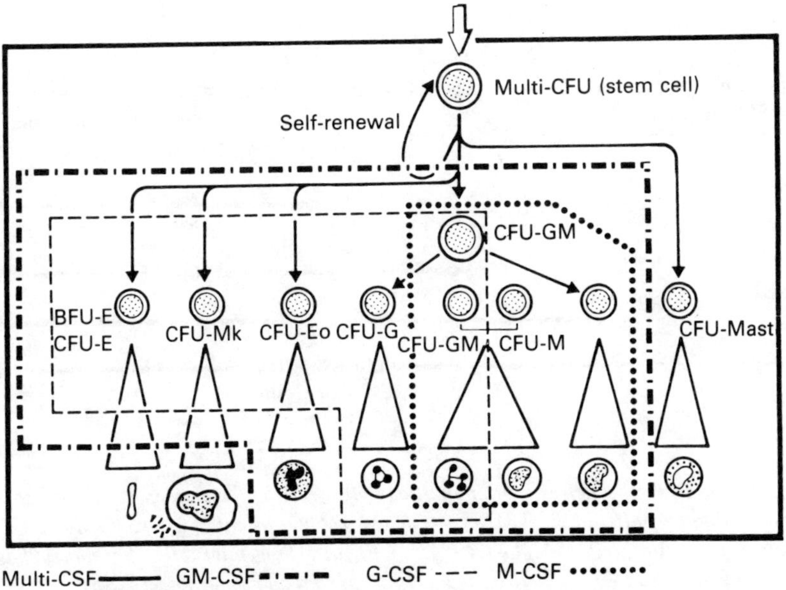

Fig. 2. *Site of action for haemopoietic cytokines. CFU = colony forming unit; BFU = burst forming unit; CSF = colony stimulating factor; M = macrophage/monocyte; E = erythroid; GM = granulocyte, macrophage; Eo = eosinophil; Mk = megakaryocyte; G = granulocyte.*

which will produce a multitude of research projects and inundate the medical journals with learned papers. Firstly, they may have adverse effects. This has come as a surprise to some doctors who appear not to be used to the fact that medical therapies are all toxic. The growth factors may interact (for instance with tumour necrosis factor) in a way that causes serious deleterious effects. Also, they may cause cells to proliferate in an undesirable way. An example of this is the use of G- or GM-CSF (granulocyte, macrophage colony stimulating factor) for the abrogation of neutropenia in acute myeloid leukaemia or myelodysplasia. There is a real risk that the leukaemic clone may be stimulated in the same way as it is *in vitro*. For these reasons the therapies are still experimental. The other aspect is that the various growth factors 'co-operate' *in vitro* and thus it may be necessary to use synergistic combinations to achieve the desired aim (Fig. 3).

Having said all of this, my prediction is that the use of haematopoietic growth factors will be a major therapeutic advance and that, in the future, little therapy for blood disorders will be given without at least a consideration of concomitant growth-factor therapy. The initial studies have been in the disorders where life-threatening neutropenia is paramount.[12]

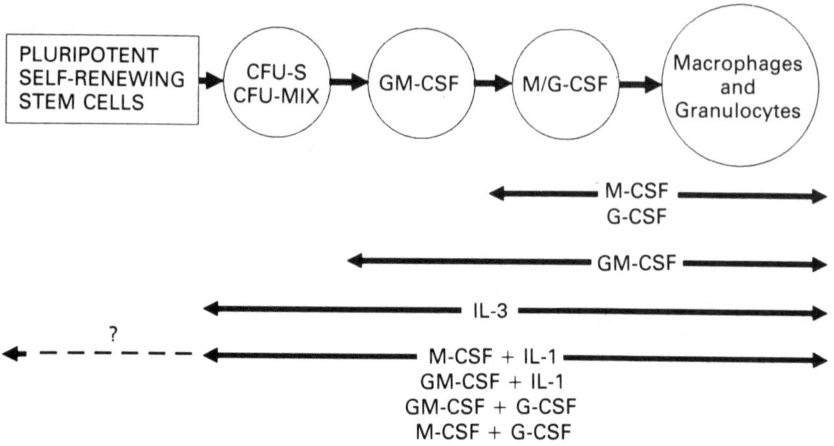

Fig. 3. *Potential synergistic combinations of growth factors. CFU-S = spleen colony forming units; CFU-MIX = mixed colony forming units; GM-CFC = bipotent progenitor cells; M/G-CFC = unipotent progenitor cells for macrophages and granulocytes. IL-1 = interleukin 1; IL-3 = interleukin 3 or multi-CSF.*

Preliminary studies of G-CSF therapy in cyclical neutropenia indicate that it will not only ameliorate the neutropenia but also increase the amplitude and frequency of oscillation of circulating progenitor cell numbers[12] (Fig. 4). Similarly G-CSF has been demonstrated to have clear benefit in severe congenital (Kostmann's) neutropenia[13] (Fig. 5). This severe disorder was usually fatal in the past unless the patient was fortunate enough to have a histocompatible sibling donor and to survive the procedure of allogeneic bone-marrow transplantation unscathed. Formal trials of larger numbers of patients are now under way in Europe and elsewhere, and it seems likely that they will confirm that this therapy is well tolerated, expensive, but cost-effective, and that these lethal disorders are at last amenable to medical management.

There are a large number of other medical areas in which the use of growth factors is being investigated at present. Whereas the problems of thrombocytopenia remain to be resolved, and may require synergistic combination therapy, neutropenia, usually induced by chemotherapy for malignant disease, looks as though it is amenable to therapy. One of the biggest bugbears of treatment for these patients is the number that still die of infection and not of the underlying disease, despite multiple antimicrobial therapy. Randomised placebo-controlled trials are in progress to assess the benefit of growth-factor therapy in various situations, the most important of which is in association with bone-marrow transplantation (BMT). Results of these trials will be available within a year and may well establish these agents as an integral part of the BMT procedure. However, that will not be the end of the story because combinations of factors may be better, especially at stimulating platelet recovery. A lot more work will also be required to establish their place in the therapy of other malignant disorders.

Acquired aplastic anaemia

Until the advent of BMT most children with severe aplastic anaemia died. Several series, including our own, confirm that two-thirds of patients are cured by allogeneic BMT[14,15] and have good quality of life. Several challenges remain, the most important of which is what to do for the two-thirds or more of children who do not have a histocompatible sibling donor. Three approaches to these problems are

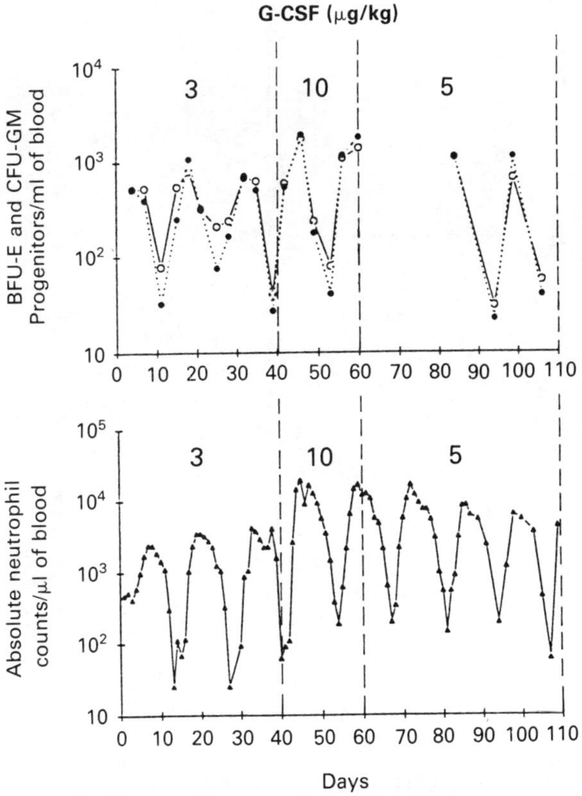

Fig. 4. *Cyclical neutropenia. Response of progenitors and neutrophils to G-CSF. (From Magliaccio (1990)* Blood, *p 1951.)*

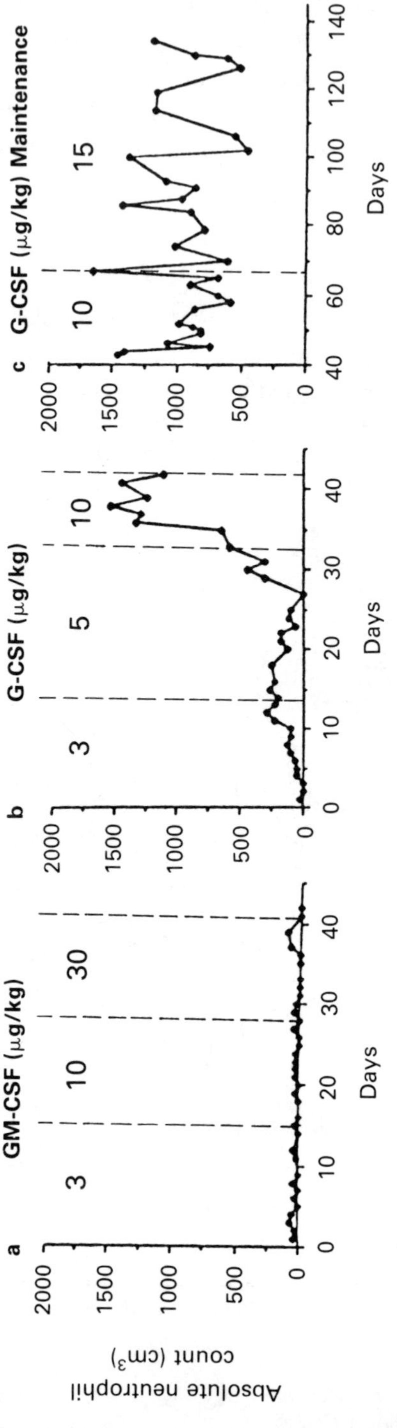

Fig. 5. *Severe congenital neutropenia differential response to GM-CSF and G-CSF. Only one out of five cases responded to GM-CSF. (From Welte (1990)* Blood, *p 1056.)*

being investigated: immunomodulation with drugs such as cyclosporin and also antilymphocyte globulin (ALG), growth-factor therapy, and matched unrelated donor transplants (MUD). The latter approach has been given a boost by the availability of large tissue-typed panels of potential donors run by the blood transfusion services and other organisations. The recent introduction of much more rapid matching procedures, eg oligonucleotide probe technology, have made feasible what previously was not. MUD transplants remain experimental, but the development of complex immunosuppressive preparative regimens has met with some success and may well be a partial answer for the future. The use of the immunosuppressive drug cyclosporin as a first-line agent for aplastic anaemia has met with some anecdotal success, and emphasises the possible role of immunological dysregulation in the aetiology of the disorder and the need for larger clinical trials of its use.

The therapeutic role of oxymethalone and ALG (separately or together) in the therapy of severe aplastic anaemia in children is still uncertain. Whereas the success rate with ALG in adults is good, children rarely respond and we are still awaiting the results of a co-operative European study of the additional use of oxymethalone. At Great Ormond Street we have recently reviewed our experience of treating aplastic anaemia over the period 1974–1988 during which 34 children were diagnosed as having this disorder. The haematological findings at presentation are shown in Table 4.

Three children had recent evidence of infection, one varicella, one non-A non-B hepatitis, and one mycoplasma; but as in other series of children about 90% were idiopathic. All presented with bruising and pallor, but only four had frank bleeding (epistaxis one, gingival/buccal two, and melaena one). Eleven were treated with oxymethalone (Table 5); two had a complete remission and two a partial response, one of these latter two eventually deteriorated and died.

Ten received ALG and seven ALG plus oxymethalone. A response

Table 4. Presenting characteristics of children with aplastic anaemia GOS 1974–1988.

Presenting haematology	N	Median	Range
Haemoglobin (g/dl)	34	7.4	3–11
Neutrophils ($\times 10^9$/l)	34	0.5	0.1–2
Platelets ($\times 10^9$/l)	34	11	1–40
Corrected reticulocyte count (%)	24	0.4	0.1–2.5

Table 5. Characteristics of children with aplastic anaemia by treatment group 1974–88.

	Oxymethalone	ALG	BMT
Number	11	17	6
Median age (years)	6	7	7
Age range (years)	3–10	2–14	1–11
Sex M : F	7:4	5:12	3:3
Disease severity Non-severe : severe : very severe	5:1:5	3:8:5	1:3:2
Haemoglobin (g/dl)*	6.5	7	7
Reticulocytes (%)*	1	0.6	0.2
Neutrophils ($\times 10^9$/l)*	0.6	0.6	0.5
Platelets ($\times 10^9$/l)*	14	16	11
Survival	3	5	5

ALG = Antilymphocyte globulin
BMT = Allogeneic bone-marrow transplantation from a family donor
*All haematology indices are mean values

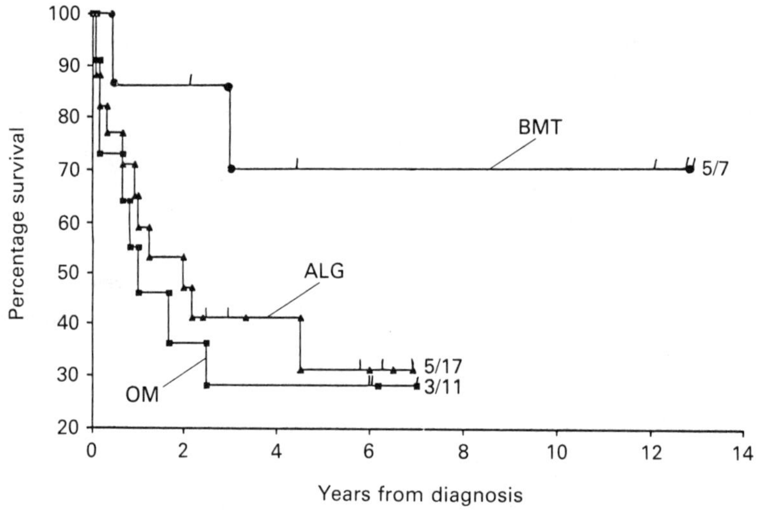

Fig. 6. *Treatment of aplastic anaemia at Great Ormond Street, 1974–1988. ALG = antilymphocytic globulin; BMT = bone marrow transplantation; OM = oxymethalone. Bars on the survival curves indicate surviving children.*

occurred in eight, three complete and five partial (of whom four deteriorated and died). Nine had no response; eight died, and one survives after a partial response to treatment with cyclosporin. Nine children had a second course of ALG and two had a partial response, one of whom is a long-term survivor with persistent neutropenia and thrombocytopenia. Nine failed to engraft and died. Of the matched BMT patients, five of the seven are alive and in normal health at two, four, 12, 13, and 13 years from BMT. No survivor has the debilitating disorder, chronic graft-versus-host disease. Figure 6 shows the survival curves of the various therapeutic groups and demonstrates 70% survival for matched BMT and extremely poor survival for the other groups. These patients all need intensive supportive care, and those who do not have a matched sibling need to be in centres which are exploring new methods of therapy if we are to make further substantial progress.

References

1. Kinnon, C., Levinsky, R.J. (1990) Gene therapy for cancer. *European Journal of Cancer*, **26**, 638–640.
2. Gibson, B. (1990) Normal and disordered coagulation. In *Fetal and Neonatal Haematology* (eds Hann I., Gibson, B., Letsky, E.), pp. 123–187. London: Baillière Tindall.
3. Meyers, J. (1988) Management of cytomegalovirus infection. *The American Journal of Medicine*, **85** (suppl 2A), 102–106.
4. Darby, S.C., Rizza, C.R., Doll, R. *et al.* (1989) Incidence of AIDS and excess of mortality associated with HIV in haemophiliacs in the United Kingdom: report on behalf of the directors of haemophilia centres in the United Kingdom. *British Medical Journal*, **298**, 1064–1068.
5. Gibson, B. (1990) Transfusion in the fetus and newborn. In *Fetal and Neonatal Haematology* (eds Hann, I., Gibson, B., Letsky, E.), pp. 190–217. London: Baillière Tindall.
6. Davies, K.E., Read, A.P. (1988) *Molecular basis of inherited disease.* Oxford: ICR Press.
7. Antonarakis, S.E. (1989) Diagnosis of genetic disorders at the DNA level. *New England Journal of Medicine*, **320**, 153–163.
8. Weatherall, D.J. (1990) *The New Genetics and Clinical Practice (3rd ed).* Oxford: Oxford University Press.
9. Weatherall, D.J. (1990). Prenatal diagnosis of haematological disorders. In *Fetal and Neonatal Haematology* (eds Hann, I., Gibson, B., Letsky, E.). London: Baillière Tindall.
10. Daffos, P., Capella-Pavlosky, M., Forestier, F. (1983) A new procedure for pure fetal blood sampling *in utero*. *Prenatal Diagnosis*, **3**, 271–277.
11. Auerback, A.D., Liu, Q., Ghosh, R. *et al.* (1991). Prenatal identification of potential donors for umbilical cord blood transplantation for Fanconi's anaemia. *Transfusion*, (in press).
12. Migliaccio, A.R., Migliaccio, G., Dale, D.C., Hammond, W.P. (1990) Hematopoietic progenitors in cyclic neutropenia: effect of G-CSF *in vivo*. *Blood*, **75**, 1951–1959.
13. Welte, K., Zeidler, C., Reiter, A. *et al.* (1990) Differential effects of GM-CSF and G-CSF in children with severe congenital neutropenia. *Blood*, **75**, 1056–1063.
14. Halperin, D.S., Grisaru, D., Freedman, M.H., Sauders, E.F. (1989). Severe acquired aplastic anaemia in children: 11-year experience with bone-marrow

transplantation and immunosuppressive therapy. *American Journal of Pediatric Hematology & Oncology*, **11**, 304–309.
15. McGlare, P.B., Haake, R., Miller, W. *et al.* (1987). Therapy of severe aplastic anaemia in young adults and children with allogeneic bone marrow transplantation. *Blood*, **70**, 1325–1330.

17 | Paediatric nephrology

Richard H. R. White
The Children's Hospital, Birmingham

Introduction

Paediatric nephrology is such a fast-developing specialty that it would be impossible to provide a comprehensive overview within the allotted space. I have therefore selected for review a number of areas in paediatric nephrology which I believe have—or should have—influenced the clinical practice of both nephrologists and general paediatricians; they fall under the two headings of investigation and management.

Investigation

Imaging of the urinary tract

Intravenous urography (IVU) is invasive in that it necessitates both the intravenous injection of an allergenic contrast medium, and radiation. Good-quality radiographs require careful bowel preparation, as well as an exceptionally patient and sympathetic radiographer. This may be incompatible with the tight schedules demanded of a busy district general hospital diagnostic radiology department, and in my experience the results have sometimes been so indifferent as to necessitate repetition.[1] The need for an alternative has to a large extent been fulfilled by the advent of both radionuclides and ultrasonography.

Static radionuclide imaging by means of ^{99m}Technetium dimercaptosuccinic acid (Tc-DMSA), which is principally incorporated into the proximal tubules and not filtered by the glomeruli, may detect local areas of renal tissue rendered ischaemic by either acute pyelonephritis or the scarring that may result, especially in the presence of vesicoureteric reflux (VUR).[2] In experiments on piglets, a remarkably good correlation has been observed between the anatomical location of Tc-DMSA defects and scarring found at necropsy.[3] While acute pyelonephritis may resolve if treated promptly, a recent study employing repeat Tc-DMSA scans showed that 80% of initial defects persisted, indicating that renal scarring had developed.[4] Although this technique is more sensitive than IVU in detecting early scars, and requires considerably less radiation, the quality of images produced and their interpretation nevertheless varies in different units, so that a consensus has not yet been reached to recommend this as a routine diagnostic procedure.[5,6]

Ultrasonography (US), on the other hand, is uncontroversial. It requires neither venepuncture nor radiation, and the high degree of resolution afforded by a modern sector scanner has made it a worthy alternative to IVU. Because US is not dependent upon the presence of renal function, it is capable of detecting such abnormalities as a non-functioning multicystic or hydronephrotic kidney, and a non-functioning upper pole draining into an ectopic ureterocele, which an IVU would not visualise.[7] The sound beam is unable to penetrate air or bone, so that access to the kidneys anteriorly may occasionally be limited by bowel gas, and the upper poles obscured by the ribs posteriorly.

For these reasons, and because the definition of calyceal shape is relatively imprecise, it is somewhat less sensitive than IVU at detecting small scars due to reflux nephropathy. Nevertheless, simultaneous comparisons between US and IVU in children investigated for urinary tract infection have yielded promising results[8,9] and, as technology has advanced and experience increased, US is now recommended as the initial imaging procedure,[6] when it should be combined with plain abdominal radiography in order to review the lumbosacral spine and exclude urinary calculi.[1] If there remains doubt concerning the presence or absence of scarring, it should be followed by either a Tc-DMSA scan or IVU, according to local circumstances.[6] We are also learning that increased echogenic 'brightness' is usually an indication of parenchymal disease.

The routine use of US prenatally has unquestionably made a major contribution to the management of serious malformations of the urinary tract, particularly those caused by damaging obstruction.[10–12] The initial enthusiasm for intra-uterine decompression of the obstructed urinary tract[13] has waned following an appreciation of the high mortality involved, not only from the procedure itself,[13,14] but also because of the serious renal damage already sustained by the fetus. Bilateral fetal uropathy is frequently associated with lethal extrarenal defects;[15] moreover, the oligohydramnios caused by deficient urine production may result in fatal pulmonary hypoplasia.[16]

Prenatal US should therefore be employed as a means of determining whether pregnancy should be terminated, when lethal defects are detected at 17–19 weeks' gestation, and in planning the immediate postnatal management of viable neonates. However, non-lethal urological defects that may nevertheless have serious consequences in postnatal life are frequently missed during the early scan[17] and, although it is not current practice to repeat all scans routinely, because of the added cost, future research should explore the potential benefits of a further scan at around 28 weeks' gestation. Transient urinary-tract dilation is frequently observed in mid-trimester pregnancy[10–12] and an agreed definition of normality has not yet been reached. However, we have recently documented a significant correlation between the presence of calyceal (as opposed to merely pelvic) dilatation and the postnatal finding of VUR.[18] The finding of mild dilatation naturally causes anxiety, and in one recent series the false-positive diagnostic rate was as high as 52%.[19] This raises the ethical questions of how much parents should be told, and by whom; it has been suggested that the best person is a well-informed paediatrician.[10] These dilemmas are most likely to be resolved, and patients' interests best served, by referral to a regional specialist centre where a multidisciplinary team consisting of obstetrician, radiologist, paediatric nephrologist and paediatric urologist can meet on a regular basis to discuss management.[10–12,26]

Assessment of renal function

Although the renal tubules have more numerous and sophisticated functions than the glomeruli, in clinical practice it is the glomerular filtration rate (GFR) which reflects the state of health of the kidneys. Techniques for measuring GFR that depend upon accurately timed urine collections have an inherent weakness in that they fail to take into account incomplete bladder emptying, a common functional defect which is exacerbated in the presence of severe VUR.[20] Thus in-dwelling bladder catheterisation, together with the need for continuous intravenous infusion, make inulin clearance an ethically unacceptable method, and this has been replaced by determining the rate of disappearance of plasma radioactivity ('slope clearance') following a single intravenous injection of ^{51}Chromium ethylenediamine tetra-acetic acid (Cr-EDTA).[21] It has recently been demonstrated that comparable results can be obtained in children using ^{99m}Technetium diethylenetriamine penta-acetic acid (Tc-DTPA), and the closest agreement with Cr-EDTA was found when Pentetate II (Amersham International) was used.[22] This method has the advantage that, when combined with dynamic imaging of the kidneys, differential renal function can also be determined, and this is of particular importance in monitoring serial changes of function in unilateral or asymmetrical disorders such as reflux nephropathy.[23]

Although the radiation dosages employed in these methods are small, they are nevertheless comparatively invasive in requiring an intravenous injection followed by two venepunctures, which must be undertaken in a separate vein in order to obtain blood samples uncontaminated by residual isotope in the injection cannula. A slope clearance takes from three to six hours to perform and is unsuitable for outpatient use. Creatinine clearance, which estimates the GFR, also suffers from the weakness of requiring a timed urine collection. However, in the stable state, the generation of creatinine to be excreted is a function of lean muscle mass, which is proportionate to the cube of body height (Ht^3), and since it is necessary to adjust its clearance to body surface area, which correlates with Ht^2, a hypothetical relationship has been derived from the familiar formula: clearance = $U_{Cr}V/P_{Cr}$ (where U_{Cr} is the urinary concentration of creatinine, V the urine flow rate, and P_{Cr} the plasma concentration), in which the GFR becomes proportionate to Ht/P_{Cr}.[24,25] With Ht expressed as cm and P_{Cr} as μmol/l, the following formula is used:[26]

$$GFR = 40 \times Ht/P_{Cr}$$

Although not a recent advance, this simple method does not appear to have been widely adopted in clinical practice except among paediatric nephrologists, and it seems timely to draw attention to it. A more recent study has shown that Ht/P_{Cr} is acceptably precise when the GFR is significantly reduced, but has limited predictive value when renal function is normal or minimally impaired.[27] However, the main value of the method lies in its consistency in demonstrating serial changes of GFR in individual patients, particularly those with incipient chronic renal failure. Blood urea levels, which are heavily influenced by dietary protein intake, should not be relied upon.

Measurement of proteinuria

Quantitative measurement of urinary protein excretion is essential in monitoring the progress of many types of renal disease. The long-standing tradition of quantifying proteinuria in a timed, 24-hour urine collection persists in clinical practice, despite the recognition that in health and disease[28] the daytime excretion rate frequently exceeds that observed under basal conditions at night. Furthermore, the discrimination of pathological from postural proteinuria is not possible by this method—a fact appreciated by the International Study of Kidney Disease in Children in its choice of timed overnight urine collections.[29]

However, errors of timing, the variable influence of incomplete voiding, and the need to correct the excretion rate make this method cumbersome, particularly in children who have not achieved nocturnal continence. Simply measuring the urinary protein concentration is unsatisfactory because it is dependent upon the osmolar concentration of the sample tested. Since the majority of pathological proteinuria is of glomerular origin, it is logical to relate its clearance rate to that of creatinine, and Barratt *et al*[30] showed that measuring the albumin/creatinine ratio in a random urine sample could adequately predict the timed albumin excretion rate. Using the same principle, we recently determined total protein by a modification of the Coomassie Blue dye-binding method,[31] which has the advantages of simplicity and low cost, and demonstrated a close linear correlation between the early morning urine (EMU) protein/creatinine ratio (U_p/U_c) and timed overnight excretion rate.[32] We also established an upper normal limit of 20 mg protein/mmol creatinine in 377 healthy subjects aged 3–19 years.

This has proved to be a highly convenient technique, and it is now our standard practice to arrange for patients to bring a fresh EMU at each clinic visit. In having eliminated the need for overnight admission of young children, it is both cost-effective and appreciated by the patients and their parents. The Coomassie Blue method is highly sensitive at low protein concentrations,[31] and facilitates the monitoring of 'microproteinuria', which is a feature of glomerular hyperfiltration resulting from reduced functioning renal mass, to be discussed later. Using the same method, we demonstrated that, in children and adolescents with the Alport nephropathy, P_{Cr} was never raised until heavy proteinuria (EMU U_p/U_c >200 mg protein/mmol creatinine) had developed,[33] implying that these patients can be safely monitored throughout most of their childhood without the need for repeated venepunctures. Moreover, we have recently observed a significant correlation between EMU U_p/U_c and plasma creatinine concentrations in patients followed up 20 years after recovering clinically from Henoch-Schönlein nephritis (A.R. Goldstein, R. Akuse, R.H.R. White, and C. Chantler, unpublished). Whether on the basis of accuracy, cost, or convenience, there is no case for continuing to make timed, 24-hour urine collections for quantification of proteinuria in routine clinical practice.[34]

Management

Vesico-ureteric reflux

The correct treatment of vesico-uretic reflux (VUR) has been the subject of debate for many years. The associated symptoms are not caused by VUR itself but are attributable, on the one hand, to urinary tract infection and detrusor instability, and on the other, to the consequences of renal scarring.[35] Patients with reflux nephropathy are at increased risk of hypertension and, where scarring is extensive and bilateral, of chronic renal failure (CRF). While there are as yet few reliable data on the incidence of CRF developing in patients with VUR from prospective studies, preliminary figures suggest that it is about 5–6%, but this is based on only five years' observation and may be an underestimate; reflux nephropathy has been found to account for 27% of children and 21% of adults with CRF entering renal replacement programmes in Europe.[35]

The main aim of treatment must accordingly be to prevent or minimise upper-tract damage. Surgical re-implantation of refluxing ureters has a high technical success rate in the hands of paediatric urologists, and is a seemingly logical way of protecting the kidneys from ascending infection.[36,37] However, a high proportion of VUR has a tendency to resolve spontaneously with time,[38] and carefully monitored chemoprophylaxis has been advocated with equal vigour. In 1975 the Birmingham Reflux Study Group established a controlled, prospective trial in which children were randomly allocated to operative or non-operative treatment, and were reassessed functionally and structurally two and five years after entry.

The results reported from Birmingham after five years' observation confirmed and extended those observed after two years, failing to demonstrate significant differences between the two treatment modes, in either the incidence of breakthrough urinary infection, GFR, renal concentrating ability, renal growth, progression of existing scars, or new scar formation.[36,37] The correction of VUR by submucosal injection of teflon has been promoted as a less invasive alternative to open surgery,[39] but its technical success rate is lower, and it has not yet been evaluated in a controlled, prospective trial. Indeed, there is no reason to believe that abolition of VUR by this method can influence the health of the upper renal tract more favourably than conventional surgery. Properly informed, most discerning parents will choose a trial of chemoprophylaxis rather than surgery; however there will be an occasional child who, for social or other reasons, is unable to comply with prolonged medication, and for whom surgery or teflon injection may be the better option.

The poor renal growth observed in children more than five years old at entry to the Birmingham study questions whether any form of intervention is effective in older children and, indeed, whether investigation by cysto-urethrography is warranted beyond that age.[37] Using Tc-DTPA renography, Verrier-Jones *et al.*[23] demonstrated, in a study of adults who had been found to have covert bacteruria in childhood, that impaired individual kidney function occurs only in the presence of renal scarring, whether or not VUR persists, whereas radiologically normal kidneys have normal function, even in the presence of VUR. It is thus becoming increasingly evident that VUR persisting into adulthood is unimportant, and that the optimum age for preventive management is before the fifth birthday.[35] The rapidity with which the scarring process is initiated in piglets with VUR after the experimental introduction of *E. coli* into the bladder, and the observation that prompt and vigorous antibiotic treatment may ameliorate it,[40] should focus our attention on the first urinary tract infection in infants and preschool children, which deserves recognition as a medical emergency.[41]

Clean intermittent bladder catheterisation

Urinary incontinence associated with a neuropathic bladder is a major handicap in children born with meningomyelocele who reach school age. Furthermore, many afflicted children develop renal damage as a result of functional obstruction, in addition to recurrent infection due to residual bladder urine. While incontinence in boys can be controlled by a penile appliance, there is no equivalent appliance suitable for girls, and the traditional choices have included in-dwelling catheter, which carries a high risk of infection, incontinence pads, and ileal loop urinary diversion, which is not infrequently complicated by infection, stenosis, calculus formation, and upper tract dilation.

Clean intermittent self-catheterisation has proved to be a satisfactory alternative for many of these children,[42] although in one series a quarter of the children and parents found it unacceptable for a variety of reasons.[43] However, the advent of a satisfactory technique of urodynamic investigation applicable to children has led to a better understanding of the reasons for failure, and hence the selection of suitable patients.[44] The child with a compliant bladder and reasonably good sphincter tone is likely to respond admirably, and the frequency of catheterisation required can be estimated from an assessment of the void and residual volumes. On the other hand, continence can never be achieved by intermittent catheterisation if the sphincter is flaccid, and an artificial sphincter is today a better proposition.[45]

As yet there are very few paediatric urodynamic units in the UK, and current workloads indicate a need for more. Although consultant-led, the essence of a successful unit is a team of nurses skilled in catheterising boys and girls of all ages, possessing endless patience and a flair for teaching; at least one such nurse should work mainly in the community and liaise with district paediatric nurses and incontinence advisers. Boys of six years old and girls of seven who are found urodynamically suitable, as well as the parents of younger children, can be trained within two days. The technique has been revolutionised for schoolgirls by supplying them with a pack of six stainless steel catheters ('Biscath'^{R}) which can be used in succession, rinsed and stored, and resterilised at the end of each school day by baking in a domestic oven. Clean intermittent bladder catheterisation is also applicable to other causes of neuropathic bladder, such as road traffic accident and transverse myelitis, and to the rare child with detrusor instability who is so severely dyssynergic as to be at risk of renal damage from functional obstruction (C.M. Taylor, personal communication).

Acute renal failure: the haemolytic uraemic syndrome

Two important changes have occurred during recent years in the incidence of acute renal failure (ARF) in childhood. The demise of palliative surgery and its replacement by advanced techniques of primary corrective surgery for serious congenital heart disease has appreciably lessened the demands made on paediatric nephrologists for post-operative dialysis. At the same time there has been a dramatic increase in the annual incidence of the haemolytic uraemic syndrome, beginning with the West Midlands summer outbreak in 1982.[46] A collaborative study conducted jointly by the British Association for Paediatric Nephrology (BAPN) and the Communicable Disease Surveillance Centre (CDSC) reported annual notifications of 81, 97, and 110 cases during the three-year period from April 1985 to March 1988.[47] In 1989, 193 cases were reported (D.V. Milford, personal communication).

Children aged one to two years were predominantly affected, and there was a marked seasonal trend reaching a peak during the summer months. Fifty-eight percent of children required dialysis. These findings have important planning and resource implications, as we have learnt from bitter experience in Birmingham where, at the time of writing, dialysis treatments for acute and end-stage renal failure are undertaken on two different sites—a situation soon to be remedied. Seasonal fluctuations in the demand for dialysis for children with ARF are more easily absorbed when this component of the regional paediatric nephrology service is grafted on to the comparatively stable end-stage workload.

The haemolytic uraemic syndrome comprises two subgroups:[48] an increasingly common variety with a seasonal incidence, associated with a prodrome of diarrhoea, frequently bloody, and an 85% prospect of recovery; and a much rarer, heterogeneous group without a seasonal incidence or obvious prodromal illness, occasionally familial, often relapsing, 70% of whom progress to CRF. These are now conveniently referred to as 'D+' and 'D−' respectively, and it is the former group that now accounts for 95% of all cases.[49] The sudden increase in incidence, beginning in the summer of 1982, has been associated with the emergence of Verocytotoxin-producing *Escherichia coli* (VTEC),[50] frequently but by no means invariably of serotype 0157:H7. Microbiological or serological evidence of VTEC was obtained in 33% of D+ cases notified to the BAPN-CDSC survey.[47]

A disappointing finding in this survey was that only 60% of patients were diagnosed as having the haemolytic uraemic syndrome on the day of onset of oligo-anuria, and in some cases renal failure remained unrecognised for two or more days. As a consequence many were inappropriately overhydrated, and hyponatraemia was a feature in 70% of cases, significantly associated with the development of seizures.[47] It is not always easy to appreciate that oliguria has developed, particularly in toddlers who are still in nappies, but the association of bloody diarrhoea with hyponatraemia should prompt an awareness that renal function has been compromised. Fragmentation of erythrocytes in a peripheral blood film is a frequent finding, while a reduction of platelet count occurs in more than half the cases.

Although 85% of D+ cases can be expected to recover normal renal function, prediction of the outcome has for many years defied clinicians. The recent observation by Walters *et al.*[51] that a neutrophilia at onset of D+ haemolytic uraemic syndrome is associated with an adverse outcome has been substantiated in the national study, and it is now becoming accepted that a neutrophil count $>20 \times 10^9/l$ will predict a difficult course.[49] Early referral of these children to a regional paediatric nephrology unit, before severe dilutional hyponatraemia has developed, makes management easier and may favourably influence the outcome. Serial investigations on children treated in our department have demonstrated that the rate of decrease of proteinuria, measured as EMU U_p/U_c, is significantly faster in children whose outcome is favourable than in those with a poor prognosis; in all but a few of the former, the proteinuria has disappeared within one year of onset.[52] In four patients followed up for 13–20 years, who had initially regained nearly normal renal function, a late decline of GFR was heralded by proteinuria which increased progressively over a period of several years, having previously been absent in two instances. We therefore recommend that children recovering clinically from the haemolytic uraemic syndrome should have their proteinuria monitored until it disappears, even if they have already achieved a normal GFR and are normotensive.

Chronic renal failure

There is now a wealth of experience in the management of end-stage renal failure in children, accumulated over 15–25 years.[53–56] Life support is achieved by means of renal transplantation and dialysis, and there is general agreement that a well-functioning transplant rehabilitates a child more effectively than dialysis. However, dialysis is required both for children awaiting a transplant and to cope with rejection episodes. Continuous ambulatory peritoneal dialysis (CAPD) is less costly than haemodialysis, and simpler for parents to undertake at home, but requires an in-dwelling Tenkhoff catheter and is not infrequently complicated by peritonitis. Although nearly half the initial cadaveric grafts cease to function within five years, the combined treatment ensures a patient survival rate exceeding 80% over ten years or more.

These satisfying results are the outcome of a team approach to management, which extends beyond skilled and sympathetic doctors and nurses. Repeated hospitalisation interferes with normal schooling, and continuity of education requires that every major paediatric renal unit employs a teacher who can liaise with an individual child's own school and supervise his learning while in hospital. The repeated travelling demanded of parents, coupled with loss of work, may lead the less fortunate families into financial difficulties, and a social worker is an essential member of the team. Retarded growth and pubertal development, repeated separation from the family, educational handicap, and other factors such as the wearing of external appliances in CAPD, may create psychological difficulties for patients, while the seemingly endless travelling and the financial loss may strain fragile family relationships to breaking point; it is therefore important to secure the regular services of a psychiatrist. Because of the need for an energetic approach to growth and nutrition, a whole-time dietitian dedicated to the nephrology unit is indispensable. In the UK, the British Kidney Patient Association has played a major role in the care of children with chronic renal disease by providing financial aid and information leaflets to parents, and by funding both capital developments and salaries that would be unlikely to have materialised in the precarious financial state of the National Health Service.

Two major problems remain to be solved. Anaemia is a feature of CRF which persists throughout dialysis but is corrected by a functioning transplant, and the advent of recombinant human erythropoietin[57] was a breakthrough. Undoubtedly the enhanced tissue oxygenation achieved improves patient wellbeing, but the increased haematocrit is associated with an increased incidence of vascular access clotting and worsening of hypertension in some patients.[58] Moreover, the long-term effects of the haemodynamic changes, notably the reduced cardiac output, on renal perfusion and function are as yet unknown.

Growth retardation is a well-recognised aspect of CRF in childhood, and is maximal when the renal disease is either congenital or acquired in infancy. Depression of growth velocity is greatest during the two periods of normally rapid growth—the first two years of life and around the time of puberty, and between these two periods velocity may be normal, even though the actual height remains below the third centile.[59] The use of alternate-day steroid therapy, combined with either azathioprine or cyclosporin A, to prevent graft rejection, causes blunting of growth hormone and gonadotrophin pulsatility, and although increased prepubertal growth can be achieved following transplantation, the velocity still declines at the age when the normal prepubertal growth spurt would be expected, and sexual maturation is delayed.[60] Trials of growth hormone treatment are currently being planned in the UK.

However, Rees *et al.*[61] have recently demonstrated that ground can be gained during the first two years of life, before dialysis or transplantation, by an intensive approach which includes: (i) the correction of acidosis by means of sodium bicarbonate; (ii) the introduction of sodium chloride supplements in children with a salt-losing nephropathy, which is not infrequently associated with severe VUR and obstructive nephropathy; (iii) maintenance of normal plasma calcium levels by means of 1α-hydroxycholecalciferol or 1,25-dihydroxycholecalciferol, and of phosphate levels by mild dietary restriction and the use of oral calcium carbonate as a phosphate binder. Dietary energy supplements were given as either glucose polymers or fat emulsions, and the protein intake was adjusted to maintain the plasma urea concentration <20 mmol/l with a normal albumin level. Anorexic infants were tube fed. The few infants who failed to grow on this regime were mainly of low birth-weight and had dysplastic kidneys. This is a clinically important advance at a time when an increasing number of very young children are being referred for treatment as a result of both better informed doctors and parents, and antenatal ultrasound screening.

Remnant kidney

'Remnant kidney' is the term often applied to a significant reduction of functioning renal tissue which results from congenital defects or acquired disease processes. These include renal agenesis and non-functioning kidney due to multicystic dysplasia or pelvi-ureteric junction obstruction; progressive nephron destruction due to reflux nephropathy, haemolytic uraemic syndrome, congenital nephrotic syndrome, hereditary and acquired glomerulonephritis; and nephrectomy, eg for Wilms' tumour. The consequence of substantial nephron loss is anatomical and functional hypertrophy of the undamaged remnant nephrons, in an endeavour to maintain a normal GFR. The anatomical hypertrophy is perhaps best illustrated by unilateral reflux nephropathy, where the disparity in size between the diffusely scarred and normal contralateral kidneys is striking; the total GFR, as measured by Cr-EDTA slope clearance, remains normal,[62] but the difference in individual kidney GFR can be demonstrated by Tc-DTPA renography.[23]

Reflux nephropathy has been the most extensively studied human example of remnant kidney. It has long been known that increasing proteinuria accompanies declining renal function,[63] and is associated with the development of focal segmental glomerulosclerosis (FSGS) in adult patients.[64] The experimental counterpart is the rat that has undergone five-sixths nephrectomy, which similarly develops proteinuria and FSGS.[65] More recently it has been shown that this glomerular destruction is more pronounced and rapid when nephrectomy is performed in infant than in adult rats,[66] and both proteinuria[67] and FSGS[68] have been demonstrated in human adults who had undergone unilateral nephrectomy during childhood. The popular view that a single kidney is enough for a lifetime now requires reconsideration.

Until recently little was known about the early evolution of either the proteinuria or the glomerular lesion. However, we have now confirmed that FSGS may develop during childhood; moreover, we demonstrated a highly significant correlation between the magnitude of EMU U_p/U_c and the percentage of glomeruli in renal biopsy specimens affected by FSGS.[69] Like Kincaid-Smith and her colleagues,[64] we demonstrated the presence of FSGS in contralateral, radiologically normal kidneys, in the presence of proteinuria, indicating that the glomerular changes are not directly due to reflux nephropathy. Furthermore, we noted that all the segmental sclerotic lesions originated at the glomerular hilum,[69] as in nephrectomised rats, whereas similar lesions occurring in the nephrotic syndrome are of random distribution.[70] Close scrutiny of hilar vessels showed that the walls were often thickened and contained hyaline subendothelial deposits, and these changes preceded the development of proteinuria.[69]

These findings are consistent with Brenner's hypothesis that a reduced number of functioning nephrons leads to chronic renal vasodilation which, in turn, causes glomerular hyperfiltration, with increased protein flux through the capillary walls and consequent mesangial injury, progressing ultimately to sclerosis.[71] The abnormalities are not confined to reflux nephropathy; we have observed similar changes many years after clinical recovery from the haemolytic uraemic syndrome, and believe that these are associated with persistent proteinuria in the minority of patients with a poor outcome.[52] It has been demonstrated that the sclerosing process is accelerated by dietary protein loading and, conversely, retarded by protein restriction.[72] Similarly, short-term dietary protein restriction has been shown to reduce microproteinuria in children with reflux nephropathy, and there is now sufficient evidence to recommend at least the avoidance of excessive dietary protein,[73] even in the presence of normal renal function and the absence of proteinuria. Prospective three-day dietary assessments on patients under my care frequently reveal protein intakes well above the recommended daily allowances. Finally, there are theoretical grounds for considering the use of angiotensin converting enzyme inhibitors, since experimental studies, together with limited clinical observations in human adults, suggest that angiotensin II plays a role in maintaining glomerular hyperfiltration by its constrictive effect on the efferent arteriole.[74] Controlled studies are now needed in children.

Alport's syndrome

A recent advance of considerable potential importance is the localisation of the gene for Alport's syndrome on the long arm of the X chromosome.[75,76] However, hereditary nephritis is heterogeneous, both clinically and morphologically, and some of the patients included under the diagnosis of Alport's syndrome are probably variants.[33] A prerequisite to the ultimate documentation of its genetics is therefore further characterisation of the underlying glomerular ultrastructural defects, using both immunohistochemical probes for type IV collagen[77] and morphometric methods.[78] This research has not so far had a major impact on clinical practice, and in most Alport families the pedigrees justify the assumption of X-linkage; however, the prospects of carrier detection and antenatal diagnosis lie ahead.

Finale

Many of the new developments described have enabled paediatric nephrologists to provide improved standards of care for children with renal disease. The laudable aim of shared care demands that general paediatricians also take advantage of this progress. Two developments, in particular, deserve reiterating: the use of EMU U_p/U_c in monitoring renal disease, and the role of the dietitian as a member of the clinical team. District general hospital laboratories tend to respond to the needs of the majority of clinicians; unfortunately there has been a notable reluctance among adult nephrologists to replace the 24-hour urine collection with EMU,[34] and it will be necessary for paediatricians to initiate this change, which will undoubtedly also benefit adult patients. To manage children with chronic renal disease and not have the professional services of a skilled dietitian is, today, unthinkable. In 1965 the Birmingham Children's Hospital employed one dietitian; in 1987 there were four, and in 1990 there are ten! While there is no specific training in paediatric dietetics, it nevertheless seems reasonable that at least one dietitian in a district general hospital should have gained some experience in a large paediatric department, and maintain a liaison with the specialist dietitians based at tertiary referral hospitals.

References

1. White, R.H.R. (1987) Management of urinary tract infection. *Archives of Disease in Childhood*, **62**, 421–427.
2. Verber, I.G., Strudley, M.R., Meller, S.T. (1988) ^{99m}Tc dimercaptosuccinic acid (DMSA) scan as first investigation of urinary tract infection. *Archives of Disease in Childhood*, **63**, 1320–1325.
3. Arnold, A.J., Brownless, S.M., Carty, H.M., Rickwood, A.M.K. (1990) Detection of renal scarring by DMSA scanning—An experimental study. *Journal of Pediatric Surgery*, **25**, 391–393.
4. Verber, I.G., Meller, S.T. (1989) Serial ^{99m}Tc dimercaptosuccinic acid (DMSA) scans after urinary infections presenting before the age of 5 years. *Archives of Disease in Childhood*, **64**, 1533–1537.
5. Smellie, J.M. (1989) The DMSA scan and intravenous urography in the detection of renal scarring. *Pediatric Nephrology*, **3**, 6–8.
6. Research Unit of the Royal College of Physicians, Report of a Working Group. (1991) Guidelines for the management of acute urinary tract infection in childhood. *Journal of the Royal College of Physicians of London*, in press.
7. Taylor, C.M., Chapman, S. (1989) *Handbook of Renal Investigations in Childhood.* London: Butterworth & Co., pp 98–127.
8. Leonidas, J.C., McCauley, R.G.K., Klauber, G.C., Fretzayas, A.M. (1985) Sonography as a substitute for excretory urography in children with urinary tract infection. *American Journal of Roentgenology*, **144**, 815–819.
9. Lindsell, D., Moncrieff, M. (1986) Comparison of ultrasound examination and intravenous urography after a urinary tract infection. *Archives of Disease in Childhood*, **61**, 81–82.
10. Tudor, J., Whitaker, R.H. (1989) Detection and Management of the Dilated Fetal Urinary Tract. *Clinical Radiology*, **40**, 229–230.
11. White, R.H.R. (1989) Fetal uropathy. *British Medical Journal*, **298**, 1408–1409.
12. Thomas, D.F.M. (1990) Fetal uropathy. *British Journal of Urology*, **66**, 225–231.
13. Manning, F.A., Harrison, M.R., Rodeck, C. (1986) Report of the International Fetal Surgery Registry. Catheter shunts for fetal hydronephrosis and hydrocephalus. *New England Journal of Medicine*, **315**, 336–347.

14. Elder, J.S., Duckett, J.W. Jr, Snyder, H.M. (1987) Intervention for fetal obstructive uropathy: has it been effective? *Lancet*, **ii**, 1007–1010.
15. Nicolaides, K.H., Rodeck, C.H., Gosden, C.M. (1986) Rapid karyotyping in non-lethal fetal malformations. *Lancet*, **i**, 284–287.
16. Thomas, I.T., Smith, D.W. (1974) Oligohydramnios, cause of the non-renal features of Potter's syndrome, including pulmonary hypoplasia. *Journal of Pediatrics*, **84**, 811–814.
17. Helin, I., Persson, P. (1986) Prenatal diagnosis of urinary tract abnormalities by ultrasound. *Journal of Pediatrics*, **78**, 879–883.
18. Newell, S.J., Morgan, M.E.I., McHugo, J.M. *et al.* (1990) Clinical significance of antenatal calyceal dilation detected by ultrasound. *Lancet*, **ii**, 372.
19. Livera, L.N., Brookfield, D.S.K., Egginton, J.A., Hawnaur, J.M. (1989) Antenatal ultrasonography to detect fetal renal abnormalities: a prospective screening programme. *British Medical Journal*, **298**, 1421–1423.
20. Winterborn, M.H., Beetham, R., White, R.H.R. (1977) Comparison of plasma disappearance and standard clearance techniques for measuring glomerular filtration rate in children with and without vesico-ureteric reflux. *Clinical Nephrology*, **7**, 262–270.
21. Chantler, C., Barratt, T.M. (1972) Estimation of glomerular filtration rate from plasma clearance of 51-chromium edetic acid. *Archives of Disease in Childhood*, **47**, 613–617.
22. Griffiths, P.D., Drolc, Z., Green, A. *et al.* (1988) Comparison of ^{51}Cr-EDTA and ^{99m}Tc-DTPA Slope Clearances in Children with Vesicoureteric Reflux. *Child Nephrology and Urology*, **9**, 283–285.
23. Verrier Jones, K., Asscher, A.W., Verrier Jones, E.R. *et al.* (1982) Glomerular filtration rate in schoolgirls with covert bacteriuria. *British Medical Journal*, **285**, 1307–1310.
24. Schwartz, G.J., Haycock, G.B., Edelmann, C.M. Jr, Spitzer, A. (1976) A simple estimate of glomerular filtration rate in children derived from body length and plasma creatinine. *Pediatrics*, **58**, 259–263.
25. Counahan, R., Chantler, C., Ghazali, S. *et al.* (1976) Estimation of glomerular filtration rate from plasma creatinine concentration in children. *Archives of Disease in Childhood*, **51**, 875–878.
26. Taylor, C.M., Chapman, S. (1989) *Handbook of Renal Investigations in Children.* London: Butterworth & Co., pp 25–34.
27. Davies, J.G., Taylor, C.M., White, R.H.R., Marshall, T. (1982) Clinical limitations of the estimation of glomerular filtration rate from height/plasma creatinine ratio: A comparison with simultaneous ^{51}Cr Edetic acid slope clearance. *Archives of Disease in Childhood*, **57**, 607–610.
28. Ginsberg, J.M., Chang, B.S., Matarese, R.A., Garella, S. (1983) Use of single voided urine samples to estimate quantitative proteinuria. *New England Journal of Medicine*, **309**, 1543–1546.
29. Internatioinal Study of Kidney Disease in Children (1974) Prospective, controlled trial of cyclophosphamide therapy in children with nephrotic syndrome. *Lancet*, **2**, 423–427.
30. Barratt, T.M., McLaine, P.N., Soothill, J.F. (1970) Albumin excretion as a measure of glomerular dysfunction in children. *Archives of Disease in Childhood*, **45**, 496–501.
31. Bradford, M.M. (1976) A rapid and sensitive method for the quantitation of microgram quantities of protein utilising the principle of protein-dye binding. *Annals of Biochemistry*, **72**, 248–254.
32. Elises, J.S., Griffiths, P.D., Hocking, M.D. *et al.* (1988) Simplified quantification of urinary protein excretion in children. *Clinical Nephrology*, **30**, 225–229.
33. White, R.H.R. (1987) The Alport nephropathy. In *Recent Advances in Paediatric Nephroogy*, (eds K. Murakami, T. Kitagawa, K. Yabuta and T. Sakai), Amsterdam: Elsevier Science Publishers B.V. (Biomedical Division), pp 201–206.

34. White, R.H.R, Taylor, C.M., Green, A. (1990) Measurement of proteinuria. *Nephron*, **55**, 437.
35. White, R.H.R. (1989) Vesico-ureteric reflux and renal scarring. *Archives of Disease in Childhood*, **64**, 407–412.
36. Birmingham Reflux Study Group (1983) Prospective trial of operative versus non-operative treatment of severe vesico-ureteric reflux: two years' observation in 96 children. *British Medical Journal*, **287**, 171–174.
37. Birmingham Reflux Study Group (1987) Prospective trial of operative versus non-operative treatment of severe vesico-ureteric reflux in children: five years' observation. *British Medical Journal*, **295**, 237–241.
38. Edwards, D., Normand, I.C.S., Prescod, N., Smellie, J.M. (1977) Disappearance of vesico-ureteric reflux during long-term prophylaxis of urinary tract infection. *British Medical Journal*, **ii**, 285–288.
39. O'Donnell, B., Puri, P. (1986) Endoscopic correction of primary vesico-ureteric reflux. *British Journal of Urology*, **58**, 601–604.
40 Ransley, P.G., Risdon, R.A. (1981) Reflux nephropathy: effects of antimicrobial therapy on the evolution of the early pyelonephritic scar. *Kidney International*, **20**, 733–742.
41. White, R.H.R. (1990) Management of urinary tract infection and vesico-ureteric reflux in children. *British Medical Journal*, **300**, 1391–1392.
42. Ananias, C., Diokno, L., Sonda, P. *et al.* (1983) Fate of patients started on clean intermittent self-catheterisation therapy 10 years ago. *The Journal of Urology*, **129**, 1120–1121.
43. Cass, A.S., Luxenberg, M., Gleich, P. *et al.* (1984) Clean intermittent catheterisation in the management of the neurogenic bladder in children. *The Journal of Urology*, **132**, 526–528.
44. Van Gool, J., de Ridder, A.L.A., Kuijten, R.H. *et al.* (1976) Measurement of intravesical and rectal pressures simultaneously with electromyography of anal sphincter in children with myelomeningocele. *Developmental Medicine and Child Neurology*, **18**, 287–301.
45. Mundy, A.R., Stephenson, T.P. (1984) Selection of patients for implantation of the Brantley Scott artificial urinary sphincter. *British Journal of Urology*, **56**, 717–720.
46. Taylor, C.M., White, R.H.R., Winterborn, M.H., Rowe, B. (1986) Haemolytic-uraemic syndrome: clinical experience of an outbreak in the West Midlands. *British Medical Journal*, **292**, 1513–1516.
47. Milford, D.V., Taylor, C.M., Guttridge, B. *et al.* (1990) Haemolytic uraemic syndromes in the British Isles 1985–8: association with Verocytotoxin producing *Escherichia coli*. Part 1: clinical and epidemiological aspects. *Archives of Disease in Childhood*, **65**, 716–721.
48. Levin, M., Barratt, T.M. (1984) Haemolytic uraemic syndrome. *Archives of Disease in Childhood*, **59**, 397–400.
49. Milford, D.V., Taylor, C.M. (1990) New insights into the haemolytic uraemic syndromes. *Archives of Disease in Childhood*, **65**, 713–715.
50. Karmali, M.A., Petric, M., Lim, C. *et al.* (1985) The association between idiopathic hemolytic uremic syndrome and infection by verotoxin producing *Escherichia coli*. *Journal of Infectious Diseases*, **151**, 775–782.
51. Walters, M.D., Matthei, U., Kay, R. *et al.* (1989) The polymorphonuclear count in childhood hemolytic uremic syndrome. *Pediatric Nephrology*, **3**, 130–134.
52. Milford, D.V., White, R.H.R., Taylor, C.M. (1991) Prognostic significance of proteinuria at one year after onset in diarrhoea-associated haemolytic uraemic syndrome. *Journal of Pediatrics*, **118**, 191–194.
53. Chantler, C., Carter, J.E., Bewick, M. *et al.* (1980) 10 years' experience with regular haemodialysis and renal transplantation. *Archives of Disease in Childhood*, **55**, 435–445.

54. Potter, D., Holliday, M., Piel, C.F. *et al.* (1980) Treatment of end-stage renal disease in children: a 15-year experience. *Kidney International*, **18**, 103–109.
55. Broyer, M. (1987) Kidney transplantation in children: results of 383 grafts performed at Enfants Malades Hospital from 1973 to 1984. *Advances in Nephrology*, **16**, 307–334.
56. Offner, G., Aschendorff, C., Hoyer, P.F. *et al.* (1988) End-stage renal failure: 14 years' experience of dialysis and renal transplantation. *Archives of Disease in Childhood*, **63**, 120–126.
57. Winearls, C.G., Pippard, M.J., Downing, M.R. *et al.* (1986) Effect of human erythropoietin derived from recombinant DNA on the anaemia of patients maintained by chronic haemodialysis. *Lancet*, **ii**, 1175–1177.
58. Canadian Erythropoietin Study Group. (1990) Association between recombinant erythropoietin and quality of life and exercise capacity of patients receiving haemodialysis. *British Medical Journal*, **300**, 573–578.
59. Betts, P.R., Magrath, G. (1974) Growth pattern and dietary intake of children with chronic renal insufficiency. *British Medical Journal*, **ii**, 189–193.
60. Rees, L., Greene, S.A., Adlard, P. *et al.* (1988) Growth and endocrine function after renal transplantation. *Archives of Disease in Childhood*, **63**, 1326–1332.
61. Rees, L., Rigden, S.P.A., Ward, G.M. (1989) Chronic renal failure and growth. *Archives of Disease in Childhood*, **64**, 573–577.
62. White, R.H.R., Taylor, C.M. (1984) The non-operative management of primary vesico-ureteric reflux. In *Management of Vesico-ureteric Reflux* (ed J.H. Johnston), Baltimore: Williams and Wilkins, pp 117–136.
63. Bailey, R.R. (1981) End-stage reflux nephropathy. *Nephron*, **27**, 302–306.
64. Kincaid-Smith, P. (1975) Glomerular lesions in atrophic pyelonephritis and reflux nephropathy. *Kidney International*, **8**, S81–S83.
65. Shimamura, T., Morrison, A.B. (1975) A progressive glomerulosclerosis occurring in partial five-sixth nephrectomised rats. *American Journal of Pathology*, **79**, 95–106.
66. Celsi, G., Bohman, S-O., Aperia, A. (1987) Development of focal glomerulosclerosis after unilateral nephrectomy in infant rats. *Pediatric Nephrology*, **1**, 290–296.
67. Wikstad, I., Celsi, G., Larsson, L. *et al.* (1988) Kidney function in adults born with unilateral renal agenesis or nephrectomised in childhood. *Pediatric Nephrology*, **2**, 177–182.
68. Thorner, P.S., Arbus, G.S., Celemajer, D.S., Baumal, R. (1984) Focal segmental glomerulosclerosis and progressive renal failure associated with a unilateral kidney. *Pediatrics*, **78**, 806–810.
69. Morita, M., Yoshiara, S., White, R.H.R., Raafat, F. (1990) The glomerular changes in children with reflux nephropathy. *Journal of Pathology*, **162**, 245–253.
70. Morita, M., White, R.H.R., Coad, N.A.G., Raafat, F. (1990) The clinical significance of the glomerular location of segmental lesions in focal segmental glomerulosclerosis. *Clinical Nephrology*, **33**, 211–219.
71. Brenner, B.M., Meyer, T.W., Hostetter, T.H. (1982) Dietary protein intake and the progressive nature of kidney disease. *New England Journal of Medicine*, **307**, 652–659.
72. Provoost, A.P., De Keijzer, M.H., Molenaar, J.C. (1989) Effect of protein intake on lifelong changes in renal function of rats unilaterally nephrectomised at young age. *Journal of Laboratory and Clinical Medicine*, **114**, 19–26.
73. Raymond, N.G., Dwyer, J.T., Nevins, P., Kurtin, P. (1990) An approach to protein restriction in children with renal insufficiency. *Pediatric Nephrology*, **4**, 145–151.
74. Dunn, M.J. (1990) Prostaglandins, Angiotensin II, and Proteinuria. *Nephron*, **55**, 30–37.
75. Brunner, H., Schroder, C., van Bennekom, C. *et al.* (1988) Localisation of the

gene for X-Linked Alport's syndrome. *Kidney International*, **34**, 507–510.
76. Flinter, F.A., Cameron, J.S., Chantler, C. *et al.* (1988) Genetics of classic Alport's syndrome. *Lancet*, **ii**, 1005–1007.
77. Kashtan, C.E., Atkin, C.L., Gregory, M.C., Michael, A.F. (1989) Identification of variant Alport phenotypes using an Alport-specific antibody probe. *Kidney International*, **36**, 669–674.
78. Morita, M., White, R.H.R., Raafat, F. *et al.* (1988) Glomerular basement membrane thickness in children: a morphometric study. *Pediatric Nephrology*, **2**, 190–195.

18 | Paediatric cardiology

Christopher Wren
Freeman Hospital, Newcastle upon Tyne

Introduction

In its short history as a recognisably separate subspecialty of paediatrics, paediatric cardiology has been characterised by rapid development and frequent major advances which have been of great benefit to patients. The changes are such that young paediatric cardiologists are now unfamiliar with the problems presented to the previous generation. In the past ten years or so our practice has been transformed by developments such as the introduction of cross-sectional echocardiography and the use of prostaglandin for palliation of neonatal heart disease. The widespread adoption of a logical and systematic classification and description has also made life easier for the paediatric cardiologist.

The outlook for most children undergoing cardiac surgery is now so good that they face a fairly normal life-span and quality of life, and this in itself has led to the need for cardiologists able to undertake long-term care of adolescents and young adults with congenital heart disease.[1] There is a continuing, and largely unprofitable, debate about who should be responsible for these patients. It seems that those treated early on by paediatric cardiologists and cardiac surgeons in children's hospitals may be at some disadvantage if the constitution of such units does not allow them to practise lifelong care of their patients.

Any review of recent developments and likely future advances in paediatric cardiology has, of course, to be selective. I have tried to choose those subjects which have produced significant advances for patients, but obviously there are many omissions. We also recognise that many of our patients have benefited greatly from parallel advances in paediatric surgical and intensive care techniques.

Advances in cardiac imaging

Cardiac ultrasound began as a clinically useful tool with M-mode echocardiography in the 1970s. This was of most use in patients with predictably normal cardiac connections, and the most rapid development in non-invasive diagnosis of congenital heart disease came about ten years ago with the widespread introduction of cross-sectional echocardiography. In the past decade we have seen a steady improvement in image quality and this, coupled with greater expertise in use and interpretation of the technique, has firmly established cross-sectional echocardiography as fundamental in the diagnosis and assessment of patients with congenital heart disease. Echocardiography is mainly concerned with cardiac anatomy and has been greatly enhanced by the development of Doppler echocardiography which improves our assessment of cardiac function enormously. The use of pulsed Doppler, continuous-wave Doppler, and colour Doppler is now routine, and more recently has been augmented by the introduction of intra-operative and trans-oesophageal echocardiography. This last development does, however, move echocardiography away from being a routine, rapid, non-invasive investigation to one which is invasive, and requires sedation or anaesthesia and special facilities for dealing with patients, but these minor drawbacks are offset by the extra yield from trans-oesophageal echocardiography in particular circumstances.

Fetal cardiology

This rapidly expanding subspecialty is mainly restricted to diagnosis at present but holds out exciting prospects of treatment in some cases.[2–4] The technology is now such that early detection of structural abnormalities of the heart is straightforward if the scan is done at the appropriate stage of pregnancy by an experienced operator with good ultrasound equipment.[5,6] Prospective schemes aimed at detecting congenital heart disease in the fetus were initially aimed at 'high-risk' pregnancies such as those with maternal diabetes or with a family history of congenital heart disease. The risk of a fetal cardiac abnormality is even higher in the presence of an abnormality such as exomphalos, fetal ascites, or a fetal arrhythmia.

More recently, fetal cardiac scanning has been extended to population screening. A survey by Cullen *et al.*[7] has shown that only about 7% of children with serious congenital cardiac abnormalities result from so-called 'high-risk' pregnancies and that, if the remainder are to be detected, 'low-risk' pregnancies will need to be scanned as well.

The problem then becomes one of resources. If the detection rate were high one would expect to pick up two or three cases per thousand scanned if screening is confined to a four-chamber scan. The detection rate does, of course, depend upon good-quality ultrasound equipment, and on the diligence and expertise of the operator. Fetal cardiac ultrasound is not an ideal screening procedure as the equipment is expensive to provide and to run, the procedure requires great technical expertise and experience, and the sensitivity of the technique is probably not high.

As well as showing that it is technically feasible it is important to decide whether fetal scanning is justified. This decision will be made by balancing benefits against drawbacks. The benefits of fetal detection of congenital heart disease include intra-uterine treatment of fetal arrhythmias,[8,9] offering the mother the option of termination of pregnancy in the case of unsurvivable lesions, relocation of delivery in the case of likely duct-dependent abnormalities which would cause rapid post-natal deterioration, and the opportunity to look for chromosome abnormalities if appropriate.

The greatest benefit is reassurance of the mother that the scan is normal and, if there is a significant 'consumer demand' for this procedure, it is likely to come from mothers with a previously affected baby. There are also obvious drawbacks to be taken into account. There are few options for treatment and the main management decision is whether to continue or terminate the pregnancy. The second half of pregnancy may well be quite traumatic for the mother if she knows in advance of a significant cardiac lesion and elects to continue with the pregnancy. It is inevitable that no counselling will be available for the mother before a routine screening scan is performed. If the abnormality is detected on a routine scan, the mother is provided with both information and a decision to take without being asked whether she wanted either the information or to take the decision. This might be regarded as an infringement of her rights, but given the low overall incidence of heart disease pre-scan counselling is not feasible. A final problem, which fortunately is rare, is a false negative scan where the mother is inappropriately reassured.

Fetal scanning and fetal cardiology in general are still in the development phase and there is no consensus on any of these points at present. It will probably be several years before adequate audit of fetal scanning enables us to take rational decisions. Fetal screening will also have to be shown to be cost-effective if it is to have a long-term future.

Future developments in fetal cardiology are likely to include interventional catheterisation, trans-uterine pacing, and a better understanding of the trans-placental pharmacokinetics of anti-arrhythmic drugs. Trans-uterine trans-ventricular balloon dilation of the aortic valve in severe fetal critical aortic stenosis has been attempted on one occasion. There is also one report of trans-uterine fetal cardiac pacing in complete AV block.[10] In both cases the technique was shown to be feasible although it did not result in survival of the baby.

Interventional catheterisation

The pioneer in this field was William Rashkind who, in 1966, introduced balloon atrial septostomy which has been the treatment of choice for immediate palliation of the transposition of the great arteries ever since. Further developments in the field were delayed until the early 1980s, when technological advances enabled the production of polyethylene balloons able to withstand high inflation pressures without overstretching. There was then a flurry of activity as most stenotic lesions encountered in paediatric cardiology were subjected to dilatation. The past few years have seen a continuous reappraisal of the technique and some consensus on the indications for its use has emerged.[11–13]

The first lesion treated by balloon dilatation was pulmonary valve stenosis and balloon dilatation is now widely accepted as the treatment of this condition.[14] Excellent relief of stenosis can be achieved in children and adults with the common, typical form of pulmonary stenosis. The longest follow-up so far is necessarily restricted to a few years, but comparison with the results of open surgical valvotomy suggest that patients will have lasting benefit and that re-stenosis will be rare. Balloon dilatation is also effective in critical pulmonary valve stenosis in the newborn but is technically more demanding in this population and associated with some risk.[15,16] However, it is again widely recognised as preferable to surgery.[17] Balloon dilatation is unhelpful in the less common, dysplastic pulmonary stenosis where obstruction results from hypoplasia of the pulmonary valve ring and thickened space-occupying dysplastic pulmonary valve leaflets rather than from cusp fusion.[18]

Re-stenosis of coarctation of the aorta continues to be a problem despite continuing surgical advances, and is more likely to occur following neonatal repair of coarctation. Balloon dilatation is able to achieve results at least as good as re-operation at lower risk, and is therefore recommended as treatment of choice.[19–21]

Congenital aortic valve stenosis is a progressive and recurrent problem and patients with significant stenosis are likely to face the need for several interventions during their lifetime. As re-operations are complicated by the previous surgery, there is an obvious attraction in replacing the primary palliation by a non-surgical procedure. In most centres balloon dilatation is accepted as the preferred palliation for children with aortic stenosis requiring treatment.[22,23] The indications for treatment are less clear. Certainly those with symptoms or severe stenosis or marked echocardiographic and electrocardiographic evidence of ventricular hypertrophy require treatment, but the decision is more difficult in asymptomatic children with moderate valve stenosis and a gradient around 50 or 60mmHg. As balloon dilatation of aortic valve stenosis is proving to be safer and easier than surgery, it is likely that the 'threshold' for treatment will be slightly lower.

Critical neonatal aortic valve stenosis is an altogether more difficult problem. The valve morphology is severely abnormal and left ventricular function is usually poor, with left ventricular hypoplasia or dilatation and endocardial fibroelastosis. Some of these neonates have a very poor outlook whatever form of treatment is employed. Balloon dilatation in this population is technically difficult.[24,25] Introduction of the balloon catheter into the femoral artery risks damage to the vessel. Occasionally it may not be possible to cross the valve with a guidewire. One or two of those with very poor ventricular function may not tolerate transient occlusion of the outflow. The results of balloon dilatation must, of course, be compared with the results of surgery. With some surgical series it is difficult to know which patients were included and those which report only patients undergoing surgery may give an over-optimistic view. However, realistic surgical series show just as great a difficulty with treatment.[26] The choice between balloon dilatation and surgical valvotomy is best decided individually in each institution. It seems likely that similar results will be achieved whatever mode of treatment is employed.[27] The smallest, sickest babies with the most dysplastic valves and poorest ventricular function will continue to have a poor prognosis.

Balloon dilatation of unoperated coarctation of the aorta has been a contentious issue since it was first introduced. It is not recommended in infancy[28] but it can be accomplished safely and effectively in children older than 12 months.[29,30] Because relief of obstruction is achieved by disruption of the aorta intima and media there have been anxieties about the long-term effects, particularly the risk of late development of aortic aneurysm.[30,31] As with all other lesions, it is important to compare the results with those of surgery. Unfortunately, few surgical patients have been subjected to the same intensive scrutiny as those now undergoing balloon dilatation with immediate, early, and late re-investigation by catheterisation and angiography. Consequently we do not know the residual pressure gradient at catheterisation in patients undergoing surgical resection of coarctation nor the incidence of aneurysm in surgical series. Until that information is available the risks and benefits of balloon dilatation of unoperated coarctation cannot be compared directly with surgical results. However, a preliminary report of 21 children undergoing surgical repair of coarctation and 27 treated by balloon dilatation concluded that surgical repair and balloon dilatation yielded similar results in terms of residual pressure gradient and aneurysm formation in short-term follow-up.[32] Balloon dilatation of coarctation will continue to be performed in a few centres, with careful assessment of long-term results. A well-designed direct comparison with surgical treatment using the same invasive follow-up is urgently needed. Until the remaining questions are resolved balloon dilatation of unoperated coarctation will remain an experimental procedure.

After early experience showed successful relief of pulmonary valve stenosis it was logical to extend the technique to other forms of right ventricular outflow obstruction. Balloon dilatation of postoperative stenosis due to conduit obstruction has been disappointing.[33,34] In this country there has been particular interest in palliation of tetralogy of Fallot, and the largest experience has been in Liverpool and at Guy's Hospital. The series is now extensive and early results suggest it is effective in improving cyanosis, relieving hypercyanotic spells, and possibly in encouraging pulmonary artery development.[35] Further experience will be necessary before the place of balloon dilatation in the palliation of children with Fallot's tetralogy can be established.

Newer developments in interventional catheterisation have addressed problems other than those of stenoses. In the past two or three years transvenous occlusion of the persistent ductus arteriosus has been introduced in several centres, using the Rashkind double umbrella occluder device.[36–39] The procedure is applicable to children weighing more than 10kg with a restrictive ductus and normal cardiac anatomy. The primary closure rate is increasing with greater operator experience and is probably now around 90%. A small residual flow past the device is not uncommon but is likely to resolve spontaneously in most patients. Embolisation rates are now low and the procedure provides an attractive alternative to surgical ligation of the ductus. It is probably more expensive and has a lower overall success rate than surgery but involves a shorter hospital stay and avoids the pain and scar associated with operation. Other unwanted vascular connections are also amenable to transcatheter closure with detachable balloons or coils.[40,41]

Transcatheter closure of atrial septal defects is now at an advanced development stage in the United States but has not so far been performed in this country. The Lock 'clamshell' device is similar to the Rashkind double umbrella in concept but is able to fix itself in position in the atrial septal defect.[42] Most of the early technical problems have now been overcome and the procedure will be introduced to this country within the next year or two. It is likely that 70% or 80% of atrial septal defects will be suitable for closure in this way.

Transcatheter closure of a ventricular septal defect (VSD) is probably a more remote prospect for most patients. The common types of VSD are surrounded by vital structures and it is difficult to foresee any imminent development which would avoid the need for surgery.

Other future developments will include expandable wire stents which are likely to prove particularly valuable in balloon dilatation of pulmonary artery stenosis. These lesions are very elastic and the results of straightforward balloon dilatation have been generally disappointing.[43] However, a wire mesh to maintain the lumen following balloon dilatation may improve results substantially.

Other experimental procedures being evaluated include transvenous myectomy as an adjunct to balloon dilatation in palliation of Fallot's tetralogy,[44] and transvenous laser valvotomy of the pulmonary valve in children with pulmonary atresia and intact ventricular septum. The next few years are likely to see a further expansion in transcatheter treatment or palliation of congenital heart disease and are likely to prove most exciting.

Cardiac transplantation

Most congenital cardiac abnormalities are amenable to surgical correction or definitive palliation to provide a good quality of life and prolonged survival. There are, however, a small number of patients who do not stand to benefit from recent advances in conventional surgery and whose outlook is poor. For these patients cardiac transplantation has recently become a possibility.[45,46] Cardiac transplantation is limited to those patients whose lesions are immediately life-threatening or which carry a very poor prognosis and for which no conventional treatment is available (Table 1). The two main groups are children with dilated cardiomyopathy and those with severe congenital heart disease.

Table 1. Indications for heart transplantation in children.

1. Heart disease with very poor prognosis and/or very poor quality of life.
2. No suitable 'conventional' surgery.
3. Absence of contra-indications.

Dilated cardiomyopathy in infants and children has a poor prognosis. Investigation should exclude treatable causes (such as incessant tachycardia or anomalous origin of the left coronary artery). Individual prognosis is difficult to define on presentation. Griffin *et al.* found the worst prognosis in those older than two years,[47] but this has not been our experience and is not supported by other studies.[48,49]

In our practice the commonest structural heart lesion for which a transplant is required is double-inlet left ventricle with transposition of the great arteries. This is frequently associated with the development of subaortic stenosis and/or left ventricular failure with atrioventricular valve regurgitation, and the general outlook is grim. If the standard criteria of suitability for transplantation (normal pulmonary resistance, no generalised disease, etc) are satisfied, then abnormalities of venous connection or arterial connection do not present insuperable surgical problems (Table 2).[45,46] One specific structural abnormality for which cardiac transplantation may be indicated is hypoplastic left heart syndrome. This is associated with a very poor prognosis in the neonate, but pioneering work by Leonard Bailey at Loma Linda in California has shown that primary transplantation is feasible and in the short and medium term is associated with a good prognosis.[50]

Cardiac transplantation is technically fairly straightforward but there are many persisting problems. Perhaps the major one is the shortage of suitable donors. This is particularly acute for neonates, where there is a small supply and perhaps less medical awareness of the need for donors; and for older children who are competing for donors with the much larger number of adults on the waiting list. The problem of donors for neonatal transplantation was addressed by a working party of the medical Royal Colleges. They made several recommendations, which included the following.

1. Organs may be removed for transplantation from apnoeic infants with anencephaly. Apnoea and absence of a forebrain is recognised as equivalent to brain death.
2. Parents should not be pressurised to continue with a pregnancy merely to provide organs for donation.
3. The standard criteria for brain death cannot be applied to neonates younger than seven days other than anencephalics.
4. Neonatal transplantation should be confined to recognised centres.

In practice, anencephalics are unlikely to be a viable donor source in this country. Liveborn anencephalics are now rare as most are detected by mid-trimester scanning and mothers are offered termination of pregnancy. The American experience has shown that most donors are otherwise-normal infants suffering brain death, either as part of near-miss sudden infant death syndrome or after head injury.[50,51]

Problems with immunosuppression persist, although the introduction of cyclosporin A was a large step forward. Most rejection episodes occur in the first few weeks and months after transplantation, and as time goes by acute rejection becomes less common. Accelerated coronary arteriosclerosis is one of the major long-term limitations following transplantation in adults and may be a subtle form of chronic rejection. It has recently been recognised in children and is now sought prospectively by routine postoperative coronary angiography.[52]

Postoperative hypertension is common. It is related in part to cyclosporin and is also a feature of the 'big heart syndrome' seen in children where the donor heart is substantially larger than their own. Hypertension may also be related to steroid treatment for episodes of acute rejection.

Following cardiac transplantation children inevitably have to make many visits to hospital for routine evaluation as well as management of acute problems with rejection or infection. They and their families adapt very well in general, but there is inevitably some stress on the family and effect on the child's education. However, this has to be balanced against a substantial improvement in quality of life, and most children are rendered totally asymptomatic.

Residual anatomical problems of transplantation are few and will be overcome with greater surgical experience. One persisting problem, however, is that relatively few children who might benefit from heart transplantation are suitable (Table 2). A normal or near-normal pulmonary resistance is required, and yet many children who might otherwise be suitable have a raised pulmonary resistance either as part of the underlying abnormality or as a result of surgical palliation. Some of these may now benefit from the fairly recent introduction of the 'domino' operation in which the heart from a patient undergoing

Table 2. Contra-indications to heart transplantation in children.

Absolute:
raised pulmonary resistance (>6–8 units)
severe renal/hepatic disease
other severe generalised disease
significant developmental delay
Relative:
raised pulmonary resistance (4–6 units)
poor family support
active infection
? abnormal venous and/or arterial connection

heart/lung transplantation is used as a donor organ for a patient with raised pulmonary resistance. The donor heart is 'primed' by pulmonary hypertension in the donor and is able to cope with the raised pulmonary resistance in the recipient. For other children the only hope in the long term will be heart/lung transplantation or lung transplantation combined with surgical repair of the cardiac abnormality. These two techniques are still very experimental, and results will need to improve substantially before they can be more widely introduced.

Future developments in paediatric cardiac transplantation are likely to include more effective and less toxic immunosuppressive drugs, more widespread use of neonatal transplantation for hypoplastic left heart syndrome, and probably eventual trans-species transplantation which offers a solution to the problem of donor supply.

Supraventricular tachycardia in early infancy

Supraventricular tachycardia is an important cause of heart failure or cardiogenic shock in the neonate and young infant.[53] It is dangerous and potentially fatal, but if diagnosed and treated appropriately it has an excellent prognosis. It is now clear that almost all cases are caused by atrioventricular re-entry via an accessory pathway.[54,55] The incidence is probably around 1 in 15,000 live births.[53] Not all infants are in tachycardia at the time of presentation and it is important to be aware of the possibility of the diagnosis.[56] It is difficult to differentiate clinically between supraventricular tachycardia and an appropriate sinus tachycardia in an otherwise sick neonate. The upper limit of heart rate in the sickest neonate is around 220 per minute, whereas supraventricular tachycardia is almost always faster than 270 per minute.[53,55] Clinical measurement of heart rate at this level is inaccurate and unsatisfactory. Many cardiac monitors employed on neonatal and paediatric units have an intrinsic upper-rate limit of around 230 per minute, and are also unhelpful in distinguishing between sinus and supraventricular tachycardias. The only safe way is to record an electrocardiogram and measure the heart rate on paper.

Having made the diagnosis the priority is to restore sinus rhythm. Until a few years ago the recommended initial treatment was either digoxin or cardioversion. However, digoxin is not always effective and there is a substantial lag time between administration of the drug and termination of the tachycardia.[53] Cardioversion is almost always effective but requires sedation or anaesthesia, and is not easily repeated if the tachycardia recurs. Many newer forms of treatment have been proposed and have found their way into standard paediatric textbooks.

They include treatment with verapamil, disopyramide, and propranolol given intravenously.[57–59] However, the dangers of some of these treatments, particularly the use of verapamil in neonates, are now recognised.[60,61] The ideal treatment for supraventricular tachycardia in infancy (or, for that matter, at any age) would be safe, rapidly effective, easily performed or given, free from side-effects, and would ideally prevent a recurrence of the tachycardia or be easily repeatable in the event of a recurrence. None of the treatments mentioned above comes close to the ideal. Currently the safest and most effective treatment available is facial application of ice-cold water.[53] This is best achieved by facial immersion in ice-cold water and has a high success rate, is promptly effective, has no adverse effects, and is easily repeated. It does not, however, prevent a recurrence of tachycardia. The procedure is somewhat frightening for the paediatrician not familiar with it (Fig. 1). It is best performed by attaching the infant to an electrocardiographic monitor and then wrapping him in a towel. His face is immersed briefly in a bowl of ice-cold water. No attempt is made to obstruct the mouth or nostrils as the infant will be temporarily apnoeic. The face is immersed for up to five seconds and termination of tachycardia usually occurs more or less immediately or within a second or two of removal from the water.

An alternative, which is soon to be widely introduced, is intravenous adenosine. This drug produces a very transient slowing of

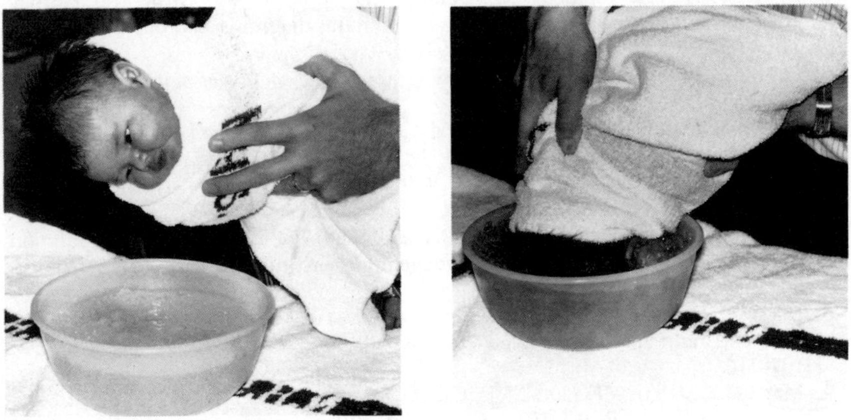

Fig. 1. *Facial immersion in ice-cold water for treatment of neonatal supraventricular tachycardia. The baby is attached to an ECG monitor and wrapped in a towel (left panel). His face is then immersed in ice-cold water for up to five seconds (right panel). Termination of tachycardia will usually occur within a second or two or sometimes immediately after he is removed from the water. No attempt is made to obstruct his nose and mouth as he will be temporarily apnoeic.*

atrioventricular nodal conduction and its rapid metabolism (the half life is around 15 seconds) means that it is not associated with significant side-effects in this age group.[62] It is given by a rapid intravenous bolus injection, starting at 50mcg/kg and increasing by 50mcg/kg/dose to a maximum of 250mcg/kg. Adenosine will not prevent recurrence of tachycardia but its rapid metabolism means that the dose can be repeated without problems. In centres where neither ice-cold water nor adenosine is felt to be suitable, cardioversion remains an effective means of restoring sinus rhythm. The few patients who suffer very frequent recurrence respond satisfactorily to intravenous and then oral flecainide, but at present experience with this drug in the newborn is not sufficient for it to be widely recommended.

Conclusion

Any account of recent advances and future developments in paediatric cardiology is necessarily selective. It would be inappropriate not to include a tribute to parallel exciting developments under way in the fields of paediatric cardiac surgery and intensive care from which many children have benefited and will continue to benefit in the future.

References

1. Somerville, J. (1989) Congenital heart disease in the adolescent. *Archives of Disease in Childhood*, **64**, 771–773.
2. Davis, G.K., Farquhar, C.M., Allan, L.D. *et al.* (1990) Structural cardiac abnormalities in the fetus: reliability of prenatal diagnosis and outcome. *British Journal of Obstetrics and Gynaecology*, **97**, 27–31.
3. Huhta, J.C. (1990) Fetal echocardiography. *Current Opinion in Cardiology*, **5**, 17–19.
4. Williams, R.G. (1989) Fetal cardiology. *Current Opinion in Cardiology*, **4**, 60–63.
5. Allan, L.D. (1988) Prenatal cardiology. *Current Opinion in Cardiology*, **3**, 50–54.
6. Wheller, J.J., Reiss, R., Allen, H.D. (1990) Clinical experience with fetal echocardiography. *American Journal of Diseases of Children*, **144**, 49–53.
7. Cullen, S., Franklin, R., Sharland, G. *et al.* (1990) Potential impact of population screening for prenatal diagnosis of congenital heart disease. *British Heart Journal*, **64**, 92.
8. Maxwell, D.J., Crawford, D.C., Curry, P.V.M. *et al.* (1988) Obstetric importance, diagnosis, and management of fetal tachycardias. *British Medical Journal*, **297**, 107–110.
9. Machado, M.V.L., Tynan, M.J., Curry, P.V.L., Allan, L.D. (1988) Fetal complete heart block. *British Heart Journal*, **60**, 512–515.
10. Carpenter, R.J., Strasburger, J.F., Garson, A. Jr. *et al.* (1986) Fetal ventricular pacing for hydrops secondary to complete atrioventricular block. *Journal of the American College of Cardiology*, **8**, 1434–1436.
11. Benson, L. (1990) Interventional cardiac catheterisation. *Current Opinion in Cardiology*, **5**, 40–44.
12. Roccini, A.P. (1989) Interventional catheterisation. *Current Opinion in Cardiology*, **4**, 93–96.

13. Deanfield, J.E. (1988) Interventional catheterisation in congenital heart disease. *Current Opinion in Cardiology*, **3**, 87–91.
14. Stanger, P., Cassidy, S.C., Girod, D.A. *et al.* (1990) Balloon pulmonary valvuloplasty: results of the valvuloplasty and angioplasty of congenital anomalies registry. *American Journal of Cardiology*, **65**, 775–783.
15. Qureshi, S.A., Ladusans, E.J., Martin, R.P. (1989) Dilatation with progressively larger balloons for severe stenosis of the pulmonary valve presenting in the later neonatal period and early infancy. *British Heart Journal*, **62**, 311–314.
16. Ladusans, E.J., Qureshi, S.A., Parsons J.M. *et al.* (1990) Balloon dilatation of critical stenosis of the pulmonary valve in neonates. *British Heart Journal*, **63**, 362–367.
17. Caspi, J., Coles, J.G., Benson, L.N. *et al.* (1990) Management of neonatal critical pulmonary stenosis in the balloon valvotomy era. *Annals of Thoracic Surgery*, **49**, 274–278.
18. Musewe, N.N., Robertson, M.A., Benson, L.N. *et al.* (1987) The dysplastic pulmonary valve: echocardiographic features and results of balloon dilatation. *British Heart Journal*, **57**, 364–370.
19. Cooper, S.G., Sullivan, I.D., Wren, C. (1989) Treatment of recoarctation: balloon dilatation angioplasty. *Journal of the American College of Cardiology*, **14**, 413–419.
20. Huhta, J.C. (1989) Angioplasty for recoarctation. *Journal of the American College of Cardiology*, **14**, 420–421.
21. Hellenbrand, W.E., Allen, H.D., Golinko, R.J. *et al.* (1990) Balloon angioplasty for aortic recoarctation: results of valvuloplasty and angioplasty of congenital anomalies registry. *American Journal of Cardiology*, **65**, 793–797.
22. Sullivan, I.D., Wren, C., Bain, H. *et al.* (1989) Balloon dilatation of the aortic valve for congenital aortic stenosis in childhood. *British Heart Journal*, **61**, 186–191.
23. Roccini, A.P., Beekman, R.H., Shachar, G.B. *et al.* (1990) Balloon aortic valvuloplasty: results of the valvuloplasty and angioplasty of congenital anomalies registry. *American Journal of Cardiology*, **65**, 784–789.
24. Ladusans, E.J., Parsons, J.M., Qureshi, S.A. *et al.* (1989) Results of percutaneous balloon dilatation for critical aortic stenosis in neonates with severe endocardial fibro-elastosis. *British Heart Journal*, **61**, 470 (abstr.).
25. Wren, C., Sullivan, I., Bull, C., Deanfield, J. (1987) Percutaneous balloon dilatation of aortic valve stenosis in neonates and infants. *British Heart Journal*, **58**, 608–612.
26. Pelech, A.N., Dyck, J.D. Trusler, G.A. *et al.* (1987) Critical aortic stenosis. *Journal of Thoracic and Cardiovascular Surgery*, **94**, 510–517.
27. Zeevi, B., Keane, J.F., Castaneda, A.R. *et al.* (1989) Neonatal critical valvar aortic stenosis. A comparison of surgical and balloon dilatation therapy. *Circulation*, **80**, 831–839.
28. Redington, A.N., Booth, P., Shore, D.F., Rigby, M.L. (1990) Primary balloon dilatation of coarctation of the aorta in neonates. *British Heart Journal*, **46**, 277–281.
29. Wren, C., Peart, I., Bain, H., Hunter, S. (1987) Balloon dilatation of unoperated coarctation: immediate results and one-year follow-up. *British Heart Journal*, **58**, 369–373.
30. Tynan, M., Finley, J.P., Fontes, V. *et al.* (1990) Balloon angioplasty for the treatment of native coarctation: results of valuloplasty and angioplasty of congenital anomalies registry. *American Journal of Cardiology*, **65**, 790–792.
31. Lock, J.E. (1984) Now that we can dilate, should we? *American Journal of Cardiology*, **54**, 1360.
32. Boucek, M.M., Ruttenberg, H.D., Orsmond, G.S. *et al.* (1988) Results of balloon coarctation angioplasty versus surgical repair in children. *American Journal of Cardiology*, **62**, 508 (abstr).
33. Zeevi, B., Keane, J.F.M., Perry, S.B., Lock, J.E. (1989) Balloon dilation of

postoperative right ventricular outflow obstructions. *Journal of the American College of Cardiology*, **14**, 401–408.
34. Ensing, G.J., Hagler, D.J., Seward, J.B. *et al.* (1989) Caveats of balloon dilatation of conduits and conduit valves. *Journal of the American College of Cardiology*, **14**, 397–400.
35. Qureshi, S.A., Kirk, C.R., Lamb, R.K. *et al.* (1988) Balloon dilatation of the pulmonary valve in the first year of life in patients with tetralogy of Fallot: a preliminary study. *British Heart Journal*, **60**, 232–235.
36. Rashkind, W.J., Mullins, C.E., Hellenbrand, W.E., Tait, M.A. (1987) Nonsurgical closure of patient ductus arteriosus: clinical application of the Rashkind PDA occluder system. *Circulation*, **75**, 583–592.
37. Dyck, J.D., Benson, L.N., Smallhorn, J.F. *et al.* (1988) Catheter occlusion of the persistently patent ductus arteriosus. *American Journal of Cardiology*, **62**, 1089–1092.
38. Wessel, D.L., Keane, J.F., Parness, I., Lock, J.E. (1988) Outpatient closure of the patent ductus arteriosus. *Circulation*, **75**, 1068–1071.
39. Musewe, N.N., Benson, L.N., Smallhorn, J.F., Freedom, R.M. (1989) Two-dimensional echocardiographic and color flow Doppler evaluation of ductal occlusion with the Rashkind prosthesis. *Circulation*, **80**, 1706–1710.
40. Reidy, J.F., Jones, O.D.H., Tynan, M.J. *et al.* (1985) Embolisation procedures in congenital heart disease. *British Heart Journal*, **54**, 184–192.
41. Perry, S.B., Radtke, W., Fellows, K.E. *et al.* (1989) Coil embolisation to occlude aortopulmonary collateral vessels and shunts in patients with congenital heart disease. *Journal of the American College of Cardiology*, **13**, 100–108.
42. Lock, J.E., Rome, J.J., Davis, R. *et al.* (1989) Transcatheter closure of atrial septal defects. *Circulation*, **79**, 1091–1099.
43. Jan, J.S., Marvin, W.J., Bass, J.L. *et al.* (1990) Balloon angioplasty—branch pulmonary artery stenosis: results from the valvuloplasty and angioplasty of congenital anomalies registry. *American Journal of Cardiology*, **65**, 798–801.
44. Qureshi, S.A., Parsons, J.M., Tynan, M. (1990) Percutaneous transcatheter myectomy of subvalvar pulmonary stenosis in tetralogy of Fallot: a new palliative technique with an atherectomy catheter. *British Heart Journal*, **64**, 163–165.
45. Bove, E.L. (1990) Congenital heart surgery. *Current Opinion in Cardiology*, **5**, 45–51.
46. Laks, H. (1989) Surgery. *Current Opinion in Cardiology*, **4**, 97–103.
47. Griffin, M.L., Hernandez, A., Martin, T.C. *et al.* (1988) Dilated cardiomyopathy in infants and children. *Journal of the American College of Cardiology*, **11**, 139–144.
48. Chen, S., Nouri, S., Balfour, I. *et al.* (1990) Clinical profile of congestive cardiomyopathy in children. *Journal of the American College of Cardiology*, **15**, 189–93.
49. Guntheroth, W.G. (1990) Congestive cardiomyopathy in children. *Journal of the American College of Cardiology*, **15**, 194–195.
50. Boucek, M.M., Kanakriyeh, M.S., Mathis, C.M. *et al.* (1990) Cardiac transplantation in infancy: Donors and recipients. *Journal of Pediatrics*, **116**, 171–176.
51. Mavroudis, C., Harrison, H., Klein, J.B. *et al.* (1988) Infant orthotopic cardiac transplantation. *Journal of Thoracic and Cardiovascular Surgery*, **96**, 912–924.
52. Pahl, E., Fricker, J., Armitage, J. *et al.* (1990) Coronary arteriosclerosis in pediatric heart transplant survivors: Limitation of long-term survival. *Journal of Pediatrics*, **116**, 117–183.
53. Sreeram, N., Wren, C. (1990) Supraventricular tachycardia in infants: response to initial treatment. *Archives of Disease in Childhood*, **65**, 127–129.
54. Benson, D.W., Dunnigan, A., Benditt, D.G. *et al.* (1983) Transoesophageal study of infant supraventricular tachycardia: electrophysiologic characteristics. *American Journal of Cardiology*, **52**, 1002–1006.
55. Zales, V.R., Dunnigan, A., Benson, D.W. Jr. (1988) Clinical and electrophysiologic features of fetal and neonatal paroxysmal atrial tachycardia resulting in congestive heart failure. *American Journal of Cardiology*, **62**, 225–228.

56. Gikonyo, B.M., Dunnigan, A., Benson, D.W. Jr. (1985) Cardiovascular collapse in infants: association with paroxysmal atrial tachycardia. *Pediatrics*, **76**, 922–926.
57. Roberton, N.R.C. (1986) *Textbook of Neonatology*. Edinburgh: Churchill Livingstone, p. 379.
58. Milner, A.S., Hull, D. (1984) *Hospital Paediatrics*. Edinburgh: Churchill Livingstone, pp 120–1.
59. Roberton, N.R.C. (1986) *Manual of Neonatal Intensive Care*. London: Edward Arnold, pp 163–4.
60. Epstein, M.L., Kiel, E.A., Victorica, B.E. (1985) Cardiac decompensation following verapamil therapy in infants with supraventricular tachycardia. *Pediatrics*, **75**, 737–740.
61. Garson, A. Jr (1987) Medicolegal problems in the management of cardiac arrhythmias in children. *Pediatrics*, **79**, 84–88.
62. Till, J., Shinebourne, E.A., Rigby, M.L. *et al.* (1988) Efficacy and safety of adenosine in the treatment of supraventricular tachycardia in infants and children. *British Heart Journal*, **62**, 204–211.

19 | Child care in general practice

Denis Pereira Gray
Director, Postgraduate Medical School, University of Exeter

Introduction

It is a special pleasure to be able to consider general practice at a time when it is so important for general practitioners and paediatricians to learn to understand each other better and to work together more effectively.

This chapter is divided into three parts: the first describes what have been called the 'fundamental features' of general practice; the second traces the history of child care in general practice and its relationship to developments in paediatric practice; and the third discusses aspects of general practice which have given rise to misunderstandings with paediatricians.

1. Fundamental features of general practice

The brief, which was to concentrate on the past five years, has deliberately been stretched because personal experience of discussion between consultants and general practitioners suggests that recent developments should always be considered in the context of earlier developments in general practice.

There are six fundamental features of general practice which are valid all over the world. The proportions vary according to the culture, system of organisation, and system of health care, but all are relevant everywhere.

1. Primary care

General practitioners normally see everything first. There are obvious exceptions, but numerically they are very small.

2. Family care

In Britain most members of an individual family register with the same general practice. There are many variations and exceptions but it is still the norm.

3. Domiciliary care

It is an important tradition in British general practice that family doctors do home visits—a tradition which has been lost in the USA. It is, however, especially important for children and for the aged.

4. Continuity of care

It is usual in Britain for children and their parents to remain registered with the same general practitioner for many years.

5. Preventive care

General practitioners are the clinicians who first integrated preventive with curative care, and are the main providers of personal preventive medicine for patients of all ages, especially children.

6. Personal care

General practitioners have special opportunities to learn about the people in their care and to make personal relationships with them. This is of particular importance with children, especially adolescents.

Primary care

Primary care for children is a key aspect of general practice. We know that a child under the age of one sees a general practitioner on average six times a year. (The average for all patients in the NHS according to the *General Household Survey*[1] is four per year.)

This contact rate is a great strength and yet poses a considerable organisational challenge for a service that is indeed the 'Front Line of the Health Service'. General practice has to meet the needs of families by providing a doctor for every problem, from maternal anxiety (which is very common) to meningitis (which is very rare), in the surgery and in the home, day and night, around the year.

General practitioners manage most conditions for most of the time. In Britain, most children never see a paediatrician after they are born: only a small minority of children are ever referred to a consultant. It is easy to forget the huge mass of common conditions, such as otitis media, chest infections, behavioural problems, asthma, and fits, which are the bread and butter of general practice. A great many children are taken to general practitioners when they are not seriously ill but a member of their family fears that they are. Prompt and accurate re-assurance is one of the great benefits of primary care.

It is the role of general practice to support the patient and the family on a constant basis and to do as much as it properly can. It is the role of secondary care to support general practice and to do as much as it properly can. It is the role of tertiary care to support secondary care.

These roles work well as long as they are understood and observed and as long as each player is competent in his own field. It is important that tertiary care does not seek to duplicate secondary care and that secondary care does not duplicate primary care, otherwise services become not only unnecessarily expensive through duplication, but also inefficient and confusing for patients.

Family care

Strangely enough, although the commonest single alternative name for general practitioners is 'family doctor', the scientific basis of family medicine is little taught and even less understood. Huygen[2] from the Netherlands has written a delightful book describing the medicine of families and showing with comprehensive statistics how illness in one member of a family significantly affects other members. This book is a classic, and is virtually required reading for family doctors. Family doctors believe that you can *only* understand a child and the illness when you understand the parents and the home. It is a fascinating experience to watch an anxious mother transfer her anxiety to her child and use the child and its behaviour as a means of presenting her own feelings. This can have most unfortunate results if, perhaps after attending the casualty department, the child comes to be seen separately and to be perhaps needlessly and extensively investigated for no real reason.

Family doctors can find this work very difficult, and we need to remind ourselves of two useful pieces of research done by Howie in Edinburgh. In 1972[3] he showed that there was no correlation between the treatments given by general practitioners and the diagnoses they made! The diagnostic labels had no real meaning, especially when they were pseudo-scientific with 'itis' endings, such as laryngitis or pharyngitis. Treatment did, however, correlate with the symptoms and signs. General practitioners are pragmatists; there is consistency about what is seen, heard, and felt, but we have to recognise that the diagnostic labels at present available in primary care are simply not yet adequate.

Secondly, Howie and Bigg[4] showed in a neat little study that the children of parents receiving psychotropic drugs were more likely to receive antibiotics. Despite the advantage of knowing the families, practitioners still respond to parental anxiety as they feel the heat of worry from the parent.

Domiciliary care

The home is the base for the family, and the insights that family doctors gain from home visiting are considerable. Family doctors have long been interested in the home and its relationship with health. As early as 1960, Hodgkin showed[5] that certain diseases were related to certain categories of home; and the next year Carne[6] documented some of the problems of that time in the homes of his patients in London.

According to the *General Household Survey*,[1] about 10% of all contacts between the British population and their general practitioners still take place in the home, with proportionately more for children and the elderly.

Pereira Gray[7] spelt out the case for the value of home visiting, and his analysis remains. Beale[8] has taken the work further, and modern home visiting is concentrated particularly on the very old. Children are a common cause of out-of-hours visits.

Continuity of care

Continuity of care has been treated in the literature as a qualitative feature of primary care. As such it is harder to grasp, and a more quantitative approach can clarify what it offers patients. First, how long does continuity last? It can, in fact, be measured arithmetically from the dates of registration and deregistration with the practice. Two figures have emerged: Cartwright and Anderson[9] produced an average of nine years, with 30% having continuity for 15 years or more, and Difford in Bristol[10] found an average of 12 years' continuity with the same practice.

Given the well-known contact rate of four consultations per patient per year, which is relatively constant, and taking the lesser figure of nine years' continuity, it is easy to calculate that the average general practitioner will see the average patient 36 times, and therefore the average family with two parents and its 2.1 children 144 times in all. Even this figure understates the contact, as virtually all small children are accompanied by a parent, usually the mother, with whom doctors naturally discuss the problem, and on many home visits other members of the family are seen as well.

One powerful piece of evidence for continuity are the findings of Douglas *et al.*[11] who showed just how important was disturbance in early childhood and how the effects could be traced to adolescence and adult life. For example, separation of the parents in the child's early years is associated with behavioural problems in the late teens. The child is indeed the father of the man. Family doctors have the very special privilege of actually seeing these events unfold with the families they know, sometimes over generations.

Despite the mobility of the population, despite an annual turnover in our practice in Exeter of about 20%, it is still true as far as my own personal list of 1420 patients is concerned that one-quarter of all the mothers in my weekly antenatal clinic were born in our practice, and I can remember delivering many of them personally. In 5% of all my under-fives I have personally treated four generations of their families. Twenty per cent of all the under-fives on my list have a grandparent registered with the practice at the same time (who, of course, chats about them and often gives us very valuable information).

I describe these figures for two reasons: first, they are little discussed, and second, they contribute to the immense job satisfaction of being a family doctor. It is not really possible to teach or fully understand families until one has worked in person with members of a family over at least two generations.

Preventive care

My grandfather, who founded our practice, spent virtually his whole life providing what social workers today would call 'crisis intervention'. Preventive medicine in Britain really only started between the wars, and general practice gained greatly from the thinking of the distinguished school of British epidemiologists/community physicians. After the second world war principles of Cochrane[12] and McKeown[13] greatly influenced general practice.

Family doctors were the first clinicians to achieve the crucial synthesis of preventive care and curative care, and to integrate the two in ordinary day-to-day practice over all age-groups. It is this integration that has become a particularly interesting feature of British general practice in the past 15 years. The theoretical model of the consultation which describes this is the Stott and Davis model[14] which emphasised the opportunity that arises in every consultation to offer 'opportunistic' health education or personal preventive medicine.

Long before the recent introduction of the new contract of employment many practices were offering a huge amount of preventive medicine—far more than is generally recognised. I calculated a few years ago that if we added together immunisations, child care surveillance, teenage boosters and counselling, preconceptual counselling, *several hundred* patients coming regularly for contraceptive advice, cervical cytology, antenatal care, anti-smoking advice, anti-coronary advice, including diet and cholesterol screening, a huge amount of advice for travellers, and geriatric screening, the second commonest reason for a patient in our practice coming through the door was for some form of health promotion. This background is important, as it sets the scene as to why child surveillance is a natural part of general practice.

Personal care

Far and away the most interesting, yet far and away the most difficult, aspect to analyse and measure of all the fundamental features of general practice is personal care. Opinions vary, from those which deny its existence to those which regard it as the be-all and end-all of general practice.

The word 'personal' is the first adjective of the job definition for the general practitioner of the Royal College of General Practitioners,[15] and also the European job definition devised by the Leeuwenhorst Group.[16] It has also been, since 1948, a key word in the general practitioner's contract in the NHS. Indeed the term 'personal doctor' is an alternative for the term 'family doctor'.

Many books have been written, mainly by psychiatrists like Balint[17] or by general practitioners like Browne and Freeling,[18] on the doctor–patient relationship. The topic has been more researched and written about by general practitioners than by any other specialty because it is a feature of continuity of care, and because it is more observable in general practice than anywhere else and especially important to both patients and doctors in that setting.

First, at the superficial level, it is easily observed. Why do patients wait so amazingly long when their own (personal) doctor is away, say on holiday (or giving lectures)? Why do they consistently decline to see locums, trainees, or partners? When they are asked about this, the reply is always much the same: 'Doctor X knows me . . . Dr X understands me . . . I've told Dr X the whole story and I don't want to go through it all again with someone else . . . I know how he ticks and he knows how I tick'. Marsh and Kaim-Caudle[19] in an early survey of patient preferences found a very high expression of preference for 'a doctor I know' *as well as* for a 'doctor who knows me'. It is apparently reassuring to be seen by a familiar face and to have some understanding of how the doctor is likely to react.

At the formal research level it was paediatricians in the USA who first tested whether the personal link between patient and doctor affected compliance (Charney *et al.*)[20] They found that the mothers of children who had a good relationship with the doctor were more likely to give the child the antibiotic as prescribed than those who did not.

Ettlinger and Freeman[21] followed this up in Britain when they contrasted the compliance between the patients of one practice which operated a personal list system and those of a similar practice in the same area which did not, and where the patients saw any doctor available. Compliance was significantly better in the practice with the personal list and was associated with the patients responding positively to the statement that they had a doctor who understood them and with whom they could identify.

In terms of patient education, Pereira Gray[22] produced figures which suggested that personal list care led to a reduction in the amount of trivial illness through education and support for patients by the same doctor.

Personal care does of course provide problems in organisational terms both as far as availability is concerned and the increasing trend towards group practice and larger numbers of partners. However, the so-called 'personal list' system[22] does make it possible for patients to see the same doctor most times, and Marsh and Kaim-Caudle[19] have reported that the very high figure of 85% of all attendances by the larger-than-average number of patients on their list were seen personally over a year. Other doctors can rarely equal this, but 75% is feasible and certainly over 80% can be sustained in all months without a holiday.

At present about one-quarter of general practices use the personal list system,[23] but a bigger proportion of training practices do so.[24] It remains to be seen how this will develop.

It is always difficult to know just how personal a personal doctor is, and general practice is indebted to Ann Cartwright's research which has started to provide some measures. In a random sample of NHS patients in Britain, Cartwright and Anderson[25] found that 80% of all patients 'regard doctor as easy to talk to', and as many as 32% 'consider the doctor to be something of a personal friend'.

2. General practice and paediatrics

General practice and paediatrics have long shared an interest in preventive work for children. At one time one discipline has taken the lead and at other times the other. In 1960 Professor Illingworth[26] produced his classic work on normal and abnormal child development which has become essential reading for a whole generation of general practitioners and paediatricians. By 1969 Egan and his colleagues[27] had written their work on developmental screening.

The 1970s were a particularly important time. My own Hunterian

Essay on the role of the general practitioner in the care of the handicapped child was published in 1971,[28] and stressed the role of the family and the family doctor. The same year the Royal College of General Practitioners produced a child record card designed to fit within a general practitioner's ordinary NHS record, which was a model of its kind. I have used it for years, and wonder if all the later versions are really any better.

The next year the Royal College of General Practitioners published one of its most important books, certainly the most important of that decade: *The Future General Practitioner*[15] was exceptionally influential because for family doctors it not only created, in effect, a syllabus for family medicine, but it went so far as to set it out in terms of educational objectives. For paediatricians, the book was important because it classified general practice into five 'areas', one of which was 'human development'. In this way one of the major perspectives of the family physician was integrated into the theory of general practice—one, incidentally, which went across all the age groups.

This concept built a great bridge with paediatrics because developmental awareness and the use of percentile charts and records have been very important and have helped us greatly.

Meanwhile in paediatrics Davie, Butler, and Goldstein's *From Birth to Seven*[29] represented the invaluable cohort approach to paediatric research. Margaret Pollak wrote *Today's Three-Year-Olds in London* in 1972.[30] In 1973 most of us were greatly helped by Mary Sheridan who documented the milestones of development and whose booklets were very useful.[31] Colour blindness was the subject of an editorial in the *Journal of the Royal College of General Practitioners* as early as 1974,[32] when, incidentally, it was suggested that it was a significant social handicap. In 1975, Starte,[33] a general practitioner in Guildford, studied two-year-olds and showed that there was a significant correlation between delayed language development and psychosocial development.

The next year, 1976, was a landmark year. The British Paediatric Association and the Royal College of General Practitioners jointly published their first report, *The Paediatric Training Required by the General Practitioner*.[34] This was generally welcomed and was republished as Appendix J in the Court Report of the same year. It was written in the light of the then fast-developing introduction of vocational training for general practice. Of course, the main event of that year was the Court Report.[35] Much, indeed most, of this report was an immensely valuable review of the subject, including an excellent international comparison, and there was a whole set of recommendations. However, there was an intense reaction from the Royal College of General Practitioners and from the General Medical Services Committee of the British Medical Association, both on the same basis, namely that general practitioners valued the care of children too highly to allow it to be given up to a partner who would be a semi-specialist. One of the earliest statements for developmental surveillance in general practice came from Curtis Jenkins.[36]

In 1977 in the RCGP James Mackenzie Lecture it was suggested that preventing illness was the highest responsibility of the doctor—the 'supreme activity', and the same year Hart's *Child Care in General Practice* was published.[37] In 1978, the Council of the Royal College of General Practitioners formally adopted a major policy statement that comprehensive care for children, that is including anticipatory preventive surveillance, should be offered to children in this country through the medium of general practice. The same year the famous Alma-Ata Declaration of the World Health Organisation was published.[38] This put great emphasis on preventive medicine and, in particular, on the primary health care team. It proposed that in future the main emphasis in health services all over the world should be on primary health care. In 1979 Margaret Pollak produced a second text, with her *Nine Years Old*,[39] and later moved from general practice to become a consulant paediatrician.

The Royal College of General Practitioners decided to form its own working party on the care of children, whose report was published in 1982 as *Healthier Children—Thinking Prevention*;[40] this was the last and best selling of the series of Preventive Medicine Reports from General Practice, published between 1980 and 1982. Professor Freddie Brimblecombe played an important part in that and did much to foster co-operation between paediatricians and family doctors. Two years later the College reached agreement with the General Medical Services Committee of the BMA, and the *Handbook of Preventive Care for Preschool Children* was published jointly,[41] the College producing the text and the BMA the record card. A second edition followed in 1988.

More recently still, Hall's *Health for all Children* was published in 1989[41] and represents the result of a multidisciplinary working party from the British Paediatric Association, the General Medical Services Committee of the BMA, the Health Visitors Association, the Royal College of General Practitioners, and the Royal College of Nursing. The same year saw the publication of the government White Paper *Working for Patients*[43] and the introduction of the new general practitioner contract, which included an option to participate in child health surveillance. In 1989 the Royal College of General Practitioners and the British Paediatric Association once again worked together to construct an agreed set of national guidelines, since both organisations thought this was a professional matter and should remain a professional responsibility. These were issued at the end of 1989 in the name of both organisations.[44] Subsequently they have been jointly amended, once in the summer of 1990 to include the membership examination of the Royal College of General Practitioners, the Diploma of Child Health, and the Diploma of Community Child Health. Now another working party has been established with membership similar to the Hall one—this time under the chairmanship of Colin Waine. It is likely to report in 1991.

3. Aspects of general practice

In the third and last section I would like to describe one or two topics of current interest to paediatricians which have arisen in previous meetings.

Target net remuneration and fees for general practitioners

The way in which general practitioners are paid in the NHS is now so complicated that anyone not personally involved can be forgiven for not being familiar with the arrangements. The principle of target net remuneration is important, however, because it throws new light on the 'fees' paid: for example, for child health surveillance under the 1990 general practitioner contract. To those who receive salaries, fees are assumed to be extra and additional payments over and above the salary. The curious feature of the remuneration of general practitioners is that this is true for any individual general practitioner, but is not true for general practitioners as a whole. The difference is of great importance to the costs of the NHS.

Take, for example, contraceptive advice. This is not required under the main contract, but about 95% of general practitioners choose to provide it, and 70% of all patients receiving advice do so through general practice. There are two different fees: one for contraceptive care involving advice, a cap, or the pill; and a higher fee for fitting an intra-uterine contraceptive device.

Now practitioners providing this care with this advice for many patients may earn several hundred pounds a year in extra income. However, each year the Review Body for Doctors' and Dentists' Remuneration calculates an average 'target net remuneration' for all general practitioners in the NHS. All fees are then adjusted to fit this, so the totality of general practitioner remuneration is well known in advance. Thus, it is now clear that the net effect is that general practitioners pay themselves for this work! The contraceptive fees are within the target figure so that, however much they are, the remaining fees are that much less. Of special importance to the NHS is that no extra cost at all is falling on the Treasury for contraceptive care for 2.5 million people (Department of Health).[45] The public argument about costs of family planning clinics and general practice is thus based on a misconception: it is vastly more expensive to the NHS to provide separate clinics outside general practice, whether for family planning or for children.

Cost-effectiveness

One of the certainties in the NHS of the future is that there will be much greater awareness of costs and relative values. It is thus instructive to compare costs across the hospital/general practice boundary. The Government's figures for British general practice in 1985/86 were that the average cost per patient of all general practitioner care, including all the doctor's income, tax-declared expenses, nurses' salaries, premises, cars, stationery, stamps, and drugs came to £47 per year.

In 1987 the cost of a single admission in a non-teaching hospital was £744, and the cost of a single out-patient case was £105. The day-and-night, round-the-year cost of a child's total medical care in general practice is therefore about half the cost of a single out-patient case in a hospital (Department of Health)[45].

Microcomputers

As a final and up-to-date comment on developments in general practice, I would like to describe briefly the rapid, indeed dramatic, developments in general practitioner microcomputing. The word 'revolution' is nowadays over-used, but I think is well deserved in this case, initiated by a small band of pioneers, starting with Preece *et al.*:[46] Preece was the first general practitioner in the world to go on-line with a general practice record. Growth has been so fast that the Department of Health[44] found this year that as many as half of all British general practitioners were now working with one, and the annual rate of increase is an astonishing 93% a year.

The main applications are repeat prescribing, age-sex analyses, diagnostic registers, and recording personal preventive medicine. This has great potential in child care as we can identify all immunisations at any time, especially children *not* immunised, those due for review at any date for any reason, and the incidence and prevalence of any condition in a precisely defined population group. The research opportunities are obvious, and the applications in ordinary day-to-day care are of even greater importance.

General practice has in the past, for a variety of reasons, not played its full part in research on the care of children. The new emphasis on research being led by the RCGP, the arrival of a generation of vocationally trained family doctors, and now the introduction of microcomputers, sets the scene for much more research in the future.

I hope this will mean, in the years ahead, much more co-operation and partnership between paediatricians and family doctors, as the two groups of doctors with a special and complementary interest in children.

References

1. Office of Population Censuses and Surveys (1989) *General Household Survey 1987*. London, HMSO.
2. Huygen, F.J.A. (1978) *Family Medicine: the Medical Life History of Families*. Nijmegen, Dekker and Van de Vegt. (Republished 1990 by the Royal College of General Practitioners).
3. Howie, J.G.R. (1972) Diagnosis—the Achilles heel. *Journal of the Royal College of General Practitioners*, **22**, 310–315.
4. Howie, J.G.R., Bigg, A.R. (1980) Family trends in psychotropic and antibiotic prescribing. *British Medical Journal*, **280**, 836–838.
5. Hodgkin, G.K.H. (1960) Caravans as homes. *British Medical Journal*, **2**, 854–855.
6. Carne, S.J. (1961) Housing in London. *British Medical Journal*, **2**, 1556–1559.
7. Gray, D.J. Pereira (1978) Feeling at home. James Mackenzie Lecture 1977. *Journal of the Royal College of General Practitioners*, **28**, 121–125.
8. Beale, N. (1991) Daily home visiting in one general practice: a longitudinal study of patient-initiated workload. *British Journal of General Practice*. (in press).
9. Cartwright, A., Anderson, R. (1979) *Patients and their Doctors 1977*. *Journal of the Royal College of General Practitioners*. (occasional paper 8).
10. Difford, F. (1988) Personal communication.
11. Douglas, J.W.B., Keirnan, K.E., Wadsworth, M.E.J. (1977) A longitudinal study of health and behaviour. *Proceedings of the Royal Society of Medicine*, **70**, 530–532.
12. Cochrane, A.L. (1972) *Effectiveness and Efficiency*. London, Nuffield Provincial Hospitals Trust.
13. McKeown, T. (1976) *The Role of Medicine—Dream, Mirage or Nemesis?* Rock Carling Fellowship 1976. London, Nuffield Provincial Hospitals Trust.
14. Stott, N.C., Davis, R.H. (1979) The exceptional potential in each primary care consultation. *Journal of the Royal College of General Practitioners*, **29**, 201–205.
15. Royal College of General Practitioners (1972) *The Future General Practitioner—learning and teaching*. London: British Medical Journal.
16. Leeuwenhorst Working Party (1977) The work of the General Practitioner: Statement by a working party of the second European Conference on the teaching of general practice. *Journal of the Royal College of General Practitioners*, **37**, 117.
17. Balint, M. (1964) *The Doctor, the Patient, and the Illness*. London, Pitman Medical.
18. Browne, K., Freeling, P. (1976) *The Doctor–Patient Relationship* (2nd edn). Edinburgh, E & S Livingstone.
19. Marsh, G., Kaim Caudle, P. (1976) *Team Care in General Practice*. London, Croom Helm.

20. Charney, E., Bynum, R., Eldridge, D. (1967) How well do patients take oral penicillin? *Pediatrics*, **40**, 188–195.
21. Ettlinger, P.R.A., Freeman, G.R. (1981) General practice compliance study: is it worth being a personal doctor? *British Medical Journal*, **282**, 1192–1193.
22. Gray, D.J. Pereira (1979) The key to personal care. *Journal of the Royal College of General Practitioners*, **29**, 666–678.
23. Gude, R., Bradley, N. (1990) *Survey of general practitioners in Devon and Cornwall*. Tavistock, Devon Local Medical Committee and Tamar Faculty of the Royal College of General Practitioners.
24. Gray, D.J. Pereira (1990) *Personal communication*. From Regional Advisers' Office, Devon and Cornwall.
25. Cartwright, A., Anderson, R. (1981) *General Practice Revisited*, London, Tavistock Publications, (Table 26).
26. Illingworth, R.S. (1960) *The Development of the Infant and Young Child: Normal and Abnormal*. Edinburgh, J & A Churchill.
27. Egan, D.F., Illingworth, R.S., MacKeith, R.C. (1969) *Developmental Screening 0–5*. London, William Heinemann Medical Books.
28. Gray, D.J. Pereira (1971) The care of the handicapped child in general practice. Hunterian Society Gold Medal Essay. *Transactions of the Hunterian Society*, **28**, 121–125.
29. Davie, R., Butler, N., Goldstein, H. (1972) *From Birth to Seven*. Edinburgh, Churchill Livingstone.
30. Pollak, M. (1972) *Today's Three-Year-Olds in London*. London, Spastics International Publications.
31. Sheridan, M. (1973) *Children's Developmental Progress*. London, NFER.
32. Editorial (1974) Confusion of colour—a significant social handicap. *Journal of the Royal College of General Practitioners*, **24**, 791.
33. Starte, G.D. (1975) The poor-communicating two-year-old and his family. *Journal of the Royal College of General Practitioners*, **25**, 880–887.
34. British Paediatric Association (BPA) and Royal College of General Practitioners (RCGP) (1976) The paediatric training required by the general practitioner. *Journal of the Royal College of General Practitioners*, **26**, 128–136.
35. Court, S.D.M. (Chairman) (1976) *Fit for the Future*. Report of the Committee on Child Health Services. London, HMSO.
36. Curtis Jenkins, G.H. (1976) The case for the developmental and medical surveillance of the pre-school child. *Update*, **12**, 777–786.
37. Hart, C. (1977) *Child Care in General Practice*. Edinburgh, Churchill Livingstone.
38. World Health Organisation and UNICEF (1978) Declaration of Alma-Ata. *Lancet*, **2**, 1040–1041.
39. Pollak, M. (1979) *Nine Years Old*. Lancaster, MTP Publications.
40. Royal College of General Practitioners (1982) *Healthier Children—Thinking Prevention*. Report from General Practice—22. London, RCGP.
41. British Medical Association (BMA), and Royal College of General Practitioners (RCGP) (1984) *A Handbook of Preventive Care for Pre-School Children*. London, General Medical Services Defence Fund and RCGP.
42. Hall, D.M.B. (ed) (1989) *Health for all Children*. Oxford, Oxford University Press.
43. Department of Health (1989) *Working for Patients*. London, HMSO.
44. British Paediatric Association (BPA) and Royal College of General Practitioners (1989) *Guidelines for the Training and Accreditation of General Practitioners in Child Health Surveillance*. London, British Paediatric Association and Royal College of General Practitioners.
45. Department of Health (1990) *Health and Personal Social Services Statistics for England*. London, HMSO.
46. Preece, J.F., Gillings, D.B., Lippman, F.O., Pearson, N.C. (1970) An on-line record and retrieval system in general practice. *International Journal of Biomedical Computing*, **1**, 4.

Reports of the Royal College of Physicians

Fraud and misconduct in medical research: causes, investigation and prevention

Compensation for adverse consequences of medical intervention

Cystic fibrosis in adults: recommendations for care of patients in the UK

Health services for adults with physical disabilities: a survey of district health authorities 1988/89

Training in infectious diseases

Teaching genetics to medical students

Research involving patients

Guidelines on the practice of ethics committees in medical research involving human subjects

Stroke: towards better management

Prenatal diagnosis and genetic screening: community and service implications

Hay fever (including abridged version)

Medical audit: a first report — what, why and how?

Care of elderly people with mental illness: specialist services and medical training

Fractured neck of femur: prevention and management

Medical care of the newborn in England and Wales

Resuscitation from cardiopulmonary arrest: training and organisation

Links between exposure to ultraviolet radiation and skin cancer

The sun on your skin (*an abridged version of the above Report*)

Computer-based sources of information in medicine

Physical disability in 1986 and beyond

The young disabled adult

Research on healthy volunteers

The relationship between physicians and the pharmaceutical industry

A great and growing evil: the medical consequences of alcohol abuse